THE NATURE
OF STUTTERING

PRENTICE-HALL INTERNATIONAL, INC., *London*
PRENTICE-HALL OF AUSTRALIA, PTY. LTD., *Sydney*
PRENTICE-HALL OF CANADA, LTD., *Toronto*
PRENTICE-HALL OF INDIA PRIVATE LIMITED, *New Delhi*
PRENTICE-HALL OF JAPAN, INC., *Tokyo*

Social psychological and emotional aspects

THE NATURE
OF STUTTERING

CHARLES VAN RIPER
Western Michigan University

PRENTICE-HALL, INC., ENGLEWOOD CLIFFS, N.J.

Book indexed by Earlyn Church.

13-858969-0

Library of Congress Catalog Card Number: 4-137895
Printed in the United States of America

Current printing (last number):

10 9 8 7 6 5 4 3 2 1

DEDICATION

To my next book, *Stuttering: Its Treatment,* the present volume having been viewed (before its monstrous growth) as the introductory chapter thereof.

PREFACE

In this volume we have tried to assemble and to organize most of the information concerning the nature of stuttering. If ever the problem of stuttering is to be solved, someone should make a comprehensive survey of the disorder, chart its major topographical features, and map its territorial unknowns. This we have tried to do.

CONTENTS

THE PROBLEM AND
ITS UNIVERSALITY

Stuttering has been called a riddle. We do not like the term because it implies a pat verbal answer and because it fails to do justice to the complexity of the disorder. Stuttering is more than a riddle. It is at least a complicated, multidimensioned jig-saw puzzle, with many pieces still missing. It is also a personal, social and scientific problem whose equation has not yet been stated completely, a problem with many unknowns. As such it has challenged men of many lands and times to find its solution, for riddles and puzzles and problems are always viewed as being potentially soluble. These solutions have ranged all the way from Francis Bacon's prescription of hot wine to thaw a presumably frozen tongue to that of the Tlahoose Indian who required the stutterer to put his mouth to a knot hole and recite "I give my stuttering to you," as the witch doctor banged the board from the other side (Lemert, 1953) or to the modern therapist's momentary deafening of his client with masking noise.

Stuttering has probably received more attention than any other speech disorder because of the way in which it dramatically exposes many of the unpleasant sides of social living. It is the dark mirror of speech, reflecting man's frustrations in communicating with his fellows. It portrays his fears of social penalties; it reveals his shame for deviancy; it is the hallmark of man's inability to communicate with his fellows. Nuttall (1937) in his "Memoir of a Stammerer," said that anyone who could solve the problem of stuttering could solve all the important troubles of the human race.

It is difficult for those who have not possessed or been possessed by the disorder to appreciate its impact on the stutterer's self-concepts, his roles, his way of living. Once it has taken hold, after a period of insidious growth, almost every aspect of the person's existence is colored by his communicative disability. Ease in verbal communication is a vital prerequisite for more than marginal existence in any modern culture such as ours. Stuttering is not merely a speech impediment; it is an impediment in social living. Lemert (1951), the sociologist, summarizes his evaluation of the stutterer as a deviant in these words. "The stutterer finds himself at a distinct loss in a culture where such a large proportion of adjustments are predominantly verbal and where competitive success in many areas depends upon the ability of the person to manipulate others through verbal controls. The stutterer simply does not possess the effective speech through which the more important roles are implemented" (p. 171). Even those who manage to cope with the disorder can do so only by continual vigilance, most stutterers feeling that they have been sentenced to endure a life of verbal hard labor. The very intermittency of the disorder compounds the problem. One of our clients said it well: "I can't get used to it. I can't get used to it. I wish I were blind or deaf or crippled. Then I'd always be that way and though it would be hard I could finally accept it. But the way it is, I talk all right for a bit and then get clobbered. I hope I can talk; I fear I can't; sometimes I can; sometimes I can't. I'm always torn." Wendell Johnson (1930) in his autobiography, puts it even more vividly: "I am a stutterer. I am not like other people. I must think differently, act differently, live differently—because I stutter. Like other stutterers, like other exiles, I have known all my life a great sorrow and a great hope together, and they have made me the kind of a person I am. An awkward tongue has molded my life" (p.1). Stuttering is more than a verbal riddle. It can be a devastating personal problem.

It is also and perhaps primarily a puzzle, the pieces of which lie scattered on the tables of speech pathology, psychiatry, neurophysiology, genetics, and many other disciplines. At each of these tables, workers have painstakingly managed to assemble a part of the puzzle, shouting "Eureka" while ignoring the pieces of their own or other tables which fail to fit. Regretfully but hopefully we suspect that some of the essential pieces are not merely misplaced but still missing. Nevertheless, in this book we shall try to put together as many as we can.

STUTTERING IN FORMER TIMES

One portion of the puzzle of stuttering is concerned with its apparent universality. The disorder has evidently been with us for a long time and has existed in all the corners of the earth. Clay tablets found in Mesopotamia dating from centuries long before the birth of Christ testify to its ancient history (Van Riper, 1963, p. 306). Laotze, in China mentions stuttering in a poem written 2500 years ago: "The greatest wisdom seems like stupidity. The greatest eloquence like stuttering." Moses has often been mentioned as having stuttered although the original Hebrew uses a term that means "heavy mouthed or slow and sluggish of speech" but there is an old tradition that he had difficulty in enunciating the labial sounds which are rarely a problem in articulatory disorders.

> "Moses, when a child, was one day taken by Pharaoh on his knee. He thereupon grasped Pharaoh's crown and placed it upon his head. The astrologers were horror-struck. 'Let two braziers be brought,' they counselled, 'one filled with gold, the other with glowing coals, and set them before him. If he grasps the gold, it will be safer for Pharaoh to put the possible usurper to death.' When the braziers were brought, the hand of Moses was stretching out for the gold, but the angel Gabriel guided it to the coals. The child plucked out a burning coal and put it to his lips and for life remained 'heavy of speech and heavy of tongue' " (Hertz, 1938, Exodus 4, Footnote, pp. 10–17).

At any rate, for one reason or another, Moses protested to the Lord that his speech problem did not fit him to lead the Jews out of Egyptian captivity, and he had his brother Aaron read the ten commandments to the Israelites after he came down from the mountain, both fairly typical behaviors on the part of a stutterer. In the Koran. (Surah: Taha, 25-32), we find this report: "Moses said: My Lord, relieve my mind and ease my task for me, and loose the knot from my tongue that they may understand my saying."

Whether Moses really stuttered or not we do not know, but we do know that the disorder was known to Isaiah whose verse is clear: "And the tongues of stammerers shall be ready to speak plainly (Isaiah: xxviii, 11)." Clark and Murray (1965) report that hieroglyphics representing the word "nit-nit" were used for stuttering in the twentieth century B.C. The ancient Greeks too were well acquainted with the disorder. Aristotle distinguished such a speech disorder as lisping ("the inability to master a letter") from stuttering hesitancy or phthongophobia. Demosthenes who has been reputed to have been cured of his speech impediment by placing pebbles in his mouth and leaden plates on his chest as he climbed the mountain or orated to the surf may really have had an articulatory problem and a weak voice instead of or in addition to stuttering. Satyrus, the actor, was his therapist, the first one of our profession unless we count the Oracle of Delphi who prescribed a change of environment (exile forever) to a stutterer named Battos, son of Polymestros.

During Roman and medieval times, handicapped persons were often known by the name of their affliction. Thus Balbus, referring to stuttering, became the surname of all members of a plebeian family named Blaesus during the Roman Republic, and a Frankish king named Ludwig the Stutterer lived and probably spoke briefly in the ninth century. Avicenna, the

Arabian poet and physician who lived from A.D. 980-1037, described the disorder clearly and stated its cause and treatment. In Moezogothic, an early Germanic dialect, *stamm* evidently referred to stuttering, and the same term is found in Anglo-Saxon but *stommettan* was also used. At one time in northern England *stoter* meant to stumble while *stammer* referred to staggering. In Germany the wheels of a machine were said to *stotter* when they moved jerkily. Although at present in England *stammering* is preferred to its usual synonym, *stuttering,* in 1598 John Skelton composed this pretty little verse:

> Her tonge was verye quicke,
> But she spak somewhat thicke;
> Her felow did stammer and stutt
> But she was a foul slut.

There are also sufficient historical figures who attest to the presence of stuttering as an old affliction of the human race. To list but a few of these we have not mentioned: Virgil, Erasmus, King Charles I and Edward VI of England, Charles Darwin, Charles Lamb, Charles Kingsley, Leigh Hunt, and Aneurin Bevan all stuttered. The references by Emerick (1966) and French (1966) have some fascinating accounts of the effect of stuttering on the lives of some of these individuals.

These are mere tidbits from a smorgasbord of historical items referring to the disorder of stuttering, and we must resist the temptation to put more on the plate than the reader can consume without indigestion. It is perhaps enough to say that stuttering has been with us throughout recorded history.

UNIVERSALITY OF STUTTERING

The universality of stuttering may also be demonstrated by its present occurrence in widely varying cultures. Although the lack of a word for stuttering can hardly be said to prove that no such disorder exists, the presence of such a term helps to corroborate its occurrence as an entity. The short list of terms referring to stuttering which we provide is illustrative, not exclusive. The disorder is so widely distributed that it is apparently found in almost all people and all cultures.

WORDS REFERRING TO STUTTERING

European
Finnish: ankyttää
German: stottern
French: begaiement
Portuguese: gagueira

Swedish: stamming
Italian: balbuzie
Spanish: tartamundear
Yugoslav (Slovene): jeclijati
Latvian: stostisanas

Estonian: tölpkeel
Hungarian: dadogó
Czech: koktani
Russian: zaikatsia; zaikanie
Esperanto: babuti

American Indian, etc.
Salish: sutsuts
Nanaimo: skeykulskwels
Tlahoose: ha'ak'ok
Haida: kilekwigu'ung
Chocktaw: isunash illi
Asage: the'-ce u-ba-ci-ge
Cherokee: a-da-nv-te-hi-lo-squi
Sioux: eye-hda-sna-sna; iyi-tag-tag
Eskimo: iptogetok

Pacific
Fiji: kaka
Hawaiian: uu uus

Eastern
Persian: locknatezaban
Hebrew: gimgeim
Arabic: yutamtem; rattat
Egyptian: tuhuhtuhuh; nit-nit
Hindi: khaha
Hindustani: larbaraha
Chinese (Cantonese): hau hick;
  kong'-tak-lak-kak
Japanese: domori; kitsuon
Turkish: kekeke mek
Vietnamese: su noi lap

African
Xhosa: ukuthititha
Luganda: okukunanagira
Ghana (Twi): howdodo
Nigeria (Ibo): nsu
Shangaan: manghanghamela
Somali: wùu haghaglayyá

A few glimpses of this universality may illustrate:

Douglass (1953) provides the following report from a Canadian psychiatric social worker's visit to the Southhampton Island's Eskimo population:

> On Southhampton, none of the present population stutters except for the Hudson Bay Company Clerk who stutters in English but not in Eskimo. The only known cases were a father and son who are not now on the island. They spent about ten years on the island, however, and were observed by my informant at the beginning and end of that period. On both occasions their stuttering was unchanged. The father, originally seen at the age of 25 was named Okarlooktook—one who has difficulty in speaking. His symptoms consisted of the repetition of initial sounds of words, particularly the *ah* sound, facial distortions in speaking and marked head movements. The son's symptoms were essentially the same. He was described as laboring when trying to speak. The Eskimos made no attempt to treat the ailment and had no notions as to its cause except to regard it as natural since Okarlooktook apparently was a stutterer from birth. The defect didn't bother him especially. Indeed it gave him status as the comedian of the community. He had a reputation for telling jokes which he used to enhance his reputation. His stuttering was the same in all situations.

Stuttering appears to be fairly prevalent in Japan, and mention of the disorder has appeared in their literature for centuries. One of their most famous doll plays, the Domo Mata, tells of an artist named Domo Matahei who stuttered very severely. Despite his talent he was much penalized by his wife. She, Otoku, says to him:

> "I am sorry for you, Matahei, but you must give up your cherished de-

sires. You have two hands with ten fingers, but it is unfortunate that you stutter." She tells Matahei that the only thing he can do to gain fame is to commit suicide, but to paint his greatest masterpiece on a stone fountain before he dies. She brings him his brushes and prepares the ink, and Matahei draws his own portrait on the stone. The Shogun who owns the fountain is enraged and cleaves the stone with his sword only to find that miraculously the portrait is also visible in the cleft, that it has penetrated the stone. And just as miraculously Matahei regains his speech. There is a touching scene in which he recites the vowels of the Japanese syllabary to convince himself that he no longer stutters. Then great rejoicings and honors and all ends well. The Domo Mata play was first performed in Osaka in 1752. Another more recent real life drama occurred in 1950 when, to the horror of all art loving and patriotic Japanese, a stutterer burned down the ancient Temple of the Golden Pavilion. (Scott, 1955, p. 274.)

In testimonial to the universality of stuttering, we jump across the Pacific to South Africa where we find Aron (1958) describing the stuttering of Bantu and Zulu children. She concludes that "Generally it might be said that the stuttering patterns, devices, and struggle responses that are presented by our African subjects *do not differ* to any great extent from the stuttering patterns that are exhibited by European subjects" (p. 129). And she adds this interesting observation:

Many of the click sounds that were noticed in the speech of African children were situated in the medial position in the words and presented no difficulty to the stutterers. Where the clicks appeared in the initial syllable of the word, in *no* instance was stuttering noticed on the click itself. There was either a pause before the click (usually in the case of predominantly non-

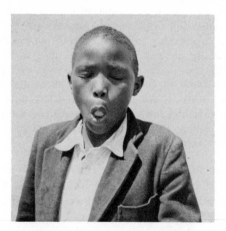

Figure 1. The universality of stuttering: Zulu Boy stuttering. (*From Aron, 1958, by permission.*)

vocalized stutterers); an accessory sound was used before the attempt on the word; the consonant or vowel preceding the click was repeated or prolonged; or there was no stuttering at all on the particular word including the click sound" (p. 127).

Without further belaboring our case for the universality of stuttering by citing the many other available examples of its occurrence in widely varying cultures, we should perhaps examine the alleged exceptions. Ignoring the dubious data procured by questionnaire and correspondence in the studies by Bullen (1945) and Morgenstern (1953) in which informants claimed never to have seen a stutterer among such exotic peoples as the Patamanas of British Guiana, the Kelabits of Borneo, and the Australian aborigines, we turn to the American Indians, the Utes, Bannock and Shoshones, made famous by Wendell Johnson (1944) and by his students Snidecor (1947) and Stewart (1959) who claimed that these Indians had no stuttering in part because they had no word for it. When these investigations are scrutinized carefully from the point of view of a cultural anthropologist, the possibility of methodological error seems obvious. According to Johnson (1946, p. 443) Snidecor appeared before a tribal council, demonstrated stuttering (perhaps excluding the simple repetitions of syllables or sounds because they did not fit the Iowa definition), and asked the Indians, who were "highly amused" at the white man's antics, whether they knew any member of the tribe who talked like that. They said no! (We might get the same response from a group of businessmen in Chicago depending upon the sample of stuttering exhibited.) Snidecor also reports interviewing a total of 800 members of the tribe in his two year investigation (during which he taught full time at Idaho State College) without discovering any stutterers. Had the incidence been that usually reported for a more stressful culture such as ours (0.7%), he should have found five of them among this population. We have no description of his interviewing methods but certainly the interviews could not have been in depth. We must remember that field investigators of such Indian societies are usually met with initial suspicion and distrust. Ralph Waldo Emerson, in his biography of Thoreau, says: "Asking questions of Indians is like catechizing beavers or rabbits." Reliable information can rarely be achieved by asking specific questions through an interpreter. Even when the investigator knows the language and has lived a long time among them, information concerning personal habits must be evoked casually and is given with extreme reluctance. To establish such rapport with 800 Indians would be most difficult. Snidecor himself says:

> The adult Indians in their own culture do not speak under pressure unless they so choose. The adult Indian faced with a critical question does not feel obligated to hurry his answer. He will frequently sit and cogitate upon the problem until he is completely ready to answer, and then his reply may be spoken with little if any substantiation for his opinion (1947, p. 494).

It would take a bold ethnologist to claim that no word for stuttering exists in a given language. Who knows all the words of a language, especially of one beginning to disappear? Moreover the lack of a specific word for a disorder may not mean that the latter does not exist. The witch doctors of the primitive peoples on the Malay peninsula diagnosed diabetes by having their patients urinate near an anthill. If the ants went to the urine, the witch doctors put a taboo on certain sweet fruits, a fairly adequate treatment for excessive blood sugar. So far as we have been able to ascertain, the Malays have no word for diabetes. They do have two for stuttering: "peicha-kapan" and "gagap." In the particular Indian tribes surveyed by Snidecor, the languages have few specific words. The phrase, not the word, is the smallest utterance. To be asked what the word for stuttering was would surely confuse such Indians. Even so, according to Liljeblad (1967), there do seem to be terms for stuttering in Bannock which are inflections of the stem *pybya-*. For example, *"pybyacacadu.a"* means "he stutters when he talks," and *"ynyy-pybyanna-kaibisa-nanaka"* means "He stutters so severely one can't hear him very well." There is another verb stem too which evidently refers to the tonic form of stuttering: *"kycajji."* Thus *"kygycajji-wynny"* means "he stutters continuously."

What is more, despite Snidecor, there are also some stuttering Indians among the Bannock and Shoshone speaking peoples as reported by Liljeblad (1967), an anthropologist who has spent years among them. The work of Stewart (1959) has often been cited as another study supporting the thesis that there exists another American Indian society, the Utes, which is entirely free from stuttering. Essentially this study provides a comparison of only 30 Cowichan (Vancouver Island) Indian households with 30 households of the Utes in terms of language, child-rearing, and other cultural activities, at best a fairly small sample. Moreover, Stewart's own protocols indicate that in two families the mother informed him that one of her children had stuttered. He justifies his selection of the Utes as his nonstuttering society in these words:

> The selection of the Ute as the "nonstuttering group" followed from reports obtained by Wendell Johnson in interviews with two physicians who stated that they had investigated the Ute community near Vernal, Utah, with relative thoroughness and had concluded that there was no stuttering within the group. Substantiation of this point, and the verification of the absence from the Ute language of a term equivalent to "stuttering" was obtained by the present investigator in communications with a Ute tribal official (p. 68).

The original statement by Johnson that the "Indians have no word for it" made an excellent title for a very important statement of his position but we now know that American Indians do have such words or phrases and at least a few members who possessed the disorder. If we have perhaps given too much space to these investigations of the alleged nonstuttering societies, we have done so only because far too few of us have examined the meager evidence upon which the denial of the universality of stuttering has been based. Perhaps this quotation from Kluckhohn (1954), the noted anthropologist, may serve also to set things straight:

> However, the fact that I have been unable to find a single unequivocal case of the complete absence of stuttering among a people suggests that biological or idiosyncratic life history factors can be productive of stuttering in all cultures. On the other hand, impressive differences in degree of incidence suggests that cultural influences are operative. The matter needs much more careful and systematic examination . . . (p. 944).

The apparent universality of stuttering must hold some clue as to its nature. If the disorder is to be considered a neurosis, it must be one shared by many diverse cultures with many different value systems. It would have to be based upon conflicts common to all human beings. Stein (1949) has presented some interesting speculations concerning stuttering as a disorder which can be understood as a regression to atavistic behaviors such as the primitive clicks which were alleged to be common in the infancy of human speech and also as a regression to the babbling and sucking movements which all persons of every race employ during the first years of life. In this latter connection, he writes: "The stammerer unconsciously wishes to remain a suckling. The patient, owing to anxiety, unconsciously reverts to the suckling stage and so replaces consonants with clicks." Others, notably the psychoanalysts, have used similar explanations which, with some stretching, seem to account in some small way for the universality of stuttering.

If stuttering is to be viewed only as learned behavior, the necessary antecedents and consequences should also be common to all races and times if the universality of the disorder is to be explained. If it is a problem due to excessive parental concern or high standards and parental misdiagnosis, these concerns and standards must be common to all cultures. If it is established and maintained by secondary gains or other reinforcements, these too must be present in all people. Doubtless a case can be made for such an explanation but no one has yet made it.

Finally, if stuttering is viewed as a coordinative disorder, one in which the intricate timing of simultaneous and successive muscular contractions required for fluent utterance tends to become disrupted under stress, its universality should not surprise us. The automatic control of the motor sequences of speech is universal and so is stress. It would indeed be astonishing, when we consider the intricacies of the servosystem which monitors speaking, if stuttering disruptions did not occur.

COMMENTARY

The external world becomes little more than a shadowy domain whose chief importance is as a source from whence comes the occasion for nervous tension and the precipitation of blockage. The real world in which one's whole endeavor is immersed is the inner world of the self. Or rather one's attention is concentrated on that limited portion of the inner self which reflects the struggle associated with stuttering. [The stutterer's] being is wracked by the tension which has been built up through years of nervousness when in the presence of the stuttering situations. This condition carries with it a hyperesthetic perception of certain words, of letters of the alphabet, of certain situations, of certain persons whose presence may lead to stuttering. One wanders perpetually on the edge of the vortex of stuttering and at intervals is drawn into it (Gustavson, 1944, p. 467).

And Moses said unto the Lord, O my Lord, I am not eloquent, neither heretofore, nor since Thou hast spoken unto thy Servant: But I am slow of speech and of a slow tongue.
And the Lord said unto him. Who hath made man's mouth? or Who maketh the dumb, or deaf, or the seeing, or the blind? have not I the Lord?
Now therefore go, and I will be with thy mouth, and teach thee what thou shalt say.
And he said, O my Lord, send, I pray Thee, by the hand of him whom Thou wilt send (Exodus: 4:10–14).

Stewart (1960), in his detailed monograph, suggested that stuttering is unknown in the Colorado Utah Indians. He related this to permissive child-rearing practices and resulting tolerance of nonoptimal verbal skills. Unfortunately the significance of his work is somewhat limited because in his criteria for diagnosis he included, as three essentials, the speaker's nonfluency, the culture's sensitivity and unfavorable reaction to such speech, and the speaker's consequent sensitivity and concern. Thus one who stuttered but was unconcerned about it would hardly be considered a stutterer. It is not surprising, therefore, that in a permissive culture Stewart found a low incidence of people concerned about stuttering (Andrews and Harris, 1964, p. 8).

A volunteer team, in an attempt to obtain knowledge of problems related to speech disorders and related oral and facial pathologies, had compared results of speech evaluations and otolaryngological examinations of 2,894 Indian and 3,111 non-Indian children in the state of South Dakota. The incidence of stuttering among the Indian children was high as compared to what is considered "normal" for the general population, averaging 1.97% . . . as compared to an overall average of .85% in the non-Indian population. (Clifford, 1965, p. 60).

In general our findings conflict with reports by Johnson, Snidecor, and Bullen of an absence of stuttering among American Indians. We encountered (1) both stuttering speech and persons regarded as stutterers among the contemporary coastal Indians, (2) evidence of precultural existence of this type of speech disorder, and (3) well defined concepts of stuttering and stutterers in the language and cultures of all the bands we came to know (Lemert 1953, p. 194).

A fifth, not uncommon, speech defect among the Nootka is stuttering. Stutterers, like all other persons who have something queer about their speech, are derided by being imitated. . . . The most Northern Nootka tribe . . . are said to be all stutterers and are accordingly imitated in jest (Sapir, 1915).

Two Ute informants, numbers 0043 and 0049, also used the term *stutter* in describing nonfluency in their children's speech (Stewart, 1960, p. 43).

stutter (to): "the'-ce u-ba-ci-ge." "I stutter," "The'-ce u-ba-ci-ge." "You stutter," "the-ce u-thi-ba-ci-ge (La Flesche, *Osage Dictionary*, Bureau of American Ethnology, Bulletin 109, 1932).

BIBLIOGRAPHY

Andrews, G., and M. Harris, *The Syndrome of Stuttering*. London: Heinemann, 1964.

Aron, M., "An Investigation of the Nature and Incidence of Stuttering Among a Bantu Group of School-Going Children." Master's thesis, University of Witwatersrand, South Africa, 1958.

Bullen, A. K., "A Cross Cultural Approach to the Problem of Stuttering," *Child Development*, XVI (1945), 1–87.

Clark, R. M., and F. M. Murray, "Alterations in Self Concept: A Barometer of Progress in Individuals Undergoing Therapy for Stuttering." In D. E. Barbara (ed.), *New Directions in Stuttering*. Springfield, Ill.: Thomas, 1965.

Clifford, S. "Stuttering in South Dakota Indians," *Central States Speech Association Journal*, XVI (1965), 59–60.

Douglass, E., personal communication, 1953.

Emerick, L., "Bibliotherapy for Stutterers: Four Case Studies," *Quarterly Journal of Speech*, LII (1966), 74–79.

French, P., "The Stammerer as Hero," *The Encounter*, XXVII (1966), 67–75.

Greene, J. S., "Hope for the Stutterer," *Hygeia*, XXIV (1946), 120–21.

Gustafson, C. G., "A Talisman and a Convalescence." *Quarterly Journal of Speech*, XXX (1944), 465–71.

Hertz, J. H., *The Pentateuch and the Haftorahs*. London: Soncino Press, 1938.

Johnson, W., *People in Quandaries*. New York: Harper, 1946, p. 443.

———. "The Indians Have No Word for It: Stuttering in Adults," *Quarterly Journal of Speech Disorders*, XXX (1944), 330–37; 456–65.

———. *Because I Stutter*. New York: Appleton-Century-Crofts, 1930.

Kluckhohn, C., "Culture and Personality." In G. Lindzey (ed.), *Handbook of Social Psychology*. Cambridge, Mass.: Addison-Wesley, 1954.

Lemert, E. M., *Social Pathology*. New York: McGraw-Hill, 1951.

———. "Some Indians Who Stutter," *Journal of Speech and Hearing Disorders*, XVIII 1953, 168–74.

Liljeblad, S., "The Indians Have a Word for It." Unpublished paper read to Nevada State Speech Association, May 6, 1967.

Morgenstern, J. J., "Psychological and Social Factors in Children's Stammering." Doctoral dissertation, University of Edinburgh, 1953.

————. "Socio-Economic Factors in Stuttering," *Journal of Speech Disorders,* XXI (1956), 25–33.

Nuttall, W., "The Memoir of a Stammerer," *Psyche,* XVII (1937), 151–84.

Sapir, E., *Abnormal Types of Speech in the Nootka.* Ottawa, Canada: Dept. Mines. Geological Survey Memoir 62, Anthropological Series, 1915.

Scott, A. C., *The Kabuki Theatre of Japan.* London: Allen and Unwin, 1955.

Skelton, J., *Elynour Rummynge.* 1598.

Snidecor, J. C., "Why the Indian Does not Stutter," *Quarterly Journal of Speech,* XXXIII (1947), 493–95.

Stein, L., *The Infancy of Speech and the Speech of Infancy.* London: Methuen, 1949.

Stewart, J. L., "Problem of Stuttering in Certain North American Indian Societies," *Journal of Speech and Hearing Disorders, Supplement VI* (1959), 1–87.

Van Riper, C., *Speech Correction: Principles and Methods,* 4th Ed. Englewood Cliffs, N.J.: Prentice-Hall, 1963, p. 306.

Waley, A., (trans.), *Laotze: The Way and the Power.* London: Allen and Unwin, 1927.

two

STUTTERING:
ITS DEFINITION

DEFINITIONS

Many very good minds have attempted definitions of stuttering, but the variability among them makes clear that this complex and variable disorder is hard to delimit. Some of its complex behaviors always seem able to evade capture. Some of the definitions are merely statements of the authors' points of view with respect to the cause or nature of the disorder. To cite some examples we find such statements as these: "Stuttering is a psychoneurosis caused by the persistence into later life of early pregenital oral nursing, oral sadistic, and anal sadistic components (Coriat, 1943)." "Stuttering is a psychological difficulty and should be diagnosed and described as well as treated as a morbidity of social consciousness, a hypersensitivity of social attitude, a pathological social response (Fletcher, 1943, p. 33)." "Stuttering is a symptom in a psychopathological condition classified as a pregenital conversion neurosis (Glauber, 1958, p. 78)." "Stuttering is an evaluational disorder. It is what results when normal nonfluency is evaluated as something to be feared and avoided; it is, outwardly, what the stutterer does in an attempt to avoid nonfluency (Johnson, 1946, p. 452)."

Some definitions are so broad that they fail to provide proper limitations, something a good definition always tries to do. For example: "Stuttering is a deviation in the ongoing fluency of speech, an inability to maintain the connected rhythms of speech." "Stuttering is a disorder of rhythm." Such definitions would suggest that there are no normal speakers—unless the word "deviation" is further characterized. We all deviate at times from perfection in fluency. Normal speech is far from being connected, many studies having shown that frequent breaks occur in verbal continuity. Goldman-Eisler (1967) for example, found that 30 per cent of her speakers' talking time was spent in filled or unfilled pauses. Normal fluency does not mean uninterrupted flow.

Conversely, there are definitions which are so restrictive that they exclude many persons who would be commonly called or would call themselves stutterers. Wendell Johnson preferred to restrict *stuttering* to designate the speech of only those individuals who were showing "anticipatory hypertonic avoidance reactions" due to misevaluations of normal disfluencies. This definition by exclusion was most convenient in supporting his semantogenic theory, but Johnson was never quite able to persuade all of us, or even most of us, that we must never use the label of stuttering except in his restricted sense. Brutten and Shoemaker (1967, p. 61) also use what seems to us to be an unduly restrictive definition. They say: "Stuttering is that form of fluency failure that results from conditioned negative emotion." Their provision that every moment of stuttering must involve negative emotion does not seem to fit the facts—as we shall see later in this text. Theorists often take care of the exceptions to their theory by defining them out of existence.

Other definitions are frankly descriptive lists of behaviors, overt or covert, shown by different stutterers. Such catalog descriptions are always incomplete, and all stutterers do not show all the behaviors listed. Finally there are the definitions consisting of descriptions of phenomena which seek to identify the essential speech characteristics that differentiate stuttering behavior from other phenomena with which it could be confused. These try to describe the behaviors common to all stutterers, and to indicate the kinds of accessory behaviors shown only by some. Wingate's definition will illustrate this.

> The term "stuttering" means: I. (a) Disruption in the fluency of verbal expression, which is (b) characterized by involuntary, audible or silent, repetitions or prolongations in the utterance of short speech elements, namely: sounds, syllables, and words of one syllable. These disruptions (c) usually occur frequently or are marked in character and (d) are not readily controllable. II. Sometimes the disruptions are (e) accompanied by accessory activities involving the speech apparatus, related or unrelated body structures, or stereotyped speech utterances. These activities give the appearance of being speech-related struggle. III. Also, there are not infrequently (f) indications or report of the presence of an emotional state, ranging from a general condition of "excitement" or "tension" to more specific emotions of a negative nature such as fear, embarrassment, irritation, or the like. (g) The immediate source of stuttering is some incoordination expressed in the peripheral speech mechanism; the ultimate cause is presently unknown and may be complex or compound (Wingate, 1964, p. 498).

The differential diagnosis of stuttering from normal disfluency is not at all difficult when the disorder is severe or in its advanced stages. Diagnostic difficulty arises mainly when the disorder is very mild or in its earliest stages of development. This is to be expected. Hearing loss, asthma, allergies, a hundred other of the ills that plague the human race are hard to identify in their incipient stages or minor manifestations. Just because stuttering is occasionally difficult to distinguish from normal disfluency in its early or minor forms (and we must remember that stutterers also have normal disfluencies) we need not deny that stuttering exists as an entity. The insistence of millions of stutterers and their listeners that there is something wrong with the way they talk is difficult to disregard.

With some reluctance, we provide our own definition. It is at least shorter: *a stuttering behavior consists of a word improperly patterned in time and the speaker's reactions thereto.* Such a definition may cause many readers to bristle at first, but we hope they will consider our following remarks in its support. When we stutter on a word, we temporally disrupt the unity of its motor patterning. The disruption of the word may be due to time distortions of the component sounds or of the syllables which comprise the word. A word can be broken by repetitions or prolongations or gaps or the insertions of other inappropriate behaviors into its motor pattern, and when these occur, the person may be said to speak that word stutteringly. In this sense, all of us "stutter" occasionally. Whether we have the disorder called stuttering or conceive of ourselves as stutterers is quite another matter.

One might wonder why all this material on definition has been presented. Has the definition of stuttering any major importance? We think it does. The erroneous definition of stuttering may lead to unfortunate consequences as illustrated in the following accounts:

> All through his previous years at school he had been known, not merely as a normal speaker, but as a definitely superior speaker. He had won a number of speaking contests, had served as chairman of several student groups. Then one day a "speech correction teacher" examined him in the course of a school survey, and for some reason, told him that he was a *stutterer,* and advised him to "watch" his speech and be careful when he talked. Within a few months he would have been regarded as a stutterer and a fairly severe one by anyone professionally familiar with this type of speech problem. In reacting to the diagnosis—to the diagnosed characteristics of his speech, the interruptions of one sort or another which are normally found in the speech of everyone, but which in his case had been called *stuttering*—he developed muscular tensions, facial contortions, and apprehensiveness about speaking. In short, that teacher made him into a stutterer (Johnson, 1949, p. 175).

And here is a letter from a classroom teacher quoted in another article from Johnson:

In our school we have a speech correctionist who comes once a week, takes the children out to a special class for thirty minutes. I did not send one little girl, six and one half years of age, from my first grade because she has spoken perfectly all year and does not have a speech defect. But her mother called the principal about her and the speech therapist came to my room to get her. "Why" I asked. "Because she stutters," was the reply. "But she has never stuttered yet in school," I said.

The speech correctionist insisted it would please the mother to have the child have the advantages of the speech correction program so I sent the child to the speech clinic room. When she returned we heard her falter and hesitate for the first time. Upon her return we were having a "sharing time" about Thanksgiving experiences. This little girl got up as usual, began with a smile, then blocked completely on the word "turkey." She struggled quite a while, then broke into tears and sobbed to her classmates: "I can't say it because I stutter" (Johnson, 1939, p. 38).

What is perhaps of greater importance is that by defining stuttering we immediately come to grips with its basic nature. There is an old Finnish proverb which says that sin has a thousand faces but all of them are evil. Stuttering also has a thousand features and our task in defining it is to find the characteristics which seem common to all.

THE SEMANTICS OF THE TERM STUTTERING

Some of the difficulty in defining stuttering results from the way the term is used. When we use the verb *to stutter* or the phrase *a moment of stuttering* we refer to certain kinds of behaviors. When we use the noun *stuttering* categorically we designate a disorder. When we employ the word *stutterer* we refer to a role or special kind of deviant. Two early investigations, one by Voelker (1942) and the other by Villareal (1945), explored the semantics of the terms referring to stuttering by asking a large number of *normal* speakers these questions and getting these positive replies:

	Voelker	*Villareal*
1. Have you ever had a stuttering defect in speech?	10.4%	14.0%
2. Have you ever been called a stutterer?	4.2	6.7
3. Have you ever been said to have been stuttering?	30.2	29.1
4. Have you ever thought you had the habit of stuttering?	1.0	1.8
5. Have you ever thought you have spoken stutteringly?	72.9	76.0
6. Have you ever called yourself a stutterer?	6.3	9.9

Sander (1963) found similar evidence that the terms *stuttering* and *stutterer* may refer to quite different patterns of behavior. He says:

... many listeners by their usage seemed to feel that it was clearly possible to "stutter" without being a "stutterer." Listeners responded: "I don't think he stuttered enough to be called a 'stutterer.' " "He stuttered because he couldn't find the word he wanted."

In another study Sander (1965, p. 26) provides some examples of the variant usages:

> In terms of their language behavior, the responses of the listeners in this study might be grouped on a continuum beginning with "He repeated," or "He hesitated" (relatively descriptive terms), passing first to "He stuttered" (less descriptive), then to "There was evidence of a speech impediment" (something removed from the behavior heard), and finally to "He has a speech defect" (a "thing"-like quality possessed by the speaker), or "He seemed to be a stutterer" (a personification of the behavior).

Gately (1967) found much the same distinctions when he had listeners diagnose the tape recording of a mild stutterer: "Of eighty-three subjects who noted that the speaker 'stuttered' or exhibited 'stuttering' only thirty-five judged him to be a 'stutterer.' "

STUTTERING AS BEHAVIOR

The studies we have just reviewed indicate the necessity for some precision in definition. We feel that our operational definition of the stuttering act as a temporally disrupted word has real utility. It enables us to count stutterings in diagnosing severity. It permits an operant therapist to program his reinforcements contingently. It pinpoints the behavior to be modified.

The lack of precision in definition has led to much confusion, as the following researches demonstrate. Tuthill (1946) played recordings of the speech of adult stutterers and normal speakers to groups of stutterers, speech therapists, and lay listeners, asking them to mark on the reading passage those words on which stuttering had occurred. Only 37 per cent of the stuttered words were so identified by *all* the listeners. Stutterers classified more words as stuttered than did the speech therapist, and the lay listeners marked the fewest. Williams and Kent (1958) tape recorded a speech which had 52 instances of simulated disfluencies of various types. Although they discovered generally that their lay listeners were more consistent in labeling syllable repetitions and prolongations as stuttering, they found much disagreement as to which words were stuttered. Moreover, by varying their instructions to the listeners, they demonstrated how subjective definitions can be controlled by set:

> When subjects were instructed to listen to the recorded speech and mark stuttered interruptions, they marked many of the same interruptions that they marked when instructed to listen to the same speech and mark normal interruptions. They tended to hear what they were instructed to listen for

at the time. . . . The group of subjects first marked as stuttered those they first marked as normal. Conversely, the groups instructed to mark normal interruptions first marked more as normal than they subsequently marked as stuttered (p. 130).

What support is there for our arbitrary statement that stuttering behaviors should be confined within morphemic boundaries? Is it true that the core behavior of stuttering consists of temporally distorted sounds, syllables, or whole words and not disrupted phrases or sentences? To put it more generally, is it the words which are broken when we stutter or is it the phrases or sentences? We shall consider only a few representative contributions here since Wingate (1964) has reviewed most of the literature and concluded that stutterers show more intra-word disfluencies than normal speakers.

In one of the first studies Voelker (1944) compared the fluency breaks of stutterers with those of normal speaking children. They differed only in that the stutterers had significantly more prolongations of sounds and more repetitions of syllables and words. Wyrick (1949) showed that syllabic repetitions comprised only an insignificant fraction of the total number of disfluencies shown by normal speakers. In the study mentioned previously, Williams and Kent (1958) reported that "syllable repetition and prolongation of sounds were more consistently responded to as stuttered interruptions" than were interjections, word or phrase repetitions, or revisions. Boehmler (1958) in a very careful investigation found that sound and syllable repetitions were judged to be moments of stuttering significantly more often than were word repetitions, phrase repetitions, or other types of disfluency and that this held true for naive as well as professional judges. Although stressing the overlap between his normal and stuttering groups, Johnson (1961) showed conclusively in another study that "of all the types of disfluency, part word repetitions are more likely to be classified by listeners, at least in our general culture, as 'stuttering' and that certain other kinds of disfluency, most notably perhaps interjections, revisions, and phrase repetitions, are more commonly considered as 'normal' disfluencies." McDearmon (1968) showed the same finding in his reanalysis of Johnson's *Onset of Stuttering* data (1959). Young (1961) demonstrated that "the types of speech disfluency that appear to be associated with ratings of severity of stuttering are syllable or sound repetitions, sound prolongations, broken words, and words involving apparently unusual stress or tension."

STUTTERING AS A DISORDER

The term *disorder* to many people implies a disease. It may well be, however, that the medical model does not fit the problem of stuttering in all of its varieties. Strong cases have been made for viewing it merely as a group of learned maladaptive responses. In this text we see stuttering as a disorder the same way we see reading disability as a disorder.

A single cough has little significance; frequent spells of coughing may indicate emphysema, tuberculosis, or other disorders. A few sneezes are part of normal living; continual sneezing may mean hay fever or even a brain tumor. The characteristics of the cough or sneeze are scrutinized by the physician in determining if a true disorder is present. Also the conditions under which coughing or sneezing occur may help determine the diagnosis. We use these analogies to introduce the concept of stuttering as a disorder. Stuttering behaviors, broken words, constitute a disorder when they are diagnosed as such by the speaker or by his listeners based upon the scrutiny of their frequency, their characteristics, and the conditions under which they occur.

As a disorder, stuttering is identified by a process of differential diagnosis. The speech must appear to be outside the norms of the culture for speech production. It must also be differentiated from other forms of speech deviancy.

Stuttering is primarily a disorder of the temporal aspects of speech, not of the articulatory, phonatory, or symbolic features. Anyone who has known many stutterers will of course recognize that some of them show abnormalities in the way they articulate or phonate a given sound or syllable. We have watched severe stutterers attempt a vowel with the mouth tightly closed, or a labial plosive with the jaws agape; we have heard them prolong a sound with a fire-siren kind of inflection; we have seen them apparently unable to produce voice. But these are not features common to all stutterers nor are they always characteristic of the single stutterer who occasionally demonstrates them. The essential feature that distinguishes a stutterer from a person with an articulatory disability is the former individual's apparent inability to perform the motor sequencing of a given sound or syllable or word at the proper moments in time. Speech is patterned in time, both motorically and acoustically; the movements, the sounds, the syllables must occur in a prescribed sequence. When this sequencing of word utterance is noticeably disrupted in a certain way and evaluated as undesirable, the person is said to possess the disorder of stuttering.

The term "disorder" implies that it is somehow unpleasant and undesirable. Any stutterer or anyone who has talked with one for some time will agree that this is true. But we have very little research bearing directly upon this feature. Perrin (1954) using a sociometric technique showed that speech defects in general tended to create isolates when school children were asked to choose partners. Giolas and Williams (1958) created three tapes of the same story, one spoken normally, one with a number of interjections (um's and ah's) and the third with the same number of stutterings. Second grade children were asked to tell which of the story tellers they would desire as their teacher. The results were not unexpected: the children chose the normal speaker first, the interjectionist second, and the stutterer third. Ro-

senberg and Curtis (1954) found that unsuspecting listeners when confronted suddenly by a stuttering talker lost their mobility and eye-contact
and reduced their speech output. Van Riper (1937) and Ainsworth (1945)
demonstrated that the breathing of listeners to stuttering was empathically
altered in an abnormal way when they listened to stuttering. Berlin and
Berlin (1964) showed that certain types of stuttering, notably a prolongation
kind, were judged as more acceptable than were the repetitive or other
types. These and other researches indicate that stuttering as a disorder is
evaluated unfavorably.

THE STUTTERING KINDS
OF DISFLUENCY

We have already shown that a special kind of disfluency serves as the criterion behavior of stuttering. Not all of the interruptions to the forward
flow of speech are signs of stuttering. Fortunately, it is possible to inhale occasionally without being referred to the speech clinic. We can repeat words
and phrases, pause silently, scratch our heads, lick our lips, utter "ah's" and
"ums" and interrupt the continuity of our speech in a hundred ways without causing our listeners to raise an eyebrow or bulge an eyeball. Such in-
terrupting behaviors do not seem to play an important role in the diagnosis
of the disorder of stuttering. According to Mahl (1956) syllabic repetitions
accounted for only six per cent of all the varieties of fluency breaks shown
by normal speakers. McClay and Osgood (1959) analyzed the spontaneous
speech of speakers at a conference to determine the kinds of repetitions
shown. Repetitions of whole words constituted 71 per cent; repetitions of
phrases, 17 per cent; and "part word repetitions" only 12 per cent. Soderberg (1967) analyzed the speech of some stutterers in the same way and
found that the proportion was reversed, that 63 per cent were part word
repetitions. It is when we have too many broken words; it is when speech
is noticeably fractured at the level of the sound, syllable, or word that we
differentially diagnose stuttering from the other acceptable kinds of fluency
interruptions.

We have said that all of us speak stutteringly at times, that is that occasionally we show a temporally disrupted word. It is certain that the frequency with which these broken words are emitted is an important factor
in the diagnosis of stuttering as a disorder. One syllabic repetition in a hundred words would have little stimulus value; 50 of them would be noticed
by any listener. This relationship of frequency to diagnosis has been demonstrated by Sander's (1963) research. He contrived recorded speech samples
having different amounts of single-unit (Sa-Saturday) and double-unit syllabic repetitions and submitted one of these to each of 240 college students
who had to describe the speech, tell whether it should be considered defective, and to decide whether the speaker was a stutterer. In essence, Sander found that the more single-unit syllabic repetitions there were in a

sample, the more frequently that sample was judged as being stuttering or the speech of a stutterer. Also fewer double syllable repetitions than single syllable repetitions yielded a stuttering diagnosis.

As we mentioned earlier according to Sapir (1915) the language of the Nootka Indians was so full of syllabic repetitions that, according to Indians of other tribes, they were all said to be stutterers. (If so, the Nootkan who failed to use reduplicated syllables often enough would probably be noticed and evaluated by his fellow tribesmen as having a speech defect!) Standards of fluency vary not only in different cultures but even within the same culture. All stuttering yardsticks are not of the same length. We Americans use a longer one for children than we do for adults. Wendell Johnson felt that the Bannock and Shoshone Indians had no yardsticks at all. Some mothers have greater tolerances for their children's broken words than other mothers. Some children seem to be able to tolerate fewer of these morphemic interruptions than other children can. Nevertheless, despite the variations in normative criteria, a speaker must keep his broken words within the frequency limits of his listeners or be noticed and judged as having the disorder of stuttering.

EVALUATION OF ABNORMALITY —FREQUENCY

Although we do not yet have objective fluency standards which are satisfactory, this does not mean that such standards do not exist. Every listener has such standards and it might be well to summarize some of the research which shows their commonality and variability. It is somewhat surprising to find that lay and unsophisticated listeners seem able to judge the severity of stuttering on a rating scale almost as well as experts according to Young (1964) and Schaef and Matthews (1954) though usually the experts tend to be slightly more influenced by frequency of disfluency than the lay listeners (Boehmler, 1958; Tuthill, 1946; and Emerick, 1960). Anxious listeners do not seem to have higher standards than unanxious ones according to Gateley (1967). Much of the research on this topic is confounded, as Sander (1963) has made clear, by variant listening instructions, lack of sufficient sampling, and no direct assessment of all the variables that normally go into the diagnosis of stuttering as a disorder. Thus, Bloodstein, Jaeger, and Tureen (1952) found that the parents of stutterers tended to make more diagnoses of stuttering than those of nonstutterers whereas Berlin (1960) failed to find any such differences when he changed the listening instructions. Bar (1967), who submitted the recording of a very severe stutterer to a large number of listeners, found that different listening instructions made little difference in the estimation of stuttering. He says:

> It may not be important for listeners to have a (formal) definition of stuttering, especially, when it is severe, in order to make accurate estimates about

stuttering. This is supported by the fact that a large majority of listeners in this study, without having any definition of stuttering, reacted relatively accurately to the amount of stuttering. This also suggests that severe stuttering is not an ambiguous stimulus event (p. 91).

OTHER DISTINCTIVE FEATURES

The diagnosis of stuttering does not depend upon frequency of disrupted words alone. Merely counting how many such words there are in a given sample of speech and determining a percentage, as in computing the Iowa Disfluency Index (Johnson, 1961), is not sufficient. Minifee and Cooker (1964), for example, found that counting all syllables, including repeated ones, and dividing them by the number of words spoken was a better measure of the severity of stuttering than this index. This makes sense. Surely a word on which the first syllable was repeated ten times or 20 times would yield an impression of greater abnormality than a word on which the first syllable was only repeated once. We have already seen that Sander (1963) found that substantially fewer instances of double-unit repetitions (Sa-Sa-Saturday) were needed to evoke judgments of stuttering than when only single-units (Sa-Saturday) were present in the samples. In differentiating stuttering from normal speech, we should also take note of how drastically the words are broken.

To our knowledge there is no research bearing directly on the duration of the internal word gaps or the prolongations of a sound or articulatory posture as related to diagnosis. All we have are the many researches which indicate that it takes a stutterer longer to read a given passage than it takes a normal speaker to do so. The wide variations in reading and speaking rate among normal speakers makes such talking-time measures rather useless when trying to decide whether a specific person has or does not have the disorder of stuttering. However, it is quite possible to measure the durations of prolonged phonemes and morphemic gaps and we hope that future researchers will do so. Our own pilot investigations have shown that 100 per cent of our listeners noticed any sound which was prolonged more than three seconds and 50 per cent of them recognized as abnormal any sound prolonged longer than two seconds. Silent pauses within the word boundaries are recognized even more easily. A silent gap of even one fifth of a second within a fractured word is enough to indicate abnormality. Silent pauses just prior to word initiation have less stimulus value (need to be longer to be recognized as abnormal) unless they are accompanied by the assumption of a visible articulatory posture. The presence of tremors or contortions or other accessory behaviors lead, of course, to immediate recognition. In general, we think we are safe in saying that the longer the duration of a sound or silent gap, the more likely it will be that a diagnosis of stuttering will be made. Any speaker who would hold the /n/ in the word "no" for 20 seconds, as some of our stutterers have done, even though it occurred only once in a thousand words, would immediately be suspected of having something wrong with him.

There are other ways in which words are temporally disrupted which cue off listeners to make (or corroborate) a tentative diagnosis of stuttering. The tempo of multiple syllabic repetitions is also important. We need to know how much faster or slower they occur than the ordinary rate of syllabic emission. If every time the speaker repeats a syllable, he does it three times faster than he emits the other syllables of his normal speech, that syllable will stand out like a third thumb. We have all known stutterers whose speech motors race in this way. However, the converse also seems to be true. If the speaker says a syllable, pauses, says it again; pauses deliberately and then says the word, most listeners would feel that he is having trouble getting that word out. This sort of behavior shows up mostly in the confirmed stutterers of the interiorized variety described by Freund (1935) and Douglass and Quarrington (1952), stutterers who often are otherwise very successful in hiding their disorder. Another clue indicating that the person either has, or is in danger of acquiring the disorder of stuttering is found in the irregularity of the syllabic repetitions. The few syllabic repetitions which normal speakers show not only occur at the same tempo as the rest of their syllables, but they occur evenly, regularly. When we find a person repeating syllables jerkily rather than smoothly, we tend to diagnose abnormality. This is only our clinical impression for the research is still to be done.

COARTICULATION FEATURES

Two other distinctive features of the stutterer's broken words as compared to the normal speaker's similar disfluencies concern coarticulation and airflow. When a normal speaker repeats syllables or prolongs a sound, the proper transitional formants appear in that syllable or sound and airflow continues. We are just beginning to get research which indicates that this may not be true of the stutterer's repetitions and prolongations, nor true for the similar kinds of behavior shown under delayed auditory feedback.

The research is not yet definitive but there are some interesting findings in terms of coarticulation and airflow. Agnello (1966) reports that the acoustic and pause characteristics of the stuttering nonfluencies of stutterers differed from their normal speech disfluencies. Some of these acoustic differences were undetectable by the ear and showed up only on the spectrograms. The normal downward shift of the second formant, usually associated with articulatory positioning, was not characteristic of the stuttering moments. The intersyllabic pauses were longer and more variable. Similarly, Stromsta (1965) demonstrated that the spectrograms of stuttered speech revealed a lack of the usual falling or rising transitions shown in spectograms of normal speech. The juncture formants were not present or were different. Nor-

mally, in the integration of a syllable, coarticulation occurs. We prepare for
the second sound while still uttering the first. The phoneticians have used
the concept of "assimilation" to indicate this essential transitional phenomenon. In servo-theory, anticipatory feedback (forward assimilation) has been
shown to be an essential controller of the automatic sequencing of complex
movements.

The stutterer who is saying "Mmmmmmmmmmmmm-other" may not seem
to be having any trouble uttering that /m/ but he will tell you that he is,
and perhaps he may not be wrong. He may be searching for the /m/ which
has the juncture characteristics that are needed for the integration of this
initial sound with its following vowel. Similarly, if the stutterer is saying
"Suh-suh-sssuh-sandwich," it is obvious that he can never say "san" so long
as he keeps saying "suh." Almost universally the schwa vowel can be heard
in the stutterer's abortive speech attempts. When a stutterer has repetitive
syllables on the word "paper" he seldom says [pe-pe-pepɛ] instead he uses
the schwa vowel in his repetitions [pʌ-pʌ-pɪ-pepɛ]. Why the schwa? Why
not "pu" or "pi" or "po?" One explanation might be that a consonant's
set of allophones (with their corresponding allopropes—to coin a word)
cluster about a pole or central tendency represented by the utterance of that
consonant in syllabic conjunction with the neutral vowel. We suspect that

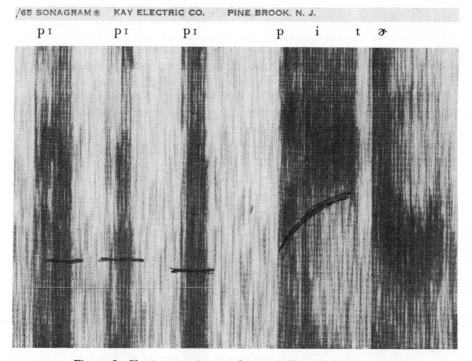

p ɪ   p ɪ   p ɪ   p   i   t   ɚ

**Figure 2. Clonic stuttering on the word "Peter" showing abrupt
interruptions and lack of juncture in three abortive syllabic
repetitions prior to successful utterance.**

even when a normal speaker tries to utter the /s/ or /m/ sounds in isolation, those isolated sounds will carry the juncture characteristics of the unspoken schwa. At any rate, when we hear the schwa vowel in repeated syllables rather than the one which should be present, we know that the proper transitions are not present and that the required coarticulation has not been achieved. Stromsta's (1965) research showed that those children whose spectrograms of disfluencies showed anomalies in coarticulation failed to "outgrow" their stuttering whereas those children whose spectrograms showed normal juncture formants had become fluent in the ten year span since the original recordings were made. Our own case studies of children whom we examined but could not treat, yet who finally acquired normal fluency, bear out Stromsta's research. We therefore feel it vitally important to determine whether or not the syllabic repetitions of the young child contain the schwa vowel. When they do, they indicate the probability of acquiring stuttering on a more permanent basis.

AIRFLOW DIFFERENCES

Another feature may also distinguish the syllabic repetitions of stutterers from those of the normal speaker. The airflow in stuttering repetitions is usually interrupted whereas in the normal speakers it usually continues during disfluencies. Moreover the interruption in stuttering repetitions is usually sudden while in contrast, the syllable of normal nonfluency shows a gradual termination before it is repeated. And there is another characteristic that seems to distinguish the abnormal from the normal syllabic repetitions: the pauses between syllables are much shorter in stuttered repetitions. It is as though the stutterer recoils while the normal speaker simply tries again. These differentiating phenomena can be seen in our exploratory sonographic and electromyographic recordings. It is possible, however, that they reflect merely the hypertensed musculatures of a confirmed stutterer in fear. We unfortunately have not been able to record many samples of the nonfluencies of the so-called primary stutterer and it may be that these are indistinguishable from normal nonfluencies. However, Stromsta (1965), again in the research quoted previously, reported findings which may throw some light on the matter. By submitting to spectrographic analysis the recordings of young stutterers which had been done ten years previously, he found that those who had continued to stutter also showed abrupt phonatory stoppages with a cessation of airflow. This blockage of phonation by the cessation of airflow may be one of the most important characteristics differentiating normal disfluency from stuttering. In assessing the disfluent behavior of any child, we should carefully scrutinize the airflow. When it is interrupted it indicates stuttering.

In the light of these observations, the commonly held belief that the core behavior of stutterers differs from normal speakers only in degree but not in kind may be viewed with less confidence. The stutterer may repeat or prolong because the sound or syllable is not motorically integrated, i.e. because he's "stuck"; the normal speaker may repeat or hold a sound or syllable for other reasons. Many of the distinguishing features we have been mentioning are difficult to identify without instrumentation and the untrained ear alone is notoriously inadequate in detecting such features. The normal speaker's syllabic repetitions may sound like those of the stutterer and yet be different. We hunger for the necessary research which will dispose of the question.

THE CONDITIONS
OF COMMUNICATION

Disfluency, both normal and abnormal, is the result of communicative stress. Most normal disfluencies result either from formulative difficulties or emotional pressures. Mahl (1956) distinguishes between them, calling the former "ah-hesitations" and the latter "non-ah hesitations." It is interesting that in the latter category he includes "stutter" as one of the less common types of normal hesitancies produced by emotional stress rather than by formulative difficulties. The loci of stuttering behaviors are much the same as those for normal hesitancies with one exception. They tend to occur on the first words of utterances which does not seem to hold true for normal disfluencies. The stutterer has trouble getting started. We therefore can use this as one more bit of information to feed into our diagnostic computer.

It also appears possible that stutterers are more vulnerable to communicative and emotional stress than normal speakers so far as the evoking of disfluency is concerned. It takes a lot of pressure before a normal speaker will show fractured words. Much less stress seems to be required to get the stutterer to stutter. Again this is a clinical impression and the basic research is lacking. However, in trying to discover whether a little child is really stuttering or is only normally disfluent, we introduce certain fluency disruptors into our interaction. We hurry him; we interrupt, contradict, and pretend to misunderstand. And do other similar things. Most normal speaking children under these conditions may show pauses, interjections, revisions, and phrase repetitions but only rarely will they demonstrate broken words. The stutterer will. The proportion of morphemic to supramorphemic disruptions will markedly increase when he feels this stress. We suspect that any final formula for the differential diagnosis of stuttering would have to include some factor to represent the communicative conditions at the time the diagnosis was made. Most of us occasionally speak "stutteringly" when communicating under great emotional stress, ambivalence, or time pressure. When these conditions do not seem to be present, whether they are or not, the diagnosis tends to be made in terms of more stringent criteria than when stress is highly evident. We make allowances.

In ordinary life, if not in the speech science laboratory, the diagnosis of stuttering is not based on short segments of tape played over and over again. A listener usually goes through a gradual checking process until enough information finally corroborates a diagnosis which at first has been only tentative. If the stuttering is highly visible in its overt struggle and other behaviors the diagnosis may of course be achieved almost instantly. But all of us have experienced enough normal nonfluency at times to make us rather conservative in applying the stuttering label indiscriminately.

ACCESSORY FEATURES

Thus far we have been considering the essential features, those common to all stutterers, the excessive repetitions and prolongations of syllables and sounds. There are also other behaviors, termed by Wingate (1964) "accessory features," which, when scanned by the listener, will swiftly give rise to the diagnosis of stuttering. Among these are the struggle behaviors, those tremors and facial grimaces, the bizarre jaw and limb and even trunk movements which appear most generally but not always in the advanced stages of the disorder's development. Since they occur in the context of the speech attempt on the syllable or sound, they tend to be viewed by the listener and by the stutterer himself as evidences of his inability to continue the flow of utterance and are hence viewed as indicating abnormality.

Also we find many avoidance behaviors, inappropriate to the normal act of speaking, such as verbal circumlocutions, stallers, and unusual interjections or substitutions of odd synonyms. These are viewed by the listener as efforts to avoid the anticipated fluency break. When they occur frequently enough or last long enough or are bizarre enough, they too lead to the diagnosis of stuttering. All these bits of information go into the listener's computer and the read-out is deviancy when their assemblage exceeds that listener's norms for fluency.

DIFFERENTIAL DIAGNOSIS
OF STUTTERING
FROM NORMAL DISFLUENCY

Since our research is still grossly incomplete, we must have recourse to clinical experience in supplementing the information we do possess in creating the guidelines for a differential diagnosis. Usually, as we have shown, no problem exists when we are confronted by a severe stutterer. The following scheme would be used when examining a person, usually a child, where the matter is in some doubt. It is the sort of information which the practicing speech therapist feeds into his internal clinical computer in assessing the child's risks or dangers of developing a full fledged disorder of stuttering.

GUIDELINES FOR DIFFERENTIATING NORMAL FROM ABNORMAL DISFLUENCY

Behavior	*Stuttering*	*Normal Disfluency*
Syllable Repetitions:		
a. Frequency per word	More than two	Less than two
b. Frequency per 100 words	More than two	Less than two
c. Tempo	Faster than normal	Normal tempo
d. Regularity	Irregular	Regular
e. Schwa vowel	Often present	Absent or rare
f. Airflow	Often interrupted	Rarely interrupted
g. Vocal tension	Often apparent	Absent
Prolongations:		
h. Duration	Longer than one second	Less than one second
i. Frequency	More than one per 100 words	Less than one per 100 words
j. Regularity	Uneven or interrupted	Smooth
k. Tension	Important when present	Absent
l. When voiced (sonant)	May show rise in pitch	No pitch rise
m. When unvoiced (surd)	Interrupted airflow	Airflow present
n. Termination	Sudden	Gradual
Gaps (silent pauses):		
o. Within the word boundary	May be present	Absent
p. Prior to speech attempt	Unusually long	Not marked
q. After the disfluency	May be present	Absent
Phonation:		
r. Inflections	Restricted; monotone	Normal
s. Phonatory arrest	May be present	Absent
t. Vocal fry	May be present	Usually absent
Articulating Postures:		
u. Appropriateness	May be inappropriate	Appropriate
Reaction to Stress:		
v. Type	More broken words	Normal disfluencies
Evidence of awareness:		
w. Phonemic consistency	May be present	Absent
x. Frustration	May be present	Absent
y. Postponements (stallers)	May be present	Absent
z. Eye contact	May waver	Normal

It is perhaps fortunate that we have run out of letters of the alphabet in creating the items of our guidelines. This list, formidable as it is, can hardly be said to be complete and we are not happy with the quality of the items nor with their lack of quantification. They are just the best indications known to those who daily confront these problems. One of the gross deficiencies is the lack of item weights. Obviously, all these items are not equal in differentiating value. The author has his own system for weighting the item probabilities, but we will not give it the presumed validity of appearing in these pages. Let each person devise his own item weights until we have the research we need so badly. We must do the best we can with what we have available to us.

CLUTTERING

Thus far we have been concerned primarily with the problems of differentiating stuttering as a disorder from the disfluencies characteristic of normal speakers. There is, however, another disorder of fluency, cluttering, which deserves consideration. A precise definition of cluttering has proved even more difficult than that for stuttering for, as usually envisaged, its symptomatology includes far more than the disordered fluency which is only one of its characteristics. The clutterer is said to show deficits or abnormality also in symbolic language development and formulation, in articulation, and in phonatory characteristics as well as in fluency. Other language functions such as reading, writing, and formulating are impaired. Since the present text is dedicated to stuttering and because cluttering has been described very adequately by other authors, notably Freund, Arnold, Luchsinger, and Weiss* we shall refer the reader to their writings and get on with our own.

COMMENTARY

A definition is like a net. It can catch one big fish—the major characteristic of the item being defined—but the little ones escape through the meshes.

Anyone who makes definitions is like a man who puts on a stove pipe hat and walks past a gang of children making snow balls. Everyone feels free to take a crack at him.

A definition is an invitation to all comers to make a better one. In Stevenson's *Treasure Island*, one of the pirates is quoted as growling, "Wot's wot? Ah, he'd be a lucky one as knowed that."

He who defines assumes the mantle of authority. He says in effect, "Hear ye, Hear ye. This is what is. I have spoken" and so immediately he becomes vulnerable.

It is interesting to note that, in spite of the multiformity of its character,

---

* See the following selected references: Freund, H., "Studies in the Inter-relationship between Stuttering and Cluttering," *Folia Phoniatrica*, IV (1952), 146–68; Luchsinger, R., and G. E. Arnold, *Voice-Speech-Language*. Belmont, California: Wadsworth, 1965; and Weiss, D. A., *Cluttering*. Englewood Cliffs, N.J.: Prentice-Hall, 1964.

even the layman, with few exceptions, is able to comprehend the various types of this disorder under one concept (Stein, 1942, p. 109).

Since "to define" means "to determine and state the nature and limits of," it may seem presumptuous to attempt a standard definition of stuttering at this time. However, the serious need for a workable definition of stuttering can be met by adhering to certain criteria. The definition should be one which: (a) identifies and emphasizes discriminative features, (b) is amenable to general application, and (c) accords with our current state of knowledge of stuttering (Wingate, 1964, p. 484).

It is a kind of St. Vitus Dance of the Tongue (Hall, 1869, p. 7).

The clinical picture of stuttering is that of a cramp-like (spasmodic) expressive neurosis in the area of oral communication stemming from a nervous reaction with a constitutional basis (Luchsinger and Arnold, 1965, p. 739).

. . . stuttering, or the disruption of normal speech fluency, is considered a disorder of . . . verbalizing deautomaticity (Mysak, 1960, p. 189).

Both introspective and objective observations convince us that most people stutter. Only a few people are sufficiently miserable over their speaking relationships, however, that they bring their problem to therapy under the label of stuttering (Travis, 1957, p. 918).

For the purposes of this study, any child was considered a stutterer who (1) showed unmistakable anxiety-tension reactions in relation to his speech nonfluencies; or (2) had been or was currently regarded as a stutterer; or (3) declared himself to be a stutterer (Johnson, 1955, p. 79).

The types of speech disfluency that appear to be associated with ratings of severity of stuttering are syllable and sound repetitions, sound prolongations, broken words, and words involving unusual stress or tension (Young, 1961, p. 53).

Prolongations of sound occur rarely in normal speech, whereas in stuttering they often form a characteristic part of the abnormality. Stuttering is an interruption in the normal rhythm of speech of such frequency and abnormality as to attract attention, interfere with communication, or cause distress to a stutterer or his audience. He knows precisely what he wishes to say, but at times is unable to say it easily because of an involuntary repetition, prolongation, or cessation of sound (Andrews and Harris, 1964, p. 1).

Revisions were primarily considered normal interruptions while syllable repetitions and prolongations were primarily considered as stuttering (Williams and Kent, 1958, p. 132).

One stutterer will make spasmodic contractions of the lips, tongue, etc., whereby a word like "berry" will be pronounced "b-b-b-b-berry." The most striking symptoms are cramps or spasms of the muscles connected with speech. . . . The lips may be pressed tightly together for a short or long time when the patient tries to say "p" or "b." The tongue may be pressed so tightly against the palate that the "t" or the "d" is two, three, or ten times too long. All the sounds may be similarly affected (Scripture, 1923, p. 1).

. . . the speech of stutterers fails not at the single sound but only at the connection between sounds (Froeschels, 1913–14).

The absurd notion, which once had a few disciples, that stammering is a disease, has nearly become obsolete; although there may be some few who still entertain the idea that it comes within the province of the physician, and will succumb to medical treatment. To characterize as a disease an improper use of the lips, tongue, breath, and lower jaw, seems quite as ridiculous, as if speaking ungrammatically, or biting one's nails, were so called. Stammering is a habit, and nothing else (Beasley, 1879, p. 21).

He closes the oral canal at one or other of the closing points according to the nature of the letter to be articulated, and this he does as well as a man who possesses the faculty of speech could do it; instead, however, of allowing the vowel to follow without delay, he presses his lips or his tongue and teeth, or his tongue and palate more firmly than is necessary (Kussmaul quoted in Wyllie, 1894).

. . . the co-movements of stutterers which indeed are not limited only to the face or breathing muscles but also overlap into the arm and leg muscles . . . (Draseke, 1921, p. 344).

There are many different forms of interruption in children's speech . . . and it is unlikely that all of them are anticipatory struggle reactions in the sense in which this term has been used here. Our thesis is simply that among the disfluencies to be heard in the speech of nearly all young children there are early prototypes of stuttering behavior which will develop into chronic and troublesome problems in a few cases. On the basis of present knowledge it would appear that among the most notable of primitive stutterings of normal children are syllable and word repetitions, and prolongations of sound (Bloodstein, Alper, and Zisk, 1965, p. 52.)

Among the possible interpretations of the data pertaining to speaker performance and listener evaluation are these: (a) a listener is more likely to classify a given disfluency as stuttering if he is set to evaluate some disfluencies as stuttering; (b) some disfluencies, particularly those associated with apparent struggle reactions, and those that are part-word repetitions even when relatively simple and effortless, are more likely than other disfluencies to be classified as stuttering by the listener; (c) the more disfluencies the speaker displays the more likely the listener is to regard him as a stutterer;

(d) the listener is more likely to classify the speaker's disfluencies as stuttering if he regards the speaker as a stutterer (Johnson, 1961, p. 15).

The frequency with which the judges applied the stuttering label varied with the rated severity of the samples. Trained judges applied the label more often than untrained judges. Sound and syllable repetitions were labeled as stuttering more often than revisions and interjections, regardless of rated severity (Boehmler, 1958, p. 139).

Half our speech time seems to issue in phrases not longer than three words, and three quarters in phrases of fewer than five words at the most. Evidently pausing is as much part of the act of speaking as the vocal utterance of words itself, which suggests that it is essential to the generation of spontaneous speech." . . . (Goldman-Eisler, 1967, pp. 119–20).

BIBLIOGRAPHY

Ainsworth, S., "Empathic Breathing of Auditors While Listening to Stuttered Speech," *Journal of Speech Disorders* IV (1939), 149–56.

Andrews, G., and M. Harris, *The Syndrome of Stuttering*. London: Methuen, 1964.

Agnello, J. G., "Some Acoustic and Pause Characteristics of Nonfluencies in the Speech of Stutterers," Technical Report National Institute of Mental Health, Grant No. 11067–01, 1966.

Agnello, J. G., and H. Goehl, "Spectrographical Patterns of Disfluencies in the Speech of Stutterers," convention address, A.S.H.A., 1965.

Bar, A., "Effects of Listening Instructions on Attention to Manner and to Content of Stutterers' Speech," *Journal of Speech and Hearing Research,* X (1967), 87–92.

Beasley, B., *Stammering: Its Treatment.* London: Hamilton, 1879.

Berlin, C. I., "Parents' Diagnoses of Stuttering," *Journal of Speech and Hearing Research,* III (1960), 372–79.

Berlin, S., and C. Berlin, "Acceptability of Stuttering Control Patterns," *Journal of Speech and Hearing Disorders,* XXIX (1964), 436–41.

Bloodstein, C., J. Alper, and P. Zisk, "Stuttering as an Outgrowth of Normal Disfluency." In D. E. Barbara (ed.), *New Directions in Stuttering: Theory and Practice.* Springfield, Ill.: Thomas, 1965.

Bloodstein, O., W. Jaeger, and J. Tureen, "Diagnosis of Stuttering by Parents of Stutterers and Nonstutterers," *Journal of Speech and Hearing Disorders,* XVII (1952), 308–15.

Boehmler, R. M., "Listener Responses to Nonfluencies," *Journal of Speech and Hearing Research,* I (1958), 132–41.

Brutten, E. J., and D. J. Shoemaker, *The Modification of Stuttering.* Englewood Cliffs, N.J.: Prentice-Hall, 1967.

Cullinan, W. L., and E. M. Prather, "Reliability of 'Live' Ratings of the Speech of Stutterers." *Perceptual and Motor Skills,* XXVII (1968), 403–9.

Coriat, I. H., "The Psychoanalytic Concept of Stammering," *Nervous Child,* II (1943), 167–71.

DeHirsch, K., and W. Langford, "Clinical Notes on Stuttering and Cluttering in Young Children," *Pediatrics,* V (1950), 934–40.

Douglass, E., and B. Quarrington, "Differentiation of Interiorized and Exteriorized Secondary Stuttering," *Journal of Speech and Hearing Disorders,* XVII (1952), 377–85.

Draseke, J. "Ueber Mitbewegungen bei Gesunden," *Deutsche Zeitschrift für Nervenheilkunde,* LXIV (1921), 340–46.

Emerick, L., "Extensional Definition and Attitude Toward Stuttering," *Journal of Speech and Hearing Research,* III (1960), 181–86.

Fletcher, J. M., "A Predisposing Cause of Stuttering," *Quarterly Journal of Speech,* XXIX (1943), 480–83.

Freund, H., *Psychopathology and the Problems of Stuttering.* Springfield, Ill.: Thomas, 1966.

———. "Ueber Inneres Stottern," *Zeitschrift Ohrenheilkunde,* LXIX (1935), 146–48.

Froeschels, E., "Pathology and Therapy of Stuttering," *Nervous Child,* II (1943), 148–61.

———. "Zur Pathologie des Stotterns," *Arch. f. Exper. u. Kleine Phonet.,* I (1913–14), 372–80.

Gateley, W. G., "Anxiety and Tension in Stuttering," convention address, A.S.H.A., 1967.

Giolas, T. G., and D. E. Williams, "Children's Reactions to Nonfluencies in Adult Speech," *Journal of Speech and Hearing Research,* I (1958), 86–93.

Goldman-Eisler, F., "Sequential Temporal Patterns and Cognitive Processes in Speech," *Language and Speech,* X (1967), 131–40.

Glauber, I. P., "The Psychoanalysis of Stuttering." In J. Eisenson ed.), *Stuttering: A Symposium.* New York: Harper, 1958, pp. 71–120.

Hahn, E., *Stuttering: Significant Theories and Therapies.* Stanford: Stanford University Press, 1943.

Hall, W. W., *The Guide Board.* London: D. E. Fisk, 1869.

Hayworth, D., "A Search for Facts on the Teaching of Public Speaking," *Quarterly Journal of Speech,* XXVI (1940), 31–38.

Johnson, W., "Language and Speech Hygiene," *General Semantics Monographs.* Chicago: Institute of General Semantics, 1939.

———. "Letter to the Editor," *Journal Speech and Hearing Disorders,* XIV (1949), 175–76.

———. "Measurements of Oral Reading and Speaking Rate and Disfluency of Adult Male and Female Stutterers and Nonstutterers," *Journal of Speech and Hearing Disorders,* Monograph Supplement 7 (1961), 1–20.

———. *The Onset of Stuttering.* Minneapolis: University of Minnesota Press, 1955.

———. *People in Quandaries.* New York: Harper, 1946.

Johnson, W., S. F. Brown, J. F. Curtis, C. W. Edney, and J. Keaster, *Speech Handicapped School Children.* New York: Harper, 1952.

Luchsinger, R., and G. E. Arnold, *Voice—Speech—Language.* Belmont, Cal.: Wadsworth, 1965.

Mahl, G., "Disturbances and Silences in the Patient's Speech in Psychotherapy," *Journal of Abnormal Social Psychology,* LIII (1956), 1–15.

McClay, H., and E. I. Osgood, "Hesitation Phenomena in Spontaneous English Speech," *Word,* XV (1959), 19–44.

McDearmon, J. R., "Primary Stuttering at the Onset of the Stuttering: A Re-examination of Data," *Journal of Speech and Hearing Research*, XI (1968), 631–37.

Minifee, F. D., and H. S. Cooker, "A Disfluency Index," *Journal of Speech and Hearing Disorders*, XXIX (1964), 189–93.

Mysak, E. D., Servo Theory and Stuttering," *Journal of Speech and Hearing Disorders*, XXV (1960), 188–95.

Perrin, E. H., "Social Position of the Speech Defective Child," *Journal of Speech and Hearing Disorders*, XIX (1954), 250–52.

Rosenberg, S., and J. Curtis, "The Effect of Stuttering on the Behavior of the Listener," *Journal of Abnormal Social Psychology*, XLIX (1954), 355–61.

Sander, E. K., "Frequency of Syllable Repetition and Stutter Judgments," *Journal of Speech and Hearing Research*, VI (1963), 19–30.

———. "Assessing Cultural Speech Fluency Expectations," *Asha*, V (1963), 619–21.

———. "Comments on Investigating Listener Reactions to Speech Disfluency," *Journal of Speech and Hearing Disorders*, XXX (1965), 159–65.

———. "Frequency of Syllable Repetition and 'Stutterer' Judgments," *Journal of Speech and Hearing Disorders*, XXVIII (1963), 19–30.

Sapir, E., *Abnormal Types of Speech in Nootka*. Ottowa: Canadian Department of Mines, Geological Survey, Memoir 62, Anthropological Series, 1915.

Schaef, R., and J. Matthews, "A First Step in the Evaluation of Stuttering Therapy," *Journal of Speech and Hearing Disorders*, XIX (1954), 467–73.

Scripture, E. W., *Stuttering and Lisping*. New York: Macmillan, 1923.

Soderberg, G. A., "Linguistic Factors in Stuttering," *Journal of Speech and Hearing Research*, X (1967), 801–10.

Stein, L., *Speech and Voice*. London: Methuen, 1942.

Stromsta, C., "A Spectrographic Study of Dysfluencies Labeled as Stuttering by Parents," *De Therapia Vocis et Loquellae*, I (1965), 317–20.

Travis, L. E., "The Unspeakable Feelings of People with Special Reference to Stuttering." In L. E. Travis (ed.), *Handbook of Speech Pathology*. New York: Appleton, 1957.

Tuthill, C. E., "A Quantitative Study of Extensional Meaning with Special Reference to Stuttering," *Speech Monographs*, XIII (1946), 81–98.

Van Riper, C., "The Influence of Empathic Response on Frequency of Stuttering," *Psychological Monographs*, XLIX (1937), 224–36.

Villarreal, J. J., "Semantic Aspects of Stuttering in Nonstutterers: Additional Data," *Quarterly Journal of Speech*, XXXI (1945), 477–79.

Voelker, C. H., "A Preliminary Investigation for a Normative Study of Fluency; a Clinical Index to the Severity of Stuttering," *American Journal of Orthopsychiatry*, XIV (1944), 285–94.

———. "On the Semantic Aspects of Stuttering in Nonstutterers," *Quarterly Journal of Speech*, XXVIII (1942), 78–80.

Williams, D. E., and L. R. Kent, "Listeners' Evaluations of Speech Interruptions," *Journal of Speech and Hearing Research*, I (1958), 124–36.

Wingate, M. E., "A Standard Definition of Stuttering," *Journal of Speech and Hearing Disorders*, XXIX (1964), 484–89.

———. "Evaluation and Stuttering," *Journal of Speech and Hearing Disorders*, XXVII (1962), 106–15; 244–57; 368–77.

Wyllie, J., *The Disorders of Speech*. Edinburgh: Oliver and Boyd, 1894.

Wyrick, D. R., "A Study of Normal Non-Fluency in Conversation." Master's thesis, University of Missouri, 1949.

Young, M. A., "Identification of Stutterers from Recorded Samples of Their 'Fluent' Speech," *Journal of Speech and Hearing Research,* VII (1964), 291–303.

————. "Predicting Ratings of Severity of Stuttering." *Journal of Speech and Hearing Disorders,* Monograph Supplement 7, (1961) 31–54.

three

THE PREVALENCE AND
INCIDENCE OF STUTTERING

One of the neglected pieces of the stuttering puzzle is its incidence. How many stutterers are there in the general population? How many of us have passed through a period of stuttering and have recovered? Are there subpopulations, special groups, in which the disorder is found very frequently or others in which it appears rarely? Is the incidence of stuttering declining? The answers to these question may contribute to the solution of its mystery.

Unfortunately, the extensive literature on the subject is not very illuminating. We have critically surveyed most of it and we find so many omissions of criteria, such vague descriptions of survey procedures, and so obviously inadequate samplings that any conclusions seem premature. The curious thing about these studies of incidence, however, is that the magical number of one per cent seems to occur over and over again, most of the incidence figures seeming to cluster about this value. We also find higher incidences reported for the younger age groups and, without exception, more males are reported as having the disorder than females.

There are many hazards lying in wait for the investigator who concerns himself with a study of the incidence of stuttering. First of these is the matter of definition. As we saw in the preceding chapter, definitions vary widely, especially when incipient stuttering is considered. The differential diagnosis of abnormal from normal disfluency is not always easily accomplished. Moreover, as Voelker (1942) pointed out long ago, and others have since, the same people who feel that they have spoken "stutteringly," or have "stuttered" are very insistent that they have never been "stutterers." Another difficulty is that the disorder is intermittent. In the early stages of its development, temporary remissions seem to be the rule rather than the exception. Some young stutterers are certain to be missed because their stuttering appears in waves. Moreover, we now have enough solid evidence (Sheehan and Martyn, 1966; Dickson, 1969) that self-recovery is more common than had formerly been believed. It is clear that some individuals would have been classified as stutterers at one age but not at another. This is an important point in differentiating between the concepts of incidence and prevalence. True incidence figures will always be higher than the prevalence ones reported in cross-sectional studies.

INCIDENCE VERSUS PREVALENCE

Although the results of many of the older surveys were reported as incidence figures, they really reflect *prevalence* rather than the true incidence of stuttering. They state how many stutterers were found in a given population at a certain time. Only longitudinal studies can reflect the true incidence of stuttering, i.e., can tell us how many individuals in a thousand would have been classified as stutterers at some time in their lives. To our knowledge, only one careful longitudinal study bearing on the true incidence of stuttering has yet been performed. It was carried out in the city of Newcastle-on-Tyne in England and has been reported by Morley (1957) and by Andrews and Harris (1964). It shows both the onset of stuttering and its remission or disappearance in about 1000 children followed from birth through age 15. Most of the cases of stuttering began before the age of five, and no new cases were discovered after the age of 11. About a third of the stuttering children seemed to pass through a period of marked nonfluency (developmental stuttering) between 2–4 years; another third (the "benign stutterers") began to stutter rather later (mean age of onset 7.5 years) and the stuttering in this group, as in the first group, lasted an average of only two years. The final third of the stuttering children began to stutter between the ages of 3–6 years and continued to stutter thereafter.

The important contribution made by this longitudinal research is that it permits us, for the first time, to compare total incidence figures with the prevalence of stuttering at certain ages. The incidence, i.e., the percentage of children who went through a period of stuttering which lasted six months or more was three per cent. If children are included who passed through a period of stuttering which lasted less than six months are added to this group, then the total incidence was 4.5 per cent. In contrast, the prevalence figures (how many were stuttering each year) shows a variation from 0.5 per cent at the age of three, reaching a maximum of 1.6 per cent at the age of eight, and stablizing at 1.1 per cent at age 12.

STUDIES OF PREVALENCE

Most of our information on the number of stutterers comes from cross-sectional surveys of school children. The methods used vary from investigator to investigator. Some used questionnaires; some used referrals only; a few personally examined each child, although we rarely know how extensively or thoroughly. All of them contain sources of error. Different age ranges are covered in different studies. One of the first surveys in this country was conducted by Wallin (1916), who sent questionnaires to school principals, and he reported that 0.7 per cent of 89,000 school children stuttered. Two years later, Carrie (1918) surveyed all the school children in Hamburg, Germany, and found a prevalence of 0.84 per cent. He also reported two earlier surveys, one in the Berlin parochial schools in 1886 in which 1.0 per cent of 155,000 school children stuttered and another in Amsterdam, Holland, in 1910 where 1.19 per cent of the Dutch children stuttered. All of these were studies in which questionnaires were sent to teachers. Perhaps the most ambitious of these questionnaire surveys was that reported in the first White House Conference Report of 1931 where the results of 44 questionnaire surveys of children and youths (ages 5-21) were pooled to yield a population of 3,800,000 of whom 1.2 per cent were said to be stuttering.

We have three reports of prevalence in which children were examined individually. The first of these were performed by Voelker (1943) who, with his assistants, claimed to have screened a total of 101,020 individuals, 50 per cent of whom were under 19 years of age. His article is difficult to evaluate but he reported an incidence of 1.87 per cent for dysrhythmia and, from his other writings, the term refers to stuttering. The second study, by Mills and Streit (1942), seems well designed and carefully performed. They personally interviewed 4685 children in the first through sixth grades of the Hartford, Connecticut, public schools. The screening was done carefully: "Each child was tested in an individual conference and by at least two examiners. Occasionally a third examiner was called in on a case. These conferences were held in the school building during regular school hours in order to keep the situation as familiar to the child as possible. All children old enough to read were tested in both reading and spontaneous speech." Mills and Streit found an over-all average "incidence" (prevalence) of 1.5 per cent. When their population was broken down by grades, 2.7 per cent stuttered in grades 1-3 as compared to 1.1 per cent in grades 4-6.

The third study, is the National Speech and Hearing Survey (Hull and Timmons, 1969). Mobile units with trained examiners sampled school populations in many areas throughout the United States with provision being made for reliability checks. Preliminary results indicate that the incidence of stuttering was 0.8 per cent in a sample of 38,000 elementary school children.

American

Root (1952): school children, grades 1-8; 1.2%
Burdin (1940): 3600 children in grades 1-4; 1.2% (averaged)
Louttit and Halls (1937): 200,000 Indian school children; 0.77%
Schindler (1955): examined school records of 23,000 Iowa school children; 0.55%

Foreign

McAllister (1937): 21,000 English children aged 5-18; 1.0%
Morgenstern (1956): 35,000 Scottish school children; 1.02%
Schreiber (1955): 18,000 German school children; 1.0%
Chrysanthis (1947): 1100 Cypriot school children; 1.85%
Watzl (1924): 136,000 Viennese school children; 0.6%
Seeman (1959): 26,000 school children in Prague; 0.55%
Katsovakaia (1960): preschool children of the Ukraine, Russia; 1.5%
Aron (1962): 6500 African school children; 1.26%
Toyoda (1959): 140,000 Japanese school children; 0.82%
Ozawa (1960): 7600 Japanese school children; 0.9%
Petkov and Iosifov (1960): 45,000 Bulgarian school children; 1.7%

THE AGE FACTOR IN PREVALENCE

Both the cross-sectional and longitudinal surveys reveal that the prevalence of stuttering is not evenly distributed with respect to age. Metraux (1950) provided, in her profiles of speech development, a period of hesitancy which she called early stuttering. It has also been called incipient stuttering, developmental stuttering, and, in the European literature, physiological stuttering. Wendell Johnson has insisted that this period of pronounced disfluency should not be called stuttering since it represents a fairly normal stage in the acquisition of speech. Nevertheless, it is apparent that some of these subclinical cases persist in their "stuttering." We have few studies of prevalence in the preschool years; most surveys have screened children in the elementary grades. There is some evidence that after about the age of 11, the prevalence of stuttering remains fairly stable at least during the school years. The monograph by Andrews and Harris (1964), for example, shows that of the 43 stuttering children from the thousand families in Newcastle, England, who were studied longitudinally, 34 achieved fluency but none of them "outgrew" it after age 12. A similar stabilization was shown by Mills and Streit (1942).

Many individuals who have begun to stutter seem to recover spontaneously, especially during the first 11 years of life. Milisen and Johnson (1936) found that 40 per cent of children who begin to stutter are fluent by their 12th year. The researches of Sheehan and Martyn (1966) and Andrews and Harris (1964) indicate that the figure is probably much higher, that only one out of five persons who begin to stutter continues to do so. Glasner and Rosenthal (1957) reported that 15 per cent of 996 parents of first grade children said that their children had stuttered and that half of them had overcome it without therapy. Dickson (1965) in a questionnaire study of parents of children enrolled in a campus school reported that 10 per cent of them claimed their children had stuttered between the years two and four. Spontaneous remission had occurred in 60 per cent of their children, although they had continued to stutter for a period of at least six months and up to two years. Johnson (1959), in his careful study of 46 stuttering children shortly after onset, said that three-fourths of the cases began to stutter at or before the age of three years, two months, though his oldest subject began to stutter at age nine. According to Lennon (1962) stuttering has its major peak of onset prior to six years and only 10 per cent develop it after eight years. Froeschels (1948) claimed that 80 per cent of all children go through a phase of repetitive speech he called physiological stuttering between the ages of two to four years and only about 1.5 per cent of these continue to stutter.

Generally, most of the literature indicates that the greatest prevalence of stuttering occurs in the preschool years. The attrition in the pool of stutterers which occurs thereafter (apparently because of the large proportion of children who spontaneously recover) is presumably compensated only slightly by new cases. Shearer and Williams (1965) in a questionnaire study of college students showed that this recovery did not seem to peak significantly at any one year, although a slight increase occurred around puberty. Wingate (1964) also studied spontaneous remission in college students who claimed to have been former stutterers, and he reported that 73 per cent of all recoveries occurred between the ages of 14 and 20. Dostalova and Dosuzkov (1965) studied 2000 cases of stuttering from infancy and found that 17.8 per cent of them attained or recovered normal speech by 18 years.

Were it not for the few studies we have of stuttering prevalence in adults such as that of Morley (1952) who found, in screening 33,000 college students at the University of Michigan, that one per cent of them still stuttered, we would expect that the number of stutterers would gradually decrease in the adult years either as the result of successful therapy or spontaneous recovery. A marked decrease in stuttering incidence during the adult years has indeed been shown by Shames and Beams (1956), who sent questionnaires to clergymen asking them how many stutterers they had among their parishioners and their ages, but, as the authors make clear, the sources of error in such a study are so great as to leave the matter in much doubt. We do know that some stutterers continue to stutter until they die, Somerset Maugham, the novelist, for one. We also know that a very few individuals do begin to stutter in adulthood as cited in the articles by Froeschels (1919), Kingdon-Ward (1941), Arnold (1948), and Wallen (1961), usually as the result of traumatic experiences. Nevertheless, in summary, we feel that the literature, miserable as most of it is, indicates clearly that the total *incidence* of stuttering probably amounts conservatively to about 4 per cent of the general population, and that its *prevalence* is highest in pre-school years declining thereafter to an unstable value of less than 1 per cent.

INCIDENCE IN OTHER CULTURES

As we have seen, the statistics on incidence and prevalence of stuttering in our own culture leave much to be desired, but when we look for some valid estimates of the number of stutterers in other societies, the available data is appallingly meager and its validity seems questionable. Lemert's investigation of the Salish Indian tribes on Vancouver Island gives us a prevalence figure of 1.9 per cent. Stewart (1960) found only .02 per cent in another Indian population presumably similar in child rearing practices and culture. In another field investigation using informants, Lemert (1962) reported his impression that there were more stutterers among the Japanese than among the Polynesians, attributing the difference to the beliefs held concerning the nature of the problem, and the amount of compliance demanded by the two societies, the Polynesians believing that "stutterers are born that way and nothing can be done about it" whereas the Japanese feel that the disorder "can and should be corrected." Moreover, there are fewer time pressures and conformity demands among the Hawaiian and Samoan peoples than among the Japanese. Besides these investigations by anthropologists using informants, we find in the Japanese literature several professional surveys of the prevalence of stuttering among elementary school children, yielding prevalence figures ranging from 0.8 to 1.0 per cent.

Perhaps the more a society resembles our own, the more likely it is to have the same prevalence of stuttering. Both Lemert (1953) and Stewart (1960) seem to attribute the alleged greater prevalence of stuttering among the Kwakiutl and Cowichan tribes than among the Utes and Shoshones in part to the greater competitiveness of the former societies and the resulting social pressures on the children. In the same vein, Aron (1962) found a prevalence of 1.26 per cent among Bantu school children in South Africa and attributed it to the fact that urban African children are subjected to many of the same stresses and speech conformity pressures that exist in the general European/American culture.

The prevalence of stuttering in a subculture, such as that of the Negroes in the southern states of our country, might be expected to differ from that in the main culture. Several such studies have been made. Carson and Kantner (1945) report that in the schools of Baton Rouge, Louisiana, the prevalence of stuttering among white children was 1.1 per cent, whereas that of Negro children was 60 per cent higher. Neely (1960), however, who carefully studied the parochial elementary schools in the New Orleans area found no significant differences in prevalence between White and Negro children. We also have some figures for Negro children in northern cities where presumably the factor of upward mobility pressure might be expected to be present. Waddle (1934) personally tested 1582 children in segregated schools of Topeka, Kansas, finding that a ratio of 1.7/1 existed, with Negro stutterers in the majority, and Pritchett (1966) reported a similar ratio of 1.3/1 for the East St. Louis schools. The results of these investigations indicate no major support for the commonly held belief that stuttering is much more common among Negroes as a race or sub-culture.

The prevalence of stuttering is doubtless affected by many factors, and one of those frequently cited is that of socio-economic status. It has been felt that families striving for greater status place demands on their children for excellence in speech as well as for other attributes. Also, there are many investigations, such as McCarthy's (1954), indicating that children from the lower socio-economic levels are retarded in language development, using shorter and less mature sentence forms than those of children from the upper strata of our society. Morgenstern (1956), whose study is perhaps best known in this respect, found higher percentages of stutterers in the families of semiskilled laborers than in those of middle or upper-class families. Andrews and Harris (1964), however, found little evidence to support the belief that stuttering appears more frequently in subgroups concerned with upward social mobility.

PREVALENCE OF STUTTERING
AMONG THE MENTALLY RETARDED

An intriguing facet of the problem of stuttering is that it seems to be much more prevalent among the mentally retarded than in the general population. Moreover, it is apparently found much more frequently in mongoloids than in nonmongoloid retarded individuals. If stuttering is basically a neurosis it is difficult to see why these increases in prevalence occur. Most mongoloids that we have known have been fairly happy persons, far from neurotic by nature. We would expect, if stuttering is a neurosis, that the incidence among the more severely retarded would be less than among those mildly impaired. Just the opposite seems to be true. And why, if stuttering is basically learned behavior, do we find such a high prevalence in children who find learning most difficult? Surely those who are less mentally retarded than the others should show more stuttering if this is true. Mongoloid children show organicity in many ways. Is their high prevalence of stuttering a reflection of neurological deficits which make the sequential timing of speech movements unusually difficult?

Although the research is fairly consistent in showing these trends, it is not definitive beyond question. One of the basic problems is that of definition and differential diagnosis. Is the disorder that they show stuttering or cluttering? Do they falter because of their admitted difficulty in finding and manipulating the symbols of speech? Is their stuttering or cluttering merely a reaction to language deficit? The incidence of all types of speech defects is very high among the mentally retarded. It might be merely that the temporal dimension of speech is affected equally with those of articulation, voice, or symbolization.

With Wendell Johnson's definition of stuttering as something that exists only after the person begins to react with fear and struggle to his "normal" repetitions and prolongations, then few of the severely impaired mentally retarded could be said to stutter. Most of them have short memories and little foresight. They anticipate contingencies with difficulty. With such a definition—which we feel is unduly restrictive and useful more to defend a theory than to describe the disorder—one would probably be forced to conclude that few mongoloids do stutter and that most of the mentally retarded do not either. However, if we view stuttering as a developmental disorder which usually begins with an excessive amount of repetitions and prolongations of syllables, sounds, or words and which then progresses through a series of gradual phases of reactivity until fear and frustration predominate, the mentally retarded do show an unusual amount of the earlier signs of stuttering. Typically, they have rather simple disfluencies. We rarely see the complicated patterns of avoidance behavior so characteristic of the advanced stutterer with normal intelligence. The disorder tends also to be more episodic as it does in the beginning stutterer. We find some mildly feared speaking situations but little word or phonemic fears. In our experience, the consistency in terms of stuttered words is low, and adaptation is less marked. Most of the time they do not seem to be aware that they have stuttered or are stuttering. They are ofen frustrated in trying to communicate, primarily because of word-finding and coding difficulties, but they do not seem to feel frustrated because they cannot utter a given word when they try to. We have heard a mongoloid child repeat the first syllable of his name 18 times without showing any signs of frustration.

Lerman, Powers, and Rigrodsky (1965) studied a group of 14 retardate stutterers in the Mansfield State Training School, and have this to say about their characteristics:

> The stutterers involved in this study reflected stuttering behavior which closely paralleled the early stages of development of stuttering in normal

children. Although the most obvious difference was the lack of chronic
avoidance and apprehension, it should be emphasized that fear of the speech
act can occur. The observation of the continual use of syllable repetition
in contrast to whole word repetitions may suggest that other factors are
contributing to the etiological and continuing aspects of this disorder (p. 32).

Cabanas (1954) analyzed the speech patterns of 50 mongoloids and felt
that their characteristic repetitions and distorted sounds resembled cluttering more than stuttering.

Except for automatisms which they have overlearned, such as saying
"Thank you" or "Good morning," much of the speech of the severely
mentally retarded, when it appears at all (and often they speak only under
great urging or need) shows many forms of hesitant behavior. They begin
to say something and then forget where they are going or where they have
been. Not all of them do this of course, but those that do also show many
other breaks in fluency besides stuttering. The mispronunciations and misarticulations cause listeners to show that they are not comprehending, and
this too may interrupt speech flow. It is a difficult diagnostic problem.
Perhaps the best we can say is that they seem to be speaking "stutteringly"
or "clutteringly."

As has been indicated, several of the writers on the subject insist that
what mentally retarded children show is "cluttering." If we accept Weiss'
(1964) position that all stuttering begins as cluttering (which we do not)
then the problem of differential diagnosis presents no problem—many of
these children clutter. They show the accompanying language deficits, the
misarticulations, the reversals, the lack of fear or awareness that characterizes cluttering. We do not find the tachylalia, the hurried bursts of rapid
speech, the swift revisions of whole phrases seen in most clutterers. And
we have found tonic stuttering with occasional tremors in a minority of
these children.

We do find a preponderance of fluency breaks on the syllable and
sound. If stuttering represents the final common path of a group of related
disorders, a syndrome, one of which arises in cluttering and language
disability, then this is the type of stuttering that the mentally retarded
show.

Schlanger (1953) found 20 per cent of institutionalized retardates to
be stutterers, and Schlanger and Gottsleben (1957) found 17 per cent in a
similar population. Preus (1968) surveying nine institutions in Norway
found 12 per cent. The one exception to this trend is the study by Sheehan,
Martyn, and Kilburn (1968), who found only one stutterer among the 133
mentally retardates in a California institution who could talk. We also
have, as mentioned before, studies reporting a high prevalence of stuttering
among mongoloids. Gottsleben (1955) reports 33 per cent among institutionalized mongoloids as compared to 14 per cent of institutionalized non-mongoloids. Edson (1964) found that 39 per cent of the mongoloid children
at the Parsons (Kansas) Training School stuttered. Schubert (1966) on a

smaller sample of 80 pairs found that 15 per cent of the mongoloid as compared to 8.8 per cent of nonmongoloid retardates were judged from tape recordings as stuttering. In evaluating these sparse investigations, we should keep in mind the caution of Zisk and Bialer (1967):

> Published reports leave unclear the exact nature of the problem, thus making it exceedingly difficult to speculate as to possible causes. Further research should aim at providing precise definitions and objective criteria of the behavior under consideration.

If this further research corroborates the trend of the research we now possess, this higher prevalence of stuttering among mental retardates and especially the mongoloids would seem to point to some deficiency in the motor control of the learned coordinations needed for normal speech rather than to neurotic or conditioned fear responses.

THE SEX RATIO

One of the most interesting findings concerning the prevalence of stuttering is the complete agreement (reached by all the investigators of the subject in all lands) that males show more stuttering than females. The preponderance is not minor. Though different researchers have given different ratios, most of them range about the figure of three or four to one. Why should so many more males than females stutter?

Immediately we confront a conflict situation which we shall meet many times in our study of stuttering: the differing points of view with respect to the nature and etiology of the disorder, namely that stuttering has a constitutional basis, that it is a learned behavior, or that it is a neurosis. And there is also the composite view that stuttering is a syndrome in which each of these may play a part and any one of which may create a homogeneous subpopulation, or combine with the others to form a multiple-faceted disorder, a position expounded in the present text.

Despite long search, we have been unable to find a study or report which shows that there are more female than male stutterers. The converse is consistently found. Male stutterers seem to outnumber female stutterers by about three to one and some of the available figures show higher proportions. Unfortunately, as with the studies of general incidence, the true proportion is in some doubt for several reasons. Besides the inadequacy of survey methods, most of the investigations of the sex ratio in stuttering fail to take into account the ratios of total male to female populations from which the samples were obtained. Also, several authors have held that the proportion of males to females tends to increase with age. However, the male/female sex ratio of college stutterers who reportedly had recovered from stuttering reported in Sheehan and Martyn's study (1967) was about five to one rather than the reverse, and Mills and Streit's (1942) careful survey showed no change with grade placement. In spite of all the limitations of the investigations, however, we cannot doubt that the sex ratio exists and must have some significance. A summary of some of the results of various studies follows:

McDowell: 2.9/1 (1928); White House Conference: 3.9/1 (1931) Brown: 4/1 (1932); Louttit and Halls: 3.8/1 (1936); Wepman: 4.4/1 (1939); Mills and Streit: 5/1 (1942); Schindler: 2.8/1 (1955); Morley: 4.3/1 in college students (1952); Morgenstern: 4.4/1 (1956); McCallien: 2.1/1 Ga-speaking African children (1956); Aron: 3.2/1 Bantu school children (1962); Daskalov: 3.1/1 Bulgarian clinic cases (1962); Hirschberg: 5/1 Hungarian clinic cases (1965); Dickson: 2/1 American school children (1969); Hull and Timmons: 3.1/1 (National Survey, 1969); McMahon: 4/1 Canadian school children (1969); Andrews and Harris: 2.5/1 British school children (1964); Sato: 4.5/1 Japanese nursery school children (1961).

One of the common explanations for the sex ratio is that many other types of deviancy show a similarly larger number of males. Chorea, asthma, convulsions, tetany, and epilepsy are only some of the spasmodic disorders which could be so cited. Baldness, cleft palate, and spinal bifida are just a few of many other disorders where males outnumber females. There appear to be more birth injuries and more illnesses among boys than girls. This point of view unfortunately does not tell us much that is useful, especially since the reported sex ratios for stuttering are far greater than for most of these other problems. Perhaps more explanatory, if not entirely convincing, is the belief held by Cobb and Cole (1939) and Karlin (1947) and others that there are more male stutterers because speech is learned during a period when the myelinization of the cortical areas subserving speech and language in male children is delayed when compared to that of female children. The difficulty with this theory is that no one has shown why or how this delay produces stuttering intermittently or why only a few of the many male children are so affected. So far as we have been able to ascertain, no one has done comparative autopsy studies of child stutterers and nonstutterers, either male or female. One little hint of another explanation for the sex ratio comes from DeSantis (1959). He found unusual endocrine changes in 16 of 20 male stutterers, primarily those of hypogonadins. Unfortunately no control group was employed.

A fair case has been made for the sex ratio in terms of learning theory. Since speech is learned, and almost all the research indicates that girls are more advanced in speech and language during the early years, equally disrupting pressures applied to boys and girls of the same age should presumably produce more disfluency in the boy child than in the girl. That this might possibly be true is indicated by Mahaffey and Stromsta's (1965) and Bachrach's (1964) research showing that delayed auditory feedback evidently disrupted the fluency of males more than females even at the college level. Different critical delay times required to produce maximal disruption have also been reported, the females requiring the longer delay times to create broken speech.

Another explanation of the sex ratio is that parents tend to penalize or react unfavorably to normal disfluencies in the speech of their boys more than they do to those in girls. Or that our culture does! The tests of this explanation have been negative. Bloodstein and Smith (1945) found that college students did not make more diagnoses of stuttering for samples of sexually ambiguous speech recordings when told that they were made by boys rather than girls. Mysak (1959) in a similar study with adolescent boys and girls found no significant differences in the tendency to diagnose stuttering in terms of sex identification. Quite apart from this scanty research we find it hard to believe that parents would be likely to be more tolerant of marked disfluency in their daughters than in their sons, since the gift of speech has certainly been highly prized by the fairer if not fainter sex.

One of the explanations which has never been particularly convincing to us is the one by Schuell (1946; 1947) that stuttering is due to the differential cultural treatment of the sexes in childhood. More boys are said to stutter because they are subjected to more parental pressures for excellence in speech and in social behavior at a time when they are linguistically more immature than girls. More parental pride is invested in them; more demands for conformity are brought to bear upon them. Schuell's explanation for the sex ratio has been widely quoted in the literature, but the actual evidence on which her wide reaching conclusions were based leaves much to be desired. She simply questioned 161 boys and 142 normal speaking girls about parental practices regarding praise and punishment. These subjects were taken from the fifth to seventh grades—far later than the age at which stuttering generally begins. Her questions seem inappropriately designed to elicit significant information regarding communicative pressures, and no reliability check was made. More boys than girls reported being punished for being noisy, quarreling, spending money, staying out late, being bad, procrastinating, having poor manners, and not helping with the housework. These items hardly seem pertinent to the age levels when stuttering usually has its onset. Moreover, we find it hard to believe that three or four times as much differential social pressure is focused directly on the prosody of male children to produce the sex ratio. One test of Schuell's position would be to discover a culture where boys and girls are treated very much alike during their speech-learning years. This has been reported by Eisenson (1966), who found the usual sex ratio of stuttering in the kibbutz colonies of Israel, where children are separated from their parents for most of their waking hours and both sexes are treated in the same way. Many other cultures which vary widely from our own in child-rearing practices such as the African Bantus (Aron, 1962) show the same sex ratio.

Those who believe stuttering to be a primary neurosis usually find the sex ratio very difficult to explain. It has been attributed in Freudian theory to the greater conflicts a male child has with his ever-present mother as an Oedipal love object than girls experience with their absent fathers, or to castration fears, or to great inhibitions in oral-anal smearing. In most of the non-Freudian presentations of stuttering as a neurosis, the sex ratio is ignored, perhaps because no other recognized neurosis has its onset so early or shows such a high proportion of males.

In concluding this section it would seem that the sex ratio must in some way reflect a less stable neuromuscular control system for speech in the male at least during the early years of life. The temporal organization of his speech, as well as its vocabulary, articulation, and other aspects, may be less mature than that of the female at this time and accordingly more vulnerable to disruption. We see no need to explain everything in terms of environmental or neurotic influences. Even as the male has a constitutional predisposition to have a phallus, it is perhaps possible that he also has a minor one to have an unstable system for coordinating sequential speech in his early years.

FAMILIAL INCIDENCE

We do not feel it appropriate at this point to discuss the hereditary factor in stuttering since we are considering problems of incidence and not etiology. Our question is only whether or not there is a higher incidence or prevalence of stuttering in the families of stutterers than in the families of nonstutterers—quite apart from its mode of transmission or correlation. Most of the pertinent studies indicate that the incidence is much higher in the families of stutterers. Unfortunately, many of the investigations speak of family incidence rather than actual incidence. Wepman (1939), for example, found that 68 per cent of the families of stutterers had some other members who stuttered while only 15.6 per cent of the families of nonstutterers had such members. To know the actual incidence figures we must know how many members of the families there were and for what generations. Johnson (1961) similarly reports that in the 44 families of his stuttering subjects, 37 other members had stuttered whereas in a comparable group of nonstutterers' families only eight had stuttered. Nevertheless, we can conclude that the familial incidence of stuttering is apparently higher than in the general population, as demonstrated by the following studies: Boome and Richardson (1931): 34 per cent of 522 stutterers had a family history of stuttering; West, Nelson, and Berry (1939) report an incidence of 3 per cent in families of stutterers as compared to 0.5 per cent for the relatives of the controls; Meyer (1945): ten times more stutterers in families of stutterers; Jameson (1955): 36 per cent of 69 stutterers; Mussafia (1964): 39 per cent of 241 stutterers had other stutterers in their families; Andrews and Harris (1964) found 30 per cent of their stutterers to have relatives who stuttered as compared with .02 per cent for the controls: Daskalov (1962) reports that stuttering existed in 32 per cent of the other members of the family of his clinic cases.

TWINNING

Among the subgroups in which a high incidence of stuttering has been reported are twins. Most of the evidence seems to show that it is higher in monozygotic twins than in dizygotic twins which may reflect mutual learning rather than heredity since twinning strains seem to be reflected more in fraternal than identical twin births. However, it could also reflect the observation that where stuttering occurred in one monozygotic twin it also occurred in the other twin 9 out of 10 times, but when stuttering occurred in one dizygotic twin, it occurred in the other one only one out of 15 times (Nelson, Hunter, and Walter, 1945). When stuttering occurs through several generations in twins, they tend to be fraternal. The onset of stuttering also seems to be earlier for this population. The "incidence" figures for stuttering in twins varies widely from study to study, ranging from 1.9 per cent (Graf, 1955) to 24 per cent (Nelson, Hunter, and Walter, 1945). Most of the studies report higher prevalence figures than those of Graf. Perhaps the explanation for the higher incidence is merely that these twins are usually delayed in speech and fail to organize their motor patterns early enough to avoid social pressures.

THE BRAIN-INJURED

Stuttering has been alleged to have a high rate of incidence among the brain-injured. Disregarding, for the moment, those individuals said to show minimal brain damage and concentrating on the more grossly impaired, we find higher proportions of stutterers in the cerebral-palsied population as cited by Palmer and Osborn (1938) and Rutherford (1938), both reporting twice as many stutterers in this group as among normal speakers. In a later study using a control group, Rutherford (1946) corroborated this higher incidence. Although stuttering has been viewed by some workers, notably West (1958), as a form of epilepsy and by others as an epileptic equivalent, about all we really know is that the incidence of the disorder in the epileptic population is apparently high. Gens (1951) found a stuttering prevalence of 3.2 per cent among the 1252 epileptics in a state hospital in Michigan, and Harrison (1947) on a smaller sample found an even higher percentage. Many individual case reports of stuttering behavior accompanying aphasia and other disorders resulting from brain injury occur in the literature but we have found none that provide appropriate information for incidence or prevalence studies. If future research corroborates these tentative findings, the higher incidence in the brain-injured population would support the position that the coordinative and monitoring aspects of speech are what become impaired to produce stuttering. Alternative explanations might be that the brain-injured are more emotionally disturbed as a result of their disabilities.

THE DEAF

There exists a fairly unanimous opinion that the incidence of stuttering in the congenitally deaf is very low though most of the research has been based upon questionnaire surveys of schools for the deaf. It has also frequently been stated that no stuttering ever occurs among this population but Backus (1938) found six totally deaf (not all congenitally) stutterers in questionnaire reports from 206 schools for the deaf with a population of 13,691. Harms and Malone (1939) found eight totally deaf stutterers in a population of 14,458 individuals in oral schools for the deaf and hard of hearing, also by questionnaire, and Voelker and Voelker (1937) and others have reported a few case studies which indicate that, though very rare, stuttering can occur among the congenitally deaf. The task of identifying stuttering in these individuals is not an easy one primarily because of the limited and distorted speech and other difficulties in communication. Sternberg (1946) attributes the low incidence to the fact that the deaf scan more carefully, speak more slowly and controllably, and have less social pressure. Others have explained the relative lack of stuttering to the fact that the deaf are taught to speak phonetically and voluntarily. Another possibility is that any distortions or delays of the airborne or bone-conducted auditory feedback which have been said to produce stuttering would not be present in the deaf.

THE DIABETIC

A very low incidence of stuttering in diabetics has also been frequently reported in the literature. West (1943) says, "The thirteenth part of our puzzle is one, the significance of which is particularly obscure, that no diabetic has been reported as stuttering." West speculated that the high blood sugar levels characteristic of diabetics inhibited the minor convulsions of the pyknolepsy which he felt constituted the basis of stuttering. If there were no diabetic stutterers, then such a hypothesis could be seriously considered. Hamre and Emerick (1967) reviewed the literature on pyknolepsy and concluded that West's use of the term and concept was in error. West's belief in the absence of stuttering among diabetics seems to have been based upon a master's thesis by Schuster (1936), in which more than a thousand case histories of diabetes mellitus were examined at the Wisconsin General Hospital at Madison. In all of these histories Schuster found no mention of stuttering and, when he interviewed two staff physicians, they said they had never known a diabetic stutterer. This is hardly impressive evidence. In view of the probability that hospital records of diabetics would not necessarily include a mention of stuttering even if present, the validity of this finding is to say the least, questionable. Later, another master's thesis at the same university was done by Boldon (1955) who questioned a larger number of physicians and did turn up some diabetic stutterers. We personally have examined five diabetic stutterers so we know they do exist. The incidence of stuttering among diabetics as compared to the general population remains a problem for future investigation. Again, a once promising path into the mystery becomes obscured.

INCIDENCE AMONG PSYCHOTICS

In the search for some clues as to the nature of stuttering, the hunt has even been extended into the back wards of mental hospitals. If stuttering is a character neurosis, and if a neurosis is a defense against repressed instinctual urges seeking expression, then once the individual really became psychotic, he should stop stuttering. Or, if he were basically psychotic rather than neurotic, he just should not stutter. So runs the involved reasoning. Accordingly, Barbara (1946) surveyed 7000 psychotic patients at the Central Islip State Hospital in New York and found an incidence of only 0.28 per cent. This low incidence might be said to lend some mild support for the neurotic theory of stuttering. Pitrelli (1948) found no stutterers among 300 psychotic females though three of them had stuttered prior to the advent of the psychosis. This, he felt, indicated the nature of stuttering as a neurotic defense against psychosis. This meager evidence was evaluated by Freund (1955) in the light of his own survey of another mental institution in which the incidence of stuttering was not lower than that usually found but higher (3.2 per cent). He also showed that the incidence of stuttering among institutionalized neurotics was approximately the same (4 per cent). Among our own successful cases we have never had one stutterer who became psychotic once he became fluent.

IS THE INCIDENCE OF
STUTTERING DECLINING?

To one who has worked in the field of stuttering for many years, it appears that the incidence of stuttering has been declining in the last 30 years. Milisen (1963) also holds this opinion. When the author of this text began to practice in 1934, the high schools seemed full of stutterers and there were many adult stutterers to be encountered everywhere. This does not seem to be true today. We still have adult stutterers seeking our services but most of them come from afar. The skeptical may doubtless attribute this to the clinical failures of the public school therapists—that the stutterers have lost all hope of being helped. We doubt this morbid view. We feel instead that the basic attitudes of our society toward the stutterer have changed markedly during this period. Only a few decades ago, stuttering was viewed as a bad, dirty habit to be broken by punishment or by will power. The whole field of rehabilitation had hardly made an impact. Speech therapy has drastically revised these old attitudes and practices. Stuttering is now viewed as a clinical problem. Information regarding prevention and treatment is widely available and so is therapy. All these influences must have had some impact.

Unfortunately, we have little research upon this important matter. Van Horn (1966), who conducted individual screening of all children prior to school entrance, reports that the prevalence percentage of stutterers who were found in Kalamazoo in 1962–1965 had decreased a fourth from those discovered in the same schools using the same screening methods that had been found in 1941–1944. Also we have Black's report (1966) of the percentage of stuttering in the total caseloads of public school speech therapists in Illinois. In 1950–1951 7.4 per cent of the total caseload in Illinois were stutterers; in 1964–1965 the percentage was only 3.2 per cent. This, of course, does not reflect the prevalence of stuttering in the general population, merely the number of stutterers being enrolled in speech therapy. Nevertheless, a reduction by one half in 15 years must reflect some sort of change. We hope others will explore their old records to determine the validity of this impression as has Jackson (1967) as illustrated in Figure 3.

COMMENTARY

If we accept early childhood nonfluencies as stuttering—then almost all children would be considered stutterers (Berry and Eisenson, 1956, p. 250).

Definitions of stuttering vary widely, and figures on incidence will vary with the definition used and the method of survey (Milisen, 1957, p. 254).

In some of the children there were intermittent periods of stammering. . . . Many more children than the 37 mentioned here may have passed through a period of hesitant speech (Morley, 1957, p. 41).

According to inquiries already made in earlier years in Brunswick, Potsdam, Elberfeld, Stettin, Königsberg, Zurich, and other places, at least 1 per cent of the school children stutter. In Dresden it is even 2 per cent. It would certainly be worthwhile if in other cities such similar statistics could be procured. As with the experiment, the statistic is a principal weapon of science. If the art of speech healing wishes to become an exact science in which the research cannot be doubted, it cannot do without statistics of this kind (Carrie, 1918).

Perhaps one of the most important pieces in our puzzle is a sex difference in the incidence of stuttering. The ratio of stuttering in boys and girls above 36 months varies all the way from 3/1 to 8/1, depending upon the respective ages. Very few adult females stutter (West, 1942, p. 48).

Explanations fall into two main categories: *social and psychological hypotheses* and *genetic ones*. According to the former, the sex ratio depends on specific psychological differences, on inequalities in the demands made on boys and girls, and on different methods of upbringing. If this were true, we should expect girls who stutter to resemble boys in some psychological aspect, or to have experienced the pressures to which boys are exposed. There is no indication of this, and it seems more likely that the distinction arises from inborn constitutional differences between boys and girls (Andrews and Harris, 1964, p. 139).

My work was . . . to begin with a detailed study of the articulatory process, its variations and deviations. The development of the articulatory function in children seemed a promising theme, and I got permission to carry out investigations among both normal and mentally defective children [at the West End Hospital for Nervous Diseases, London]. In a couple of years I had records of some *two million* tests, which then demanded a very lengthy and detailed statistical treatment. I never had the opportunity to complete this latter task, but a few findings of interest emerged in the four or five papers in which some of the results were incorporated. One, for instance, was that *girls use lip reading in learning to talk much more than boys, who rely almost entirely on hearing* [Italics mine.] (Ines, 1959).

Setting aside a theory of final causes, viz., that nature in order to compensate a woman for her weakness, has bestowed upon her a powerful weapon in the gift of the tongue, we must rest satisfied with the physiological fact that the vocal and articulating apparatus of woman, being more elastic and mobile than that of man, is less liable to be affected by some of the causes which produce the infirmity (of stuttering) in the male sex (Hunt, 1870, p. 37).

This difference is due to the greater tendency of small boys to pick up dirty words from their small associates and inadvertently to let these choice words slip out in the presence of the parents. Such accidents, with the resulting punishment (whipping, washing the tyke's mouth with soap, etc.) would lead to the child's watching his speech carefully and being careful about words of other categories which began with the same sounds as these tabooed words. . . . By listening to the speech of a juvenile patient and noting the sounds which gave him trouble, I have sometimes been able to tell him the dirty words he first learned (Dunlap, 1944, pp: 192–93).

The results indicate that normal speakers became disfluent when their verbalizations were punished. Males and females were similarly affected by punishment except that males were more disfluent than females as a result of 100 per cent punishment (Stassi, 1961, p. 361).

The results under the conditions of this study indicated that differences existed between males and females with respect to the effects on speech performance of altering the frequency, intensity, and time parameters of auditory feedback. As such, the results allow the tentative hypothesis that inherent differences exist in the cybernetic relationship between hearing and speech for males and females that would be related to the difference in the incidence of stuttering for the two populations (Mahaffey and Stromsta, 1965, p. 234).

The typical patterns of stuttering in this mentally retarded sample could be viewed from the following symptoms: Stuttering would occur most often in the school situation, especially when talking to teachers or teacher's aids. Stuttering would be cyclic and would depend upon the stress of the moment. Stuttering as repetitions would occur primarily on a syllable level throughout the speech attempt. There would be little word or sound fears. Some secondary release techniques would be demonstrated. Embarrassment and tension could occur following stuttering. Avoidances and apprehensions of the speech act, although occasionally observed, were noticeably deficient (Lerman, Powers, and Rigrodsky, 1965, p. 31).

In answer to the question, "Why should mongoloids show more stuttering than nonmongoloid retardates," several explanations appear to be plausible. First, if stuttering has an organic basis, it would appear that mongoloids are especially prone to a condition which predisposes the individual to be non-fluent in his speech. Karlin's theory that stuttering is caused by a delay in the myelinization of the cortical areas of the brain which are directly concerned with the control of the speech organs, could explain the prevalence of stuttering in mongoloids since Benda has found underdeveloped myelinization in all his cases of mongolism (Gottsleben, 1955, p. 216).

I have been engaged in teaching the deaf for more than fifty years and have visited many schools in this country and Europe. I must have met many thousands of this class of persons. . . . I have never known a congenitally deaf person who stammered or stuttered (Gallaudet as quoted in Bluemel, 1913, p. 234).

BIBLIOGRAPHY

Andrews, G., and M. Harris, *The Syndrome of Stuttering*. London: Heinemann, 1964.

Arnold, G. E., *Die traumatischen und konstitutionellen Störungen der Stimme und Sprache*. Vienna: Urban and Schwarzenberg, 1948.

Aron, M., "Nature and Incidence of Stuttering Among a Bantu Group of School Young Children," *Journal of Speech and Hearing Disorders*, XXVII (1962), 116–28.

Bachrach, D. L., "Sex Differences in Reactions to Delayed Auditory Feedback," *Perceptual Motor Skills*, XIX (1964), 81–82.

Backus, O., "Incidence of Stuttering Among the Deaf," *Annals of Otology, Rhinology and Laryngology*, XLVII (1938), 632–35.

Bar, A., "Investigating Stuttering in a Special Culture," *Journal of Speech and Hearing Disorders,* XXXIII (1968), 94–95.

Barbara, D. A., "A Psychosomatic Approach to the Problem of Stuttering in Psychotics," *American Journal of Psychiatry,* CIII (1946), 188–95.

Berry, M. F., and J. Eisenson, *Speech Disorders.* New York: Appleton-Century-Crofts, 1956.

Black, M. E., *Annual Report to Superintendent of Schools, State of Illinois.* Springfield, Ill.: 1966.

Bloodstein, O., and M. Smith, "A Study of Diagnosis of Stuttering with Special References to the Sex Ratio," *Journal of Speech and Hearing Disorders,* XIX (1954), 459–66.

Bluemel, C. S., *Stammering and Cognate Defects of Speech.* New York: Stechert, 1913.

Boldon, A. T., "The Coexistence of, and Certain Relationships Between Diabetes and Stuttering." Master's thesis, University of Wisconsin, 1955.

Boome, E. J., and M. A. Richardson, *The Nature and Treatment of Stammering.* London: Methuen, 1931.

Brown, F. W., "Stuttering: Its Neurophysiological Bases and Probable Causation," *American Journal of Orthopsychiatry,* II (1932), 363–76.

Bryngelson, B., "Prognosis of Stuttering," *Journal of Speech Disorders,* III (1938), 121–23.

Burdin, L. G., "A Survey of Speech Defectives in the Indianapolis Public Schools," *Journal of Speech Disorders,* V (1940), 247–58.

Cabanas, R., "Some Findings in Speech and Voice Therapy Among the Mentally Retarded," *Folia Phoniatrica,* VI (1954), 34–37.

Carrie, W., "Statistik über Sprachgebrechliche Schulkinder in den Hamburger Volkschulen," *Monatsschrift für Ohrenheilkunde,* LII (1918), 178–87.

Carson, C., and C. E. Kanter, "Incidence of Stuttering Among White and Colored School Children," *Southern Speech Journal,* X (1945), 57–59.

Chrysanthis, K., "Letter to Editor," *Lancet,* CCLII (1947), 270.

Cobb, S., and E. M. Cole, "Stuttering," *Physiological Review,* XIX (1939), 49–62.

Daskalov, D. D., [On the Problem of the Basic Principles and Methods of Prevention and Treatment of Stammering,] *Zhurnal Nevropatologii i Psikhiatrii imeni S. S. Korsakova,* LIII (1962), 1047–52.

De Santis, M., "Richerche endocrine in soggetti affetti da balbuzie," ("Endocrine Research into Cases of Stammering"), *Valsalva,* XXXV (1959), 328–33.

Dickson, S., "Incipient Stuttering Symptoms and Spontaneous Remission of Non-stuttered Speech," *Asha,* VII (1965), 370 (abstract).

————. "Incipient Stuttering and Spontaneous Remission of Stuttered Speech," convention address, A.S.H.A., 1969.

Dostalova, N., and T. Dosuzkov, "Uber die drei Hauptformen des neurotischen Stotterns," *De Therapie et Loquellae,* I (1965), 273–76.

Dunlap, K., "Stammering: Its Nature, Etiology and Therapy." *Journal of Comparative Psychology,* 37, (1944), 187–202.

Edson, S. K., "The Incidence of Certain Types of Nonfluencies Among a Group of Institutionalized Mongoloid and Non-Mongoloid Children." Master's thesis, University of Kansas, 1964.

Eisenson, J., "Observations of the Incidence of Stuttering in a Special Culture," *Asha,* V (1966), 391–94.

Forchhammer, E., "Speech Defectives in the Schools for the Mentally Retarded in the Danish Isles," *Nordisk Tideskrift for og Stemme*, XV (1955), 171–74.

Freund, H., "Psychosis and Stuttering," *Journal of Nervous and Mental Diseases*, CXXII (1955), 161–72.

Froeschels, E., "Die sprachärztliche Therapie in Kriege III das Stottern," *Monatsschrift für Ohrenheilkunde*, LIII (1919).

———. *Twentieth Century Speech and Voice Correction*. New York: Philosophical Library, 1948.

Gens, G. W., "The Speech Pathologist Looks at the Mentally Deficient Child," *Training School Bulletin*, XLVIII (1951), 19–27.

Glasner, P. J., and D. Rosenthal, "Parental Diagnosis of Stuttering in Young Children," *Journal of Speech Disorders*, XXII (1957), 288–95.

Goldman, R., "The Effects of Cultural Patterns on the Sex Ratio in Stuttering," *Asha*, VII (1965), 371 (abstract).

Gottsleben, R. H., "The Incidence of Stuttering in a Group of Mongoloids," *Training School Bulletin*, LI (1955), 209–18.

Graf, O. I., "Incidence of Stuttering Among Twins." In W. Johnson, (ed.) *Stuttering in Children and Adults*. Minneapolis: University of Minnesota Press, 1955.

Hamre, C. E., and M. E. Wingate, "Pyknolepsy and Stuttering," *Quarterly Journal of Speech*, LIII (1967), 374–77.

Harms, H. A., and J. Y. Malone, "The Relationship of Hearing Acuity to Stammering," *Journal of Speech Disorders*, IV (1939), 363–70.

Harrison, H. S., "A Study of the Speech of Sixty Institutionalized Epileptics." Master's thesis, Louisiana State University, 1947.

Hirschberg, J. ["Stuttering,"] *Orvosi Hetilap*, CVI (1965), 780–84.

Hull, F. M., "National Speech and Hearing Survey—A Preliminary Report," Convention address, A.S.H.A., 1969.

Hull, F. M., and R. J. Timmons, *National Speech and Hearing Survey*. U. S. Office of Education, Project No. 5-0978; Grant No. 32-15-0050-5010, 1969.

Hunt, J., *Stammering and Stuttering: Their Nature and Treatment*, 1870. Reprinted, New York: Hafner, 1967.

Jackson, R. M., "Stuttering Report," Convention address, California Speech and Hearing Association, 1967.

Jameson, A., "Stammering in Children," *Speech* (London), XIX (1955), 60–67.

Johnson, W., *The Onset of Stuttering*. Minneapolis: University of Minnesota Press, 1959.

Jones, E., *Free Associations: Memoirs of a Psychoanalyst*. New York: Basic Books, 1959.

Karlin, I. W., "Psychosomatic Theory of Stuttering," *Journal of Speech Disorders*, XII (1947), 319–22.

Katsovakaia, I., [The Problem of Children's Stuttering] *Proceedings Third Session Institute of Defectology* (1960), 133–34.

Kingdon-Ward, W., *Stammering*. London: Hamilton, 1941.

Lemert, E. M., "Some Indians Who Stutter," *Journal of Speech and Hearing Disorders*, XVIII (1953), 168–74.

———. "Stuttering and Social Structure in Two Pacific Societies," *Journal of Speech and Hearing Disorders*, XXVII (1962), 3–10.

Lennon, E. J., *Le Begaiement: Therapeutiques modernes*. Paris: Dion and Cie, 1962.

Lerman, J. W., G. R. Powers, and S. Rigrodsky, "Stuttering Patterns Observed in a Sample of Mentally Retarded Individuals," *Training School Bulletin,* LXII (1965), 27–32.

Louttit, C. M., and E. C. Halls, "Survey of Speech Defects Among Public School Children of Indiana," *Journal of Speech Disorders,* I (1936), 73–80.

Mahaffey, R. B., and C. Stromsta, "The Effects of Auditory Feedback as a Function of Frequency, Intensity, Time and Sex," *De Therapia Vocis et Loquellae,* II (1965), 233–35.

Martyn, M. M., and J. Sheehan, "Onset of Stuttering and Recovery," *Behavior Research and Therapy,* VI (1968), 295–307.

McAllister, A. M., *Clinical Studies in Speech Pathology.* London: U. London Press, 1937.

McCallien, C., "Problems of Speech Defect in the Accra District," *Speech* (London), XX (1956), 15–18.

McCarthy, D., "Lauguage Disorders and Parent-Child Relationships," *Journal of Speech and Hearing Disorders,* XIX (1954), 514–23.

McDowell, E., *Educational and Emotional Adjustment of Stuttering Children.* Columbia University Teachers College Contributions to Education, No. 314, 1928.

McMahon, E. M., *Report of the Three Year Survey to Assess Speech and Hearing Needs in British Columbia, 1962–1964.* (1969).

Metraux, R. W., "Speech Profiles of the Pre-School Child," *Journal of Speech Disorders,* XV (1950), 33–36.

Meyer, B. C., "Psychosomatic Aspects of Stuttering," *Journal of Nervous and Mental Diseases,* CI (1945), 127–57.

Milisen, R., "The Public Schools as a Site for Speech and Hearing," *Speech Teacher,* XII (1963), 1–9.

Milisen, R., and W. Johnson, "A Comparative Study of Stutterers, Former Stutterers and Normal Speakers Whose Handedness has Been Changed," *Archives Speech,* I (1936), 61–86.

Mills, A., and H. Streit, "Report of a Speech Survey in Holyoke, Mass.," *Journal of Speech Disorders,* VII (1942), 161–67.

Morgenstern, J. J., "Socio-economic Factors in Stuttering," *Journal of Speech and Hearing Disorders,* XXI (1956), 25–33.

Morley, D. E., "A Ten Year Survey of Speech Disorders Among University Students," *Journal of Speech Disorders,* XVII (1952), 25–31.

Morley, M., *The Development and Disorders of Speech in Childhood.* Edinburgh: Livingstone, 1957.

Mussafia, M., "The Role of Heredity in Language Disorders," *Folia Phoniatrica.* XVI (1964), 228–38.

Mysak, E. D., "Diagnosis of Stuttering as Made by Adolescent Boys and Girls." *Journal of Speech and Hearing Disorders,* XXIV (1959), 29–33.

Neeley, M. M., "An Investigation of the Incidence of Stuttering Among Elementary School Children in the Parochial Schools of Orleans Parish." Master's thesis, Tulane University, 1960.

Nelson, S. E., N. Hunter, and M. Walter, "Stuttering in Twin Types," *Journal of Speech Disorders,* X (1945), 335–43.

Ozawa, Y., [Studies of Misarticulation in Wakayama District], *Journal of Medicine: University of Osaka* (Japan) V (1960), 319.

Palmer, M., and C. Osborn, "One Thousand Consecutive Cases of Speech Defects," *Transactions Kansas Academy of Science*, XLI (1938), 16–27.

Petkov, D., and I. Iosifov, ["Our Experience in Treatment of Stuttering in a Speech Rehabilitation Colony"], *Zhurnal Neuropatologii e Psykhiatrii imeni S. S. Korsokova*, XL (1960), 903–4.

Pitrelli, F. R., "Psychosomatic and Rorschach Aspects of Stuttering," *The Psychiatric Quarterly*, XXII (1948), 175–94.

Preus, A., personal communication, 1968.

Prichett, M., "The Role of the East St. Louis Schools: A Study of the Effectiveness of the Multi-approach in Stuttering Therapy," *Proceedings Illinois Speech Association*, November, 1966.

Root, A. R., "A Survey of Speech Defectives in the Public Elementary Schools of South Dakota," *Elementary School Journal*, XXVI (1925), 531–41.

Rutherford, B., "A Comparative Study of Loudness, Pitch, Rate, Rhythm and Quality of the Speech of Children Handicapped by Cerebral Palsy," *Journal of Speech Disorders*, IX (1946), 263–71.

———. "Speech Reeducation for the Birth Injured," *Journal of Speech Disorders*, III (1938), 199–206.

Sato, N., ["Young Stutterers: Their Actual State of Affairs"], *Voice and Language Medicine* (Japan), II (1961), 40–42.

Schuell, H., "Sex Differences in Relation to Stuttering," *Journal of Speech Disorders*, XI (1946), 277–98; XII (1947), 23–38.

Schindler, M. D., "The Educational Adjustments of Stuttering and Nonstuttering School Children." In W. Johnson (ed.), *Stuttering in Children and Adults*. Minneapolis: University of Minnesota Press, 1955.

Schreiber, W., "Die Medizin in Dienst der Sprachheilfürsorge," *Psychological Abstracts*, XXIX (1955), 255 (abstract).

Schubert, O. W., "The Incidence Rate of Stuttering in a Matched Group of Institutionalized Mentally Retarded," convention address, American Association on Mental Deficiency, Chicago, 1966.

Schlanger, B. B., "Speech Examination of a Group of Institutionalized Mentally Handicapped Children." *Journal of Speech and Hearing Disorders*, XVIII (1953), 339–49.

Schlanger, B. B., and R. H. Gottsleben, "Analysis of Speech Defects among the Institutionalized Mentally Retarded." *Journal of Speech and Hearing Disorders*, XXII (1957), 98–103.

Schuster, G., "Diabetes Mellitus and Epilepsy Viewed From the Standpoint of Dysphemia. Master's thesis, University of Wisconsin, 1936.

Seeman, M., *Sprachstörungen bei Kindern*. Marhold: Halle-Saale, 1959.

Shames, G. H., and H. L. Beams, "Incidence of Stuttering in Older Age Groups," *Journal of Speech and Hearing Disorders*, XXI (1956), 313–16.

Shearer, W. M., and J. D. Williams, "Self-Recovery from Stuttering," *Journal of Speech and Hearing Disorders*, XXX (1965), 288–90.

Sheehan, J., M. M. Martyn, and K. L. Kilburn, "Speech Disorders in Retardation," *American Journal of Mental Deficiency*, LXXIII (1968), 251–56.

Sheehan, J., and M. M. Martyn, "Spontaneous Recovery from Stuttering," *Journal of Speech and Hearing Research*, IX (1967), 121–35.

Stassi, J., "Disfluency of Normal Speakers and Reinforcement," *Journal of Speech and Hearing Research*, IV (1961), 358–61.

Sternberg, M. L., "Auditory Factors in Stuttering." Master's thesis, State University of Iowa, 1946.

Stewart, J. L., "The Problem of Stuttering in Certain North American Indian Societies," *Journal of Speech and Hearing Disorders,* Monograph Supplement No. 6 (1960), 1–87.

Toyoda, B., ["A Statistical Report"] *Clinical Paediatrica,* XII (1959), 788.

Van Horn, H., "Comparative Incidence of Stuttering After Twenty Years," *Western Michigan University Journal of Speech Therapy,* III (1966), 6–7.

Voelker, C. H., "A Preliminary Investigation for a Normative Study of Fluency: a Critical Index to the Severity of Stuttering," *American Journal of Orthopsychiatry,* XIV (1944), 285–94.

———. "Incidence of Pathologic Speech Behavior in the General American Population," *Archives of Otolaryngology,* XXXVIII (1943), 113–21.

———. "On the Semantic Aspects of Stuttering in Nonstutterers," *Quarterly Journal of Speech,* XXVIII (1942), 78–80.

Voelker, E., and C. Voelker, "Spasmophemia in Dyslalia Cophotica—Case Report," *Annals of Otology, Rhinology and Laryngology,* 1937.

Waddle, E., "A Comparison of Speech Defectives Among Colored and White Children." Master's thesis, University of Iowa, 1934.

Wallen, V., "Primary Sutttering in a 28-Year-Old Adult," *Journal of Speech and Hearing Disorders,* XXVI (1961), 394–95.

Wallen, V., "Primary Stuttering in a 28-Year-Old Adult," *Journal of Speech and School and Society,* III (1916), 213–16.

Watzl, I., "Statistiches Erhebungen über das Vorkommen von Sprachstörungen in den Wiener Schulen," *Proceedings First International Congress of Logopedics and Phoniatrics,* Vienna, 1924.

Weiss, D. A., *Cluttering.* Englewood Cliffs, N.J.: Prentice-Hall, 1964.

Wepman, J. M., "Familial Incidence in Stammering," *Journal of Speech Disorders,* IV (1939), 199–204.

West, R., "An Agnostic's Speculations About Stuttering." In J. Eisenson (ed.), *Stuttering: A Symposium.* New York: Harper, 1958.

———. "The Pathology of Stuttering," *Nervous Child,* II (1943), 96–106.

West, R., S. Nelson, and M. Berry, "The Heredity of Stuttering," *Quarterly Journal of Speech,* XXV (1939), 23–30.

White House Conference on Child Health and Protection, Section 3: *Special Education: The Handicapped and the Gifted.* New York: Century, 1931.

Williams, C. Y., "Parental Attitudes and Maternal Rejection of Stuttering Children Among Southern Negroes." Master's thesis, Ohio University, 1964.

Wingate, M. E., "Recovery from Stuttering," *Journal of Speech and Hearing Disorders,* XXIX (1964), 312–21.

Zisk, P. K., and I. Bialer, "Speech and Language Problems in Mongolism: A Review of the Literature," *Journal of Speech and Hearing Disorders,* XXXII (1967), 228–41.

four

THE ONSET OF
STUTTERING

The surrealistic montage of behaviors which forms the picture of fully developed stuttering is most difficult to comprehend. We gaze upon this composition, feel its strong emotional impact, but cannot quite discern the fluctuating pattern from case to case. Perhaps if we could view stuttering at its beginnings, the design of its basic nature might be more clear. Let us seek to know when it begins, how it begins, and—what will probably be more difficult—why it begins.

AGE OF ONSET

One of the few solid bits of information we have about stuttering is that it usually begins in childhood. Very rarely we do find an occasional person whose disorder clearly began during adulthood, although when we do there is always some suspicion or even evidence to indicate that the adult stuttering was a recurrence of a problem which had shown itself much earlier in the person's life. Those who view stuttering merely as a neurosis find this early onset rather difficult to explain. Neuroses may begin at any age, but most of them first show themselves later than the preschool years. With great consistency stuttering begins early in the person's life.

Some of the evidence for this belief comes from clinical observations and surveys and some from research. While we always prefer the latter to the former, the unanimity of statements made by clinicians from many different countries has some value. To review just a few of these:

Japanese writers report the following onset data. Otsuki (1958): 55 per cent of 331 stutterers began before five years; 93 per cent before ten years; Shiraiwa (1958): 70 per cent of 70 stutterers began before age six; Fujita (1964): 40 per cent of 80 stutterers began between ages two and three years. Other Japanese writers give similar results: Takagi (1962): most stutterers begin at two and three years, a few after six years; Toyoda (1967): onset usually between two and three years.

In Africa, McCallien (1956) reports that 66 per cent of 138 children began to stutter prior to school entrance; Aron (1958) interviewed parents of African and European school children and found the average age of onset to be three years, four months, for the African, and four years, ten months, for the European stutterers.

In France, de Ajuriaguerra (1958) and his co-workers found 51 cases with onset prior to seven years and 33 cases who began later than this time. Radol'skii (1965) reports in a Russian publication that of 125 stuttering children, stuttering first appeared in 116 of them between the ages of two through five, and only in nine did it have a later onset. Seeman (1959) found that 66 per cent of the first signs of stuttering occurred in children between the ages of three through six at the time the child is mastering sentence structuring. Fritzell (1963) found that the disorder usually begins between two through four years in Sweden. Jameson (1955) intensively studied 69 English children and found that most had begun to stutter before age four. Two of the more extensive studies are by Daskalov (1962) in Bulgaria and by Hirschberg (1965) in Hungary. Daskalov gives this data on age of onset for 655 stutterers: two years—13 per cent; four years—13 per cent; five years—13 per cent; six years—9 per cent; seven years—14 per cent; eight years—12 per cent; nine years—3 per cent; ten years—1 per cent; 11 years—1.5 per cent; 12 years—2 per cent; 13 years—2 per cent. Hirschberg's data (p. 782) may be best presented in the form of a graph:

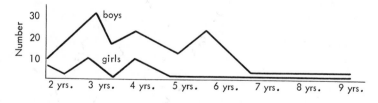

Age of the Stutterers at Onset

Figure 4. Age of stutterers at onset. (*From Hirschberg, 1965.*)

The longitudinal studies reported by Morley (1957) and by Andrews and Harris (1964) provide us with some of our best information concerning the onset of stuttering. Some of their findings may be summarized as follows:

Age in years:	3	4	5	6	7	8	9
Number of children							
Morley (1957)	1	20	12	2	2	–	–
Andrews and Harris (1964)	6	34	15	11	10	3	1

Morley also reports ages of onset for another population of 249 stutterers (p. 348) in which the same pattern of early onset was demonstrated.

The two major American investigations of the onset of stuttering were reported by Johnson (1959) and by Darley (1955), both based on intensive interviewing of parents. Earlier, Johnson (1955) found that the median age of onset was three years for 46 children. He writes:

> It is to be underscored perhaps that in three-fourths of the cases the difficulty began at or before the age of three years, two months, and that in half the cases it began sometime within an eight-months period between the ages of two years, six months, and three years, two months. The modal age of onset found in this study is somewhat earlier than that given by most writers in the field. The most important reason for the discrepancy would appear to be the fact that in the present study the case histories were obtained relatively soon after onset while memories were presumably comparatively fresh (p. 63).

Darley (1955) interviewed the mothers and fathers of his 50 stuttering children separately, hoping thereby to have some check on the validity of the information procured. The median age of onset reported by the mothers was three years, seven months (onset range=1 yr. 3 mos.–9 yrs.); and by the fathers (onset range: 18-132 months) the median age of reported onset was four years and seven months.

While this discrepancy in parental reports is hardly sufficient to make us doubt the overwhelming consensus that most stuttering begins in the preschool years, it should also make us very cautious in evaluating a reported age of onset when it is provided by an adult stutterer. Darley's and Johnson's subjects were the parents of stutterers, not the stutterers themselves, and the interviewing was done only a relatively short time after the onset of stuttering had occurred. Despite this, the parental replies were often vague and very inconsistent. Aron (1958) compared the age of onset reported by the stutterers themselves with what the stutterers said their parents had told them and with the parents' actual statements. She found huge discrepancies. Most importantly, the stutterers themselves tended to place the age of onset much later than the parents did. We must remember this when considering the validity of onset data given in such questionnaire studies as that by Martyn and Sheehan (1968) in which adult college stutterers and former stutterers served as the subjects. The difficulty of recall, the lack of precise definition, the absence of written records, all these facttors militate against placing complete confidence in such testimony.

TIME LAPSE BETWEEN ONSET
OF SPEECH AND ONSET
OF STUTTERING

In what proportion of stutterers does the onset of stuttering coincide with the onset of speech? This question is of more than casual importance. For example, Bluemel (1957) distinguished between *stuttering* as "unorganized speech" and *stammering* as "disorganized speech." Are there different kinds of stutterers—those who never attained normal fluency and those who once had it but lost it? Are the so-called "recovered stutterers" those who are recovering or convalescing from an episode of stuttering or are they discovering a fluency they never possessed? Should therapy be structured around learning or unlearning? If stuttering has a strong organic component, should not the disorder become evident as soon as connected speech appears? These are just a few of the reasons why we need to know more about the relationship between the onset of speech and the onset of stuttering.

Unfortunately our data on this important matter leave much to be desired, again primarily because of the difficulty in getting reliable information concerning the onset of both speech and stuttering. Johnson (1955) writes:

> Because of differences among parents in their extensional definitions of "word" and "sentence" and because of parental pride, as well as the relative difficulty of recall in the absence of written records, information of this kind is difficult to obtain with a high degree of precision by the interview method. We simply recognized the operation of these factors and did what we could to counteract their influence by careful interviewing (pp. 47–48).

Darley and Winitz (1961), in their extensive review of the literature concerning age of first words, have added:

> In summary, it would seem that the use of operational definitions of the first word have been so consistently different from investigator to investigator as to be an important source of error in the reported age of appearance of the first word. Coupled with it are other sources of error: the inadequacy of parental records; the fallibility of parents' memory; parents' "wishful hearing," "optimism," and pride; and the infrequency and meagerness of sampling of infants' vocalizations by observers other than parents (p. 283).

We thus have two major sources of error: the dating of stuttering onset and the dating of speech onset. Moreover, if the onset of speech is considered to occur not with the first words but instead with the first connected speech, even more vagueness and inaccuracy in parental testimony is to be expected. All we can do, therefore, is to cite what research we do possess and keep our fingers crossed in interpreting it.

Most of the meager information we have deals with the percentages of stutterers who reportedly have stuttered since the beginning of speech. Thus Berry (1938) found that 72 per cent of 500 stutterers began to stutter within the first year after onset of speech. Aron (1958) interviewed parents of 16 stuttering children and found nine of them who said the stuttering had coincided with the first speech. Of Morley's (1957) 249 stutterers, 50 claimed never to have had a period entirely free from stuttering. Andrews and Harris (1964) showed that the severe stutterers (at age ten) in general had an earlier onset of stuttering than milder stutterers. At that age, only nine per cent of the mild stutterers had stuttered since the beginning of speech while 33 per cent of the severe stutterers had always stuttered. Most of the stutterers in their population, however, had experienced a period of fluent speech before beginning to stutter.

The Iowa studies also demonstrate that the stuttering appeared only after normal fluency had been achieved. Johnson (1955) gives his findings as follows:

> If we consider the ages at which first words were spoken, the extent of the interval between first spoken words and the onset of stuttering ranged from six months to eight years. The median interval was 23 months, the 25th percentile fell at 17 months, and the 75th percentile at 32 months. The extent of the interval between the first speaking of sentences and the onset of stuttering ranged from minus ten months to plus seven years and seven months (91 months). That is, in one case the onset of stuttering was reported to have occurred ten months before the child began to speak sentences. In two other cases the onset of stuttering occurred four months and two months, respectively, before sentences were spoken. In all other cases the speaking of sentences occurred before the child was regarded as a stutterer. The median interval was 13 months, the 25th percentile fell at seven months, and the 75th percentile at 24 months (p. 63).

Darley (1955) also provides data on the interval between the age of first speaking sentences and the onset of stuttering. Using the mothers' estimates, he found that the interval ranged from a minus twelve months (i.e., that the child stuttered when in the one-word sentence stage) to 66 months, with a median interval of one and a half years between the first sentences and the first stutterings. Darley points up the significance of this finding in the following words:

> A theory of stuttering that posits any type of constitutional difference which somehow predisposes certain children to stutter must account for the apparently normal speech behavior manifested during this interval (p. 135).

We must remember, however, that other research has shown that some children do begin to stutter from the onset of consecutive speech or at least that the diagnosis was made at that time. Stuttering behaviors—temporally disrupted words—may occur very early but not be diagnosed as a disorder until later.

We have analyzed the case records of 114 children whom we saw personally and whose parents we interviewed within six months after the time of this diagnosis. Five of these we saw on the day of onset and nine within a week, and we felt fairly certain that the diagnosis was justified. Of the 61 cases, all were seen within three weeks after onset. The age-range of onset was from two years, one month to nine years, three months; the median age of onset was three years, one month.

IS THE ONSET OF STUTTERING SUDDEN OR GRADUAL?

This is a very difficult question to answer, posing as it does the problem of definition and differential diagnosis from normal disfluency. As we shall see, there are many anecdotal accounts and case reports of stuttering occurring very suddenly after a specific incident, but a search of the literature and a survey of our own cases indicates that in the large majority of instances, stuttering begins gradually. Levina (1968) states:

> Our [Russian] studies have confirmed that stammering usually begins at ages three to four. In almost all cases of stammering among children it sets in gradually, beginning with slightly interrupted speech similar to the physiological difficulties accompanying the transition to phraseological speech (p. 28).

De Ajuriaguerra (1958) and his colleagues intensively studied 51 stutterers in France, reporting that 44 of them showed a gradual onset while 15 others showed a sudden one. Three of the latter began to stutter after a period of mutism. Morley (1957) found a sudden onset in only three of 37 children in her longitudinal research. She says:

> In most of the children, however, the onset was gradual, beginning with a slight degree of occasional hesitant speech: and the age of onset, as reported to us, is probably the age at which the mother first became aware of the child's difficulty. Many more children than the 37 mentioned may have passed through a period of hesitant speech, accepted by the mother as a normal and transient stage in speech development," (pp. 41–42).

These findings are probably limited because parents find difficulty in judging the gradualness of onset. How gradually does anyone become aware that one's child is having difficulty speaking? Parents look back and remember that their child had perhaps shown other broken words at one time or another, that he had repeated syllables and spoken "stutteringly" on occasion. Perhaps this is what they mean when they say the disorder developed gradually. The diagnosis itself probably always begins with a sentence such as this: "Isn't Johnny beginning to stutter?" Then there follows a period of observation and checking until negation or confirmation is achieved. Since this too takes time, the impression is gained that the disorder is developing gradually when perhaps it is only the diagnosis which is gradual.

In this discussion we are not opposing the idea that stuttering behaviors probably show a gradual increase in frequency, duration, and a number of other significant features until they evoke a diagnosis of disorder. We think that this is what usually happens, though not in all cases. We are merely saying that there is a built-in bias in favor of the concept of gradual onset and that this bias must be considered in any theory which bases itself partly upon this matter. Bloodstein, Alper, and Zisk (1965), for example, hold that stuttering is an exacerbation and outgrowth of normal nonfluency. If the onset of stuttering is universally gradual in nature, this should support their position. Also, if there are different types of stutterers, perhaps those whose stuttering started very suddenly (and we are pretty sure that some of them do have this sort of onset) comprise a different subpopulation within the syndrome. Again we need more and better research bearing directly on this facet of the problem. In our own observations of 114 children, whom we personally were able to see within six months of reported onset, we found that in only 11 of these individuals were we fairly certain that the stuttering occurred very suddenly. One of them was the author's own daughter.

THE ONSET OF STUTTERING
IN ADULTS

Although, as we have seen, the onset of stuttering in adulthood is comparatively rare, it does seem to occur occasionally, and when it does it appears suddenly. The literature is not extensive, and much of it consists of general observations such as the following one from Freund (1966):

> Hysterical stuttering tends to have its onset later in life than the other types. It may occur in adulthood. Bizarre and hysterical forms of stuttering were observed by us and others after shell shock, head trauma, or the first parachute descents. It tends to begin suddenly rather than gradually, and these stutterers or their parents report that it began during or following trauma or cumulative stress. Histories of complete mutism as the initiating feature are not uncommon (pp. 139–40).

We will cite a few of the case reports of the onset of stuttering in adults. To illustrate Freund's view of hysterical stuttering, Smith (1921) tells of a woman who developed stuttering after administration of ether during surgery. During the hallucinatory period as she came out of the anesthesia, she dreamed that she had won a competition to collect all the glass in the world, doing harm to many people in the process who then put the curse of stammering upon her.

All of the adults who suddenly develop stuttering behaviors, however, are not hysterics. Glaser (1936) reports the onset of stuttering after injections of epinephrine were used subsequent to removal of ovaries. Eisenson (1947) and many other authors mention stuttering resulting from strokes. Head injuries, war-time or otherwise, have produced many accounts in which stuttering followed the trauma as has been reported by Kingdon-Ward (1941), Fahy, Irving, and Millac (1967) and Peacher and Harris (1946). Mochizuki (1962) tells of two adult men, aged 25 and 56, who developed stuttering as a result of the great shock caused by the atomic bomb at Hiroshima. Hirschfield (1916) found frequent instances of sudden onset of stuttering following shell explosions. Froeschels (1917) described in detail a case study of a traumatic war stutterer who began with clonic repetitions of syllables then progressed to tonic prolongations as he endeavored to cope with his frustration. In another publication, Froeschels (1916) declares that it is possible to tell the difference between traumatic and developmental stuttering by an analysis of the symptoms. Traumatic stutterers do not show starters or breathing abnormalities or inappropriate speech postures; developmental stutterers do. Finally, only a few years ago, Wallen (1961) described an adult stutterer whose speech remained repetitive:

> He first came to the attention of the medical staff when he reported in for "sick call" one morning. He was visibly disturbed—trembling, crying, and stuttering severely. . . . He stated that he had been overworking for several months, having little time to spend with his family.
>
> On admission to the hospital his speech was characterized by rapid repetitions of initial syllables of words and prolongations of vowels, especially the vowel /æ/. The disfluency was pronounced at the beginning of sentences and tapered to fluency at the end.
>
> Testing indicated that he was basically a passive-dependent person with introversion tendencies who used repression and withdrawal as primary ego defense mechanisms.
>
> Several days later [after his admittance to the hospital] the acute signs of trembling, crying, and stuttering abated and disappeared. It was noted that the patient had a mild tendency to stutter automatically and without any evidence of anxiety. He would say, for example, "I-I-I didn't like the long hours. It looks like—looks like I'll be here for a while, I never minded the re-re-re-responsibility." He denied ever being aware of any speech problem until his present hospitalization (p. 394).

As we remarked earlier, one must evaluate such accounts of adult onset of stuttering with some caution. When carefully investigated, some of them turn out to be interiorized stutterers who, under great stress, could no longer hide their disorder. Others were stutterers in their youth who recovered, and the adult onset often has all the features characteristic of ordinary relapse. Klinger (1963) reported three cases of adult onset, all of whom "showed psychiatric or neurologic signs." However, later on he found that although all three men had stated that they had not had any history of stuttering prior to examination, one of them turned out to have the notation of "speech defect" on his Army induction records and another turned out to be a "pathological liar" (Klinger, 1966). The third case was well documented and the onset of stuttering at 43 years of age was evidently genuine. We have gone over our own case records and have found seven individuals who we are fairly certain did develop their stuttering for the first time in adulthood. Three of these were highly neurotic,* one was psychotic, and the other three began to stutter suddenly and severely after head injuries. Though there was no sign of aphasia in the latter three cases, all had experienced mutism for some hours after regaining consciousness. We also had 17 other cases who reported adult onset of the disorder but for whom we were able to find earlier evidence of stuttering in their childhood. It seems surprising to us that more adult neurotics do not assume the symptomatic picture of stuttering. Stuttering is highly visible; it is easily simulated; it should serve as an excellent defense against a wide variety of intolerable realities; it can beget sympathetic consideration as well as penalty; it has its secondary gains. If it is a neurosis, why then does it appear so rarely in adulthood?

SPEECH CHARACTERISTICS AT ONSET

How do children first begin to stutter? What kind of speech behaviors do they show at the time when parents first decide that a child is having an abnormal amount of disrupted fluency? What is the child doing that impels parents to diagnose stuttering? The answers to these questions are vitally important to most theories. An impressive amount of opinion—and a little research—indicates that usually the first sign of the disorder to be diagnosed as stuttering is an excessive amount of repetitive speech, primarily of repeated syllables. Less commonly, but also of diagnostic importance, are the prolongations of silent articulatory postures (blockages) or of voiced sounds.

Hoepfner (1911) was one of the first authors to describe syllabic repetitions as the earliest features of stuttering. He attributed them to some neurological deficit in the organization of the motor sequencing of words. Froe-

---

* One of these was the author's first treatment case. He suspects that she was given to him as a patient by Dr. Bryng Bryngelson to dissuade him from entering the field of speech pathology. The woman suddenly began to stutter very severely with a monosymptomatic facial contortion during the course of her college training as a speech therapist.

schels, in a long series of publications in both German and English, also insisted that the first signs of stuttering at onset consisted of iterations (syllable and word repetitions.) Unlike Hoepfner, Froeschels viewed these repetitions as a normal phase of speech development due mainly to word-finding difficulties under communicative stress. He writes:

> The opinion that frequent iterations are the usual start of stuttering is based upon statistics on 800 cases. They consisted partly of patients which when seen by the writer did not show any signs of stuttering other than iterations, and partly of cases with other signs of stuttering whose case history revealed that the first signs of speech trouble were exclusively word- or syllable-repetitions. In order to avoid any suggestive question, the patients and/or their parents were not asked what the signs were. Only if a description of the initial state was given spontaneously was it considered a reliable scientific fact. These spontaneously delivered reports described *without a single exception iterations as the first sign of the speech trouble* (Froeschels, 1952, p. 221).

In another publication, Froeschels (1943) said that in 700 stutterers he had only found one case with a "tonic" beginning, i.e., where it began with a tensed fixation or prolongation although he mentions that H. Gutzmann, Jr., had claimed that occasionally the first sign of stuttering was tonic (with pressure) rather than repetitive. Many of the statements in the literature referring to the type of stuttering behavior at onset are just such statements so that their validity is difficult to assess.

CASE STUDIES

We also have a fair number of individual case reports such as those by Wyatt (1969), Solomon (1933), Gondaira (1960) and Schmeer (1966). In each of these reports, one child who had begun to stutter was examined and studied intensively very soon after onset. We have read most of these case reports and find it difficult, even in the best of them, to do the kind of differential diagnosis we have outlined in a preceding chapter. To provide a sample, let us give our translation from the German of Schmeer's account:

> On January 28th, 1965, Andreas was aged 4 years and 4 months. As usual, once a week that winter, he was fetched from kindergarten which he had attended since the end of May, 1964, by his grandmother with whom he was to have dinner, spend the afternoon and night, and from where he would return to kindergarten the next morning.
> The grandmother phoned me that evening and told me that Andreas had started repeating the initial syllables of his words when speaking. When she had bathed him he had been very excited and had threatened to lock her up in a prison and shoot her with a gun: Bang! Bang! etc. . . . She had never seen the child like this before; he had always been quite well behaved

and responsive to her attempts to teach him good manners. When the next day Andreas was fetched from the kindergarten by his mother, he stuttered quite obviously, repeating his initial syllables as many as 16 times. I was alarmed because I feared that Andreas would develop the same speech impediment affecting his father and three other relatives on his father's side . . . (p. 46).

These detailed case reports, of course, should not be ignored. They are a far cry from such casual observations as Fogerty's (1930): "A tramp looked in the window and frightened the twins. One began to stammer three weeks later" or Greene's (1924): "One child began to stutter at the sudden opening of an automatic umbrella; another when he fell off the sofa on his head." The better case reports are very detailed and careful observations and in some instances are those of the author's own child as in the case of Nana reported by the speech pathologist Wyatt (1969). In this sense they are probably more valid than data procured by interviewing parents, especially when the questioning is done months after onset. Unfortunately, the reports still lack enough analytical precision in description to enable us to be certain just what speech behaviors did occur. Generally, however, they indicate that the main feature of the speech at stuttering onset seems to be the presence of an excessive number of syllabic repetitions. Wyatt describes it thusly:

> These compulsive repetitions must be differentiated clearly from developmental repetitions. The linguistic units repeated under the influence of frustration or anxiety are no longer representative of the child's normal stage of language development; they are different in kind from developmental repetitions. Compulsive repetitions do not serve as building blocks in the construction of larger syntactic units. The child is no longer able to shift freely back and forth between simpler and more advanced language patterns. An example of compulsive repetition is *I-I-I wa-wa-want to, to, to, th-th-throw the c-c-clay away* (p. 87).

Not all the authors of these anecdotal studies of the onset of stuttering report this feature of compulsivity, but most of those that we have examined mention frequent syllabic repetitions, usually with many of them occurring in the same word.

INTERVIEW DATA

Taylor (1937) compiled the data procured by 12 interviewers of parents of 47 children who had begun to stutter a few weeks or months before. The interviewers had also observed the children speaking. Of the 47 children, 85 per cent exhibited only repetitions at onset; 6 per cent had sound stoppages, and 2 per cent showed prolongations. Also, of the total number, 8 per cent showed some forcings and struggle, 6 per cent accompanied their stuttering with abnormal co-movements of head and limbs, and 6 per cent seemed to have been aware of the difficulty immediately.

The most extensive interview studies of the nature of stuttering at on-set were performed by Johnson (1955; 1959) and his students. These have been often quoted as supporting the proposition that the kind of speech shown by stutterers at onset is indistinguishable from normal disfluency, a belief which Johnson sought to foster since it supported his semantogenic theory. For example, he repeatedly (and, in our opinion, unjustifiedly) lumped together repetitions of phrases and whole words with the syllabic repetitions to conclude that "the same kinds of nonfluency were reported" by the parents of stutterers and nonstutterers. Nevertheless, when these studies are rigorously examined, as they have been both by us and by Mc-Dearmon (1968), they show clearly that *syllabic* repetitions in the main and, to a less extent, prolongations of sounds, were the dominating features which distinguished the behaviors diagnosed by parents of stutterers as stutterings from those noticed by parents of nonstuttering children as be-ing normal nonfluencies. Tucked away in Johnson's formidable monograph (p. 229) is his own recognition of this finding:

> There were interesting group differences with reference to the various kinds of repetition. Sound or syllable repetitions were reported for significantly more experimental group children, phrase repetitions were reported for significantly more control group children, and there was not a significant group difference for word repetitions.

In his reanalysis of Johnson's data McDearmon (1968) gives this summary:

> (1) Among experimentals, children labeled as stutterers by at least one parent, at least 63 per cent at onset of stuttering evidenced primary stutter-ing (simple repetitions and prolongations of sound and syllables), and at least 28 per cent evidenced only normal nonfluencies (repetitions of words and phrases, and other interruptions common in children), as indicated by parents' responses to one question. (2) This primary stuttering was much more frequent, and normal nonfluency much less frequent, in experimentals at onset of stuttering than in controls; and these differences were statistically significant. (3) Slight tension was the only secondary reaction indicated in more than 15 per cent of the experimentals at onset, according to parents' responses to other questions (p. 637).

While the study did not specifically consider speech at onset, in his cross-sectional study of stuttering, Bloodstein (1960) showed that among the youngest of his cases, the 30 children aged two and four years, repetitions and prolongations were the characteristic features in 75 per cent of these children. Forty per cent showed occasional hard contacts and 33 per cent had other associated symptoms. He reports that the repetitions "are most often reported by parents as the earliest noticed symptoms of the disorder." And further:

The word and syllable repetitions described above are referred to as stuttering for several reasons. (1) They were in most cases both far more frequent and far more prolonged than the repetitions usually observed in the speech of young children. (2) In many cases, including some of the mildest who were brought for examination, the parents' and the author's evaluation of the repetitions as abnormal was apparently shared by relatives, friends, or neighbors who had referred to them as "stuttering." (3) Even in cases in which it might have been possible, by a somewhat liberal interpretation of speech adequacy, to regard the repetitions as not wholly or essentially different from those of normal children, there was often a past history of unquestionable stuttering which served to destroy the illusion of a completely typical child with normal nonfluency (p. 221).

During the years 1934–36, the author held a research appointment with the Department of Child Welfare at the University of Iowa, and his project was to discover the cause of stuttering. We advertised in newspapers and on the radio for information concerning children who had just begun to stutter and, when we heard of them, we went directly to their homes to interview their parents and associates and to observe the children carefully. Although the material was never published, the 30 case studies we obtained served as the basis for a continuing interest in the onset of stuttering, and we have since augmented the data considerably. Of the 61 cases reported in the following table, nine were seen within a week of reported onset and the others within three weeks. The kinds of behaviors shown were observed by the author:

	Observed	*Reported by Parent at Onset*
Sound and syllable repetitions:* ("s-s-s-some;" "to-to-today")	49	53
Single syllable word repetitions: ("Can-can-can-can")	43	50
Prolonged sounds: †	17	11
Prolonged articulatory postures: †		
Without tension	12	3
With tension	9	7
Broken words: (medial gaps: "v——ery")	4	0
Evidence of awareness:	9	5

* In this tabulation, we refer to syllabic or word repetitions which occurred more than three times on a single word.

† Duration had to exceed two seconds to be counted.

Note: As is evident from this table, some children showed several of these behaviors. Our data regrettably are incomplete as to repetition rate, regularity, airflow, and other features.

In reviewing all this information, it is obvious that much more needs to be done before we can be sure what actually happens at the onset of stuttering. We regret that the longitudinal studies reported by Morley (1957) and Andrews and Harris (1964) provide no data on this important matter and we hope that any future longitudinal study will do so.

CONDITIONS AT ONSET

In this section we invade a never-never land in which much of our information is suspect. The parents of stutterers, the stutterers themselves, even our casual acquaintances always ask the age old question: "What is the cause of stuttering?" When we temporize and answer that there seems to be no one cause and that stuttering is probably the end result of many forces both external and internal, both past and present, our questioners, if they do not immediately judge speech pathology to be a benighted profession, tend to ask: "Then under what conditions does it arise? What sets it off?" These too are very difficult for us to answer unhesitatingly and without stammering a little. Our own study of the literature and our long clinical experience, in which we tried very hard to come to some definite conclusions about the matter, have not yielded us any real assurance. Indeed we envy those writers of the past and present who seem so certain about the causes of stuttering. Witness this quotation from Stein (1942):

> One of my patients had a purely tonic stammer due to an extremely short frenulum which made the articulation of all dental sounds impossible. The disorder with all its anxiety and inferiority symptoms disappeared after the tongue had been freed by cutting the frenulum (p. 110).

Though the pudding has apparent therapeutic proof, we still find it difficult to swallow the alleged etiology.

We are also duly impressed but not convinced by the authoritarian statements of presumed causes which certain writers have been able to identify in their series of cases. For example, the Russian, Katsovskaia (1962) states flatly that the causes of stuttering in 200 children were found in 35 per cent of the cases to be due to psychic shocks; 27.5 per cent to the sequellae of illnesses affecting the brain; 26 per cent to delayed speech and language; 4.5 per cent to imitation and 2 per cent to forcing a premature development of speech. We also have some doubts about the Hungarian investigation in which Hirschberg (1965) summarizes his findings as follows:

Infection	11 cases
Tonsillar hypertrophy	67
Change-over of left-handed children	38
School conflicts	5
Unfavorable family background, deficient education	43

Imitation	7
Frightened by animals	23
Other psychic trauma	13
Falls, being beaten	18
Bilingualism	2

Hirschberg does qualify these results with the following statement: "We must stress that we have not been able to determine in all cases of stuttering the circumstances which were directly responsible for the stuttering or the speech neurosis." Nor have we—even for those we investigated in depth! We found some of the same circumstances (bad tonsils!) which Hirschberg mentioned but we were never sure that they were either predisposing or precipitating causes of the stuttering. All we could say was that they might have contributed.

But we must not confine these examples to the area behind the Iron Curtain for it is not hard to find many of the same ilk on our own side. Thus McAllister (1958) in England reports an etiological investigation of 139 cases of stuttering, and classifies them into four groups according to "possible causes": 1. 13.6 per cent had some abnormality in structure or functioning [sic!] of the speech organs; 2. 6.5 per cent were left-handed; 3. 5.7 per cent were due to imitation; 4. 75 per cent had emotional conflicts and complexes of many varieties.

SOURCES OF ERROR

These figures were probably obtained by scrutinizing a series of casefolders for information obtained by interviewing either the stutterers themselves or their parents. Many years have elapsed since the disorder began and truth is always diluted by time. Moreover, the alleged circumstances surrounding onset, when reported by the stutterer himself, may merely be those that occurred at the time when he became highly aware of his speech disability. Since this awareness usually occurs in situations of emotional stress, he will report that the disorder began under these emotional conditions. Whenever possible, we have tried to determine if the person showed a history of stuttering prior to the alleged emotional shock, illness, or other such reported causal experiences. The following may illustrate:

> A 16-year-old stutterer was brought to us by his mother with a clear history of onset at the age of eight years. Both the mother and the boy remembered the incident vividly. The boy was on his way home in the early darkness of a winter evening and stumbled across the body of a dead man on the sidewalk in front of the boy's home. (They had the newspaper clipping to prove it.) The boy rushed into the house, opened his mouth to speak, and was unable to do so for some minutes despite repeated attempts. His stuttering dated from this time, so they said, and it was interesting that his

major stuttering behavior was this same wide gaping mouth. The mother was absolutely convinced that the boy had been completely fluent previously. Nevertheless, we were able to find school records, and to get the testimony of his first grade teacher who remembered the boy because of his speech difficulty. It was clearly established that he had been stuttering fairly frequently and severely, though repetitively, before the incident.

This and many other similar discrepancies have taught us to evaluate with some skepticism such reports when they come to us long after onset. This is not to say that stuttering may not emerge originally from such dramatic events. We have found enough instances which we could corroborate to know that at times the disorder does arise in such an emotional context, but we are no longer naive enough to accept such testimony at face value. Parents and stutterers also are so frequently asked what caused the disorder that they have had to come up with some answer, usually one which absolves them of any responsibility. If there happens to be another child in the block who stutters, then they tell us he caught it by imitation; if the little stutterer happened to be ill prior to onset, then the cause was the illness; if he had a stuttering great aunt whom he had never met, then he inherited the disorder. And so on! Irwin and Duffy (1955) express the same point of view:

> It is natural for parents to look for some condition or experience that might account for the onset of stuttering—a physical injury, an emotional upset, a severe illness, or the appearance of a stuttering child in the neighborhood. That a severe illness might retard speech development and account for a period of nonfluency is quite possible. However, it is difficult to establish that such dramatic events are basic to the onset of stuttering. In fact, it often happens that children whose stuttering is attributed to such dramatic experience had shown hesitations, repetitions, and prolongations in their speech long before such events occurred (p. 49).

With these cautions in mind, let us review the literature on the subject of the "precipitating causes" of stuttering.

SHOCKS AND FRIGHT

The older literature is filled with accounts of stuttering beginning after a shock or frightening experience.

According to Luchsinger and Arnold (1965), Gutzmann, in 1900, found 14 per cent of his stutterers reporting the onset as being due to frightening events and these authors add: "In most cases minor physical or emotional mishaps are incriminated: a dog barked suddenly; a rooster flew onto the child's shoulder; or the child stumbled over a carpet in a department store (p. 745)." Makuen (1914) reported that 28 per cent of his 1000 stutterers "date the origin of the affection from the instant of having received a nervous shock (p. 388)." Scripture (1912) mentions terrifying experiences at amusement resorts, being frightened by someone dressed as a ghost, or severe falls. Ssikorski (1891) mentions 27 cases precipitated by severe emotional shock, six of whom showed a period of mutism prior to the onset of stuttering.

Even today we find published anecdotal accounts of the sudden onset of stuttering after shock or frightening experiences. Baba (1952) tells of a boy whose stuttering began after he fell into a river and Hastings (1966) writes:

> At 3 years of age he had been playing in a hayloft when he fell through an opening in the floor onto a metal container standing on the floor below. John's head was badly cut above the right eye and he was very shaken. The child's speech had developed normally up to this time (p. 47).

A very detailed and convincing account of stuttering following shock is given in the careful French study by Schachter (1967) of a little girl, aged 3 years, 11 months, who, after a collision with a motorized bicycle, became completely mute for four days and developed stuttering when she did again begin to talk. This brief sampling of the literature is representative. Perhaps the most important information we can glean from all this anecdotal material is that a period of mutism often precedes the onset of stuttering in these accounts of stuttering precipitated by shock or fright.

ILLNESS

Illnesses have also been often mentioned as precipitating causes of stuttering. It is highly probable that some of the illnesses which most children contract during the years when the disorder usually begins will inevitably precede its onset. Whether or not they have a causal rather than a correlative relationship is not so evident. We can be fairly certain, however, that if stuttering did appear subsequent to some illness, the parents would be prone to view it as the essential cause if only to relieve themselves of any responsibility they may feel. One mother we interviewed was very sure that her son's suffering followed a siege of scarlet fever, but in the hospital records we found that the illness had preceded her dating of the onset of stuttering by 11 months! Nevertheless, throughout the literature we find repeatedly the reference to illness as contributing to the onset of the disorder.

The causal relationship of illness to onset of stuttering is certainly not a simple one. Gutzmann (1939) found that in almost 10 per cent of his cases the stuttering followed severe attacks of infectious diseases and even intestinal infestation with worms. Berry (1938) surveyed the medical histories of stuttering children and concluded that two groups of illnesses appeared with greater frequency in stutterers than they did in normal speakers. The first group consisted of severe respiratory infections, rheumatic fever, scarlet fever, whooping cough, bronchitis, and pneumonia; the second group consisted of encephalitis, epilepsy, and convulsions. West, Nelson, and Berry (1939) reported that "from 16 to 20 per cent" of their stutterers began to stutter immediately upon recovery from one of these diseases. Again we wonder about the validity of the word "immediately," and we hunger to understand how these diseases actually triggered the stuttering if indeed they really did so. Perhaps a reasonable explanation may be found in this quotation from Luchsinger and Arnold (1965):

> The causative influence of infections or worm infestation should not be construed to represent a specific neurological damage. What is important is the general debilitation and the reduction of physical and mental resistance. Following such a breakdown of psychophysical well-being, stuttering may develop as a psychic reaction. To what extent such illnesses may alter the reactivity of the infant brain is beyond our comprehension at the present time (p. 745).

The pertinence of these remarks may be applied to Goda's (1961) account of stuttering following spinal meningitis. A seven-year-old boy had normal speech until an attack of spinal meningitis resulted in a right hemiplegia. Many of the physical activities he had formerly enjoyed were then denied him, and he had to remain an extra year in the second grade. He spoke without difficulty on his return to school, but two months later he began to stutter and with increasing severity. Was it the spinal meningitis which triggered the stuttering or the other consequences of the disease?

Fortunately we have two experiments concerned with illness and onset in which control groups were used. Johnson (1959) found no significant differences in the number of illnesses as reported by parents of stuttering and nonstuttering children fairly soon after onset, and Andrews and Harris (1964) reported that their 80 pairs of stuttering and nonstuttering children showed almost identical histories of illness. There at present the matter should rest in peace until some future investigator in this morbid boneyard unearths some better evidence.

IMITATION

As we have shown previously, the onset of stuttering has been ascribed by many writers as due to the child's imitation of some other person's stuttering. We often confront this belief in clinical practice. Many of our own stutterers have claimed that their disorder began this way. As we have seen in the studies by Van Riper (1937) and Ainsworth (1939), a listener tends to empathize with the stutterer. Many children use a kind of mockery which is not always vindictive but rather an attempt to perceive unusual behaviors. They limp when they see a lame person. They imitate a facial tic. It is their way of trying to understand what the behavior must be like. It seems logical that some children who, for other reasons, are on the verge of stuttering anyway, will develop stuttering through imitation. Parents might also find such an etiology highly convenient in absolving themselves of guilt.

The earlier literature stressed imitation as a causative factor much more than we do today. Thus Mygind (1898) found that in 13 per cent of his stutterers, usually those who had other stuttering family members, imitation was the important precipitating cause. The belief is still prevalent. In Japan, Otsuki (1958) claimed that imitation was a significant causal factor in 70 per cent of his cases, which is by far the highest guess we have discovered. Most contemporary authors place imitation as the precipitating cause in from 4 per cent (Katsovskaia, 1962) to 12 per cent (Froeschels, 1943). We suspect that Froeschels, in claiming this latter percentage, may have been involved in justifying his belief that those stutterers who show *prolongations of sounds or postures without the usual concomitant pressure or tension* must have acquired their disorder through imitation. This belief is an interesting hypothesis as yet unsupported by objective physiological research. Froeschels tells us that whenever he saw this particular behavior (which he called pseudotoni) he was able through questioning to elicit the fact that the stutterer had been in close association with some other stutterer. Although generally, the old emphasis on imitation as an essential and common cause of stuttering seems to have faded, nevertheless, we still occasionally find such case reports as that by Soufi (1960) appearing in our own journals. Soufi tells of a boy named Ricky who, previously denied much companionship, moved to an aunt's home in which the youngest boy stuttered severely.

> After ten days in this environment, Ricky stuttered in exactly the same manner as his cousin. After about two weeks of the stuttering, Ricky's mother informed him that he did not need to keep talking that way just because his cousin did. Ricky cried and said, "That's the only way I know how to say it" (p. 411).

For many years we have sought evidence for imitation as a precipitant of the onset of stuttering in every case we examined. Though we have never counted up the cases we saw in those years, they constitute a substantial number. We tried to trace every account of imitation as a source of stuttering and only in one single stuttering child do we feel fairly confident that the disorder was triggered in this way. In many cases, when we compared the stuttering behaviors of our case with those of the person he was said to have imitated (a playmate or the father), we found the stuttering patterns substantially dissimilar. These also were children whom we examined soon after onset and before other changes might have occurred. In the one case where we did feel imitation might have served as a trigger, there was a very close identification of the child with a very beloved playmate and we remembered what Blanton and Blanton (1936) said long ago: "A child might imitate dozens of stutterers and never have any difficulty in a real sense unless he selected some one *with whom he was under a compulsion to identify himself* (p. 99)." In most instances of alleged imitation that we investigated, the contact and association had been so minimal and transient that even had the behaviors shown some resemblance, which they did not, it was difficult to see how they could have been connected causally.

If imitation were a substantial factor in precipitating or creating stuttering, we should expect that each member of a pair of twins would be prone to stutter. In none of our own collection of eight pairs of twins did both individuals stutter. Although the incidence of stuttering among twins seems to be higher than that among singletons, the appearance of the disorder in both members of the pairs is surprisingly rare. Graf (1955) found that in only three of her 18 pairs of twins did both individuals stutter. In the other 15 pairs, which included six presumably identical pairs, only one of the two twins stuttered. Surely, if imitation were as potent a precipitating factor as it has been said to be, we should have expected a greater concordance of stuttering. In this connection Brodnitz (1951) reports that the two identical twins whom he studied stuttered in completely different ways.

Again, if imitation were a strong precipitating factor, one might expect that because of the greater contact, younger siblings would be more likely to stutter than older ones, and that siblings in general would show a fairly high incidence of stuttering. Our own unpublished data do not corroborate these assumptions. The only large scale study of the problem was done 30 years ago by Nadoleczny (1938) who reported that there were ten times more nonstuttering siblings in the families of his stutterers than there were stuttering siblings. In summary, we conclude that imitation is not a very important factor in the onset of stuttering and we feel Robert West's remarks on the topic well worth repeating:

> The question of whether or not imitation is a causal factor of stuttering has been responsible for perhaps more than its share of printing costs. If imitation is a factor, it is obviously not an important one, since the imitation of the stutterer's speech is an almost universal game of childhood. There is something dramatically amusing about stuttering—something that does not escape the child observer. Few children, indeed, come to puberty without witnessing the phenomenon of stuttering. If they have seen it nowhere else, they have seen it on the stage or screen. The imitation of stuttering the child has witnessed is as irresistible to him as the handling of some object that he has never before seen. If imitation were a sole cause of

stuttering, practically all children would stutter; and if it were one of the important precipitating causes of stuttering, there would be a tendency for stuttering to be "contagious," spreading from child to child until large numbers in a given school or community stuttered. Stuttering would thus spread like slang or popular songs. We would find some schoolrooms free of stuttering and others heavily spotted with it. The rather equal distribution of stuttering cases throughout the elementary schools of any given city indicates the sporadic rather than "infectious" nature of stuttering. Authorities in the field incline to the view that if imitation plays any causative role in stuttering, it is a very minor one as a precipitator of the stuttering (p. 104).

CONFLICT

More than any other etiological factor, emotional conflict has been blamed as the source of stuttering. We find this belief running throughout the literature, and it is certainly held by most of the parents of the young stutterers we have interviewed. Without prejudging the validity of the belief, we should point out that few lives are free from conflict and that most children at the typical age of onset are having a difficult time reconciling their urges and impulses with the demands for conformity that adults are then requiring. Some coincidence of the onset of stuttering with some conflict seems inevitable just because the child lives in a state of rather continual conflict at this period. As Sheehan (1958) has shown, conflicts involving ambivalence (approach-avoidance tendencies) may occur on many levels. At the word level, for example, the child is caught between conflicting urges to say a certain word or not to say it. In an old article, Dunlap (1917) illustrates such a conflict by attributing stuttering to the boy's approach-avoidance urges to say forbidden or dirty words. He says:

> The boy, in constant fear lest one of his obscene terms may slip out in the wrong company, and having experienced this dangerous tendency of words to go astray, soon comes to hesitate over every word which begins in the same way as do these dangerous words; and as the hesitation becomes a more and more fixed and noticeable habit, it extends to other types of words also. . . . The peculiar feature of stuttering, the repetition of the syllable many times, is a result of the usual method of checking the utterance of a word (p. 46).

There are many other such conflicts at the word level: trying to say unfamiliar words; trying to say the right word without being sure which one is right (Froeschel's word-finding difficulties); having to utter the unspeakable, the unacceptable word, and so on. These conflicts are not unknown even to adults; certainly they occur in young children. Our question however is this: Does stuttering begin in such word conflicts?

Conflicts can also arise at the situation-level. The onset of stuttering in four of our cases was said by the parents to have occurred when the child was asked to talk on the telephone for the first time. In these instances, the stuttering seemed to be localized only in the telephoning situation for some days before it spread to other types of communication. Another child whom we observed shortly after onset surprisingly showed a concentration of stuttering when speaking to his puppy or to some of his stuffed animals. We could not believe the parents when they told us this, but it was true. They said they had first noticed the stuttering shortly after the boy had called the puppy to him and had been knocked down by the dog. We report this reluctantly, hating to contribute any more to the fantastic folklore of the disorder, but we are pretty sure that this is what happened. Is it possible that the motor patterning of words can be so disrupted by such situation conflicts that the disorder of stuttering could result?

Conflicts of course can occur on the relationship level, and it is here that we find more testimony than for any other type of approach-avoidance conflict. It seems to us that disturbed personal relationships are alleged by parents as the cause of stuttering onset more often than any other factor. Again, however, we must be cautious in evaluating such testimony. Such disturbed relationships probably occur very frequently in the homes of nonstuttering children too at one time or another. They also probably occurred earlier in the child's home many times before the actual onset occurred. Their concurrence with the time of onset may therefore be no more than accidental. Nevertheless, the innumerable accounts reported in the literature and in our own clinical practice demand that we consider them seriously.

First let us consider some representative case reports. Solomon (1933) tells of a conflict which involved a sibling, an older brother:

> *Onset of the stuttering.* For more than a half year, since the younger child had been getting more and more active, the older one had been doing his utmost to dominate him, interfere with his free activity, play, and decisions, make him pattern after him and be obedient to his wishes. He took joy in teasing B. as much as possible. He would repeatedly call him into his room and then abruptly put him out and shut the door on him. He would offer him some toy and then purposely take it away from him. He would display his possessions to B. but at the same moment caution the latter not to touch them or would dare him to do so. He would go into B.'s room when B. was playing there alone, and begin to boss him around. He would frighten B., ridicule him, call him baby and sissy. The younger boy, although resenting the other's annoying tendencies as much as he could, also took his older brother as his hero and patterned after him to his best ability. "Ralph does this or says this and that" was his frequent remark. The parents, although not showing favoritism, had for some time done their best to control the situation diplomatically and prevent undue domination of and repression of the younger by the older son. Finally, about a month before the onset of the stuttering, the mother had independently entered upon a

persistent, vigorous and unremitting campaign to stop, once and for all, the misbehavior of the older child, so that there followed almost constant quarrelling and tense scenes, whenever the older boy was at home at the same time as his mother and younger brother, the former now annoying the latter even more than before as revenge against the mother who was pursuing him most of the time. At supper, when the whole family ate together, and conversation flew thick and fast, B. was especially excited. B. was the center about which the conflict raged.

After this had been going on for a month or more, B. began to stutter occasionally with repetition of initial consonants. This took place almost exclusively in the presence of the older boy, mainly when the latter teased him, or interfered with his play, or put him out of his room. When not excited and when his brother was not at home, there was no stuttering. One day, while at supper, with the conversation lively, B. asked for an object, seemed unable to recall its name, pointed to it and then went into a definite block. This was repeated several times during the meal, B. getting red in the face and appearing embarrassed when blocked. Thereafter occasional speech blocks as well as repetition occurred during the day when not at meals. Within a week of the onset of speech block the case was intensively studied with the unearthing of the above data (p. 40).

Many of the reported conflicts are between parents and child as one might expect at this time of growing independence and assessing limits of freedom. Usually, the mother-child relationship is cited as the basic problem, but the fathers are also occasionally implicated. Maslow and Mittelmann (1941) for example tell of a boy who was continually rejected by his father and who found it impossible to speak to him without stuttering, a behavior which further enraged the father. The boy showed no stuttering in speaking to his mother or to other children or to anyone else. Despert (1943), Baurand and Striglioni (1968), and many other authors feel that a disturbed mother-child relationship is very potent in precipitating stuttering. One illustration from Harle (1946) may suffice:

Patty was referred to the clinic at the age of three and a half by her mother who was concerned about the child's stuttering. This symptom had started three months earlier following a spanking administered by the mother after the child had run into the street and narrowly missed being run over by a car. Shortly afterward the stuttering had cleared up but a few weeks later, after a second spanking for running into the street, she again began to stutter (p. 156).

Regrettably mothers must do most of the spanking in our culture, and many children have been so punished without setting off any stuttering. In Harle's case, however, as the rest of her article makes clear, a profoundly disturbed mother-child relationship was indeed present.

Perhaps the most eloquent and convincing evidence for disturbed family relationships being productive of stuttering has been contributed by Wyatt (1969). Her series of case studies, including that of her own child, strongly supports her developmental crisis theory of stuttering. Briefly, her position is that stuttering arises when a child finds difficulty in communicating with a significant adult, especially at a critical time of developmental stress or crisis. One excerpt from her book, which is well worth reading by all students of the disorder, is as follows:

> The onset of Nana's stuttering occurred at a time when her mother, because of acute illness, had become inaccessible to the child. Nana consequently experienced a break in a previously well-established speech chain. This disruption coincided with a critical period in Nana's language development, the change from mere naming to the learning of grammatical speech patterns (p. 93).

Of course, many children experience such crises without developing stuttering, and we do not have an adequate explanation which would tell us why some do and some don't. It is at least tenable that the motor sequencing of speech breaks down when communication is overloaded by stress of any kind and certainly the kinds of interpersonal conflicts we have been describing do constitute an important stress. Glasner (1949) showed that many young stutterers demonstrated other behaviors unrelated to stuttering which appeared to be consequences of emotional overloading. He studied 70 young stutterers under five years of age and says:

> All of the children studied had exhibited some degree of emotional manifestation other than stuttering. Fifty-four per cent were characterized as "feeding problems." Twenty-seven per cent were enuretic. Twenty per cent had exaggerated sibling jealousy, nail-biting, encopresis, masturbation, emotional vomiting, and numerous others. It is realized, of course, that the "normal" child is a fiction, not a reality, but these children apparently had more than their share of behavior symptoms (p. 137).

Glasner's observations were made some time after the onset of stuttering and could therefore be effects of the disorder rather than reflections of its etiology in terms of emotional conflict, a supposition which seems supported by his comments about how the children reacted when speaking. Nevertheless, many of the children whom we studied shortly after onset showed evidence of greater emotionality than we would expect to find in the ordinary child. This clinical impression we have refused to dignify by citing any percentage figures because we had no controls. Johnson's (1959) data and that obtained by Andrews and Harris (1964) show no significant differences in the amount of emotional conflicts between the stuttering children and their normally speaking controls. Nevertheless, we have studied individual cases in which stuttering did seem triggered by such conflicts, and it is difficult for us to ignore these experiences.

COMMUNICATIVE CONFLICTS

Although it is hard to separate communicative from emotional conflicts, since no one can really tell how much emotion may have been generated in any communicative interaction, we often find accounts of stuttering beginning under such circumstances. This quotation from Duncan (1949) will illustrate:

> When I was four years old my mother took a job and put me in a day nursery. . . . We had moved to an apartment at about that time which was located on the top floor and we were required to walk up five flights of stairs to get up to it. One of my habits was to run up the five flights and upon getting into the house I would try to speak while out of breath. This is the first time I can remember "stumbling" in my speech (p. 258).

Or this from Rand, Sweeny, and Vincent (1962):

> Laughing at the child's cute accent or his imperfect pronunciation is particularly dangerous since children are unable to discriminate kinds of laughter and do not always know the laughter of indulgent amusement from that of mockery. . . . Self-consciousness or fear of ridicule as a rule produces one of two results: either it discourages effort and tends to produce silence or it provides one of the commonest causes of stuttering (p. 192).

Woolf (1957) tells of a boy who had been unduly precocious in speech and had received much praise for it. The stuttering began when the parents and an older sister gave him tongue-twisters and other difficult sentences to say. Schuell (1949) provides an example which we have found frequently in parental reports: "Sarah's trouble is that she never gets a chance to say anything. The rest of us talk all the time and she can't get anyone to listen to what she wants to say (p. 253)."

In determining the circumstances surrounding the onset of stuttering, we have our greatest trouble with those children who seem to have started to stutter very early or at the same time that they began to speak phrases and sentences. Even when the reported onset of both speech and stuttering is as late as six and seven years, the parents of these children are so concerned about the delay in acquiring any speech at all or adequate articulation or intelligibility that they tend to ignore any stuttering which may accompany the speech. Most of those we have seen at onset were children receiving therapy for delayed speech and language either in our clinic or from other clinicians. The cluttering component in these cases is often evident, and it is difficult to tell when the stuttering emerges from it. However, it is quite apparent that these children have a great burden placed upon their communicative efforts. They must acquire vocabulary, proper grammatical structures, and perfect articulation as well as some fluency. Watching such older children struggle to learn to talk, we can see how very young children may have had some of the same difficulties, but it is very difficult to pinpoint them. One of the factors contributing to the onset of stuttering in these cases seems surprisingly to be the parents' delight in the newly attained speech. Often they overpraise and overencourage the child once he begins to talk and demand more and more verbal facility. Many times we have been able to eliminate the stuttering merely by reducing these parental expectations and demands. In the same connection we occasionally find an onset of stuttering being reported as due to overcorrection of articulatory errors, but most of these turn out to have had a previous history of marked disfluency or stuttering.

By its sheer length, the previous discussion may have led the reader to believe that it is usually possible to identify one or another of the circumstances surrounding the onset of stuttering as being a significant cause. Nothing could be further from the truth. In the great majority of the children we have carefully studied soon after onset, we were unable to state with any certainty (or even with some feeling of probability) what precipitated the stuttering. In most instances there simply were no apparent conflicts, no illnesses, no opportunity to imitate, no shocks or frightening experiences. Stuttering seemed to begin under quite normal conditions of living and communicating. We cannot, of course, be sure of this. Who can look within the inner world of a child? All we can say is that usually we could not account for the onset of stuttering in terms of the conditions surrounding it. In only a fraction of our cases do we feel we identified the circumstances that might have been precipitating. If this is a confession of incompetence, then at least we are in good company—as the following quotation from Wendell Johnson (1959) would indicate:

> . . . the conditions reportedly associated with the "first" stuttering of the experimental group children were, in general, the same as those associated with the "first" nonfluencies which the control group parents said they observed in the speech of their children. The major conclusion would seem that, generally speaking, the problem of stuttering was found to develop under quite ordinary circumstances (p. 131).

COMMENTARY

At what age stuttering begins is most difficult to determine, for parents are surprisingly unable to remember early stuttering, or remember it but do not consider that it was such, especially if there has been a well period. We once examined a boy who began to stutter at 14 after a series of operations. His father assured us that he had never stuttered before. One day, however, the father mentioned that he had kept a day-by-day diary of the child from the time he was born, and when we were permitted to examine this book, we discovered that the first reference to the child's speech was to the fact that the boy stuttered, and there were forty references to stuttering within a few pages (Blanton and Blanton, 1936, p. 71).

. . . the onset of stammering has been found to be rare after the age of seven or eight years. Information concerning the exact age of onset is, however, frequently unreliable (Morley, 1957, p. 371).

At an early age, between two and three years, almost every child for a period of several weeks or months, is inclined to repeat syllables or words. These repetitions in the young child, however, are merely the result of an incongruity between the formation of thoughts and the capacity to find words to express them adequately, a discrepancy between the thought tempo and the speech tempo. . . . The difficulty [may] become a fixation and the vicious circle of imaginary difficulties and the resulting fear of the anticipated difficulty with its entire galaxy of symptoms is started. The child becomes a stutterer (Kastein, 1947, pp. 195–196).

There are two types of stuttering: (1) stuttering that dates from the first manifestations of speech and that never stopped throughout the child's language development—we may call this form "constitutional stuttering"; (2) stuttering that appeared more or less tardily, the child's language being normal during the early period (Kopp, 1943, p. 108).

The conditions surrounding the original emission and early development of nonfluencies in the speech of infants are still obscure and in need of detailed observation. It is possible that the repetitions observed in later speech may be related to the vocal behavior emitted by infants during their early speech development (babbling and chaining of syllables) (Shames and Sherrick, 1963, p. 5).

The stammer was of a special type: the first syllable, or sometimes the first two, was easily and quickly uttered; the patient then exhibited a genuine "arrest of phonation" often lasting from three to ten seconds, during which time he appeared incapable of voicing the least sound, though making strenuous expiratory efforts. After several seconds (or sooner if he deliberately abandoned his attempts at speech), a lull occurred during which another syllable or two could be uttered (Guillaume, Mazars, and Mazars, 1957, p. 60).

One of my patients, when he was five or six years old, had an unlucky fall upon his head with much loss of blood. As a result he remained speechless for a year. Then his speech returned but was made abnormal by severe stuttering which persisted until his thirty-first year (Denhardt, 1890, p. 104).

An exceptionally bright and clever boy of five showed a clonic stammer which had lasted only a few weeks. After a few introductory words, I asked the child straight away: "Tell me frankly, *why* are you stuttering?" The boy was astonished and answered: "Why do you ask me; *you* ought to know." This indeed was the answer I had expected. I then went on: "If I stammered, I should certainly know; but as it is *you* who do so, *you* ought to know." The boy became pensive and after a while said, "Really, I often don't know, but sometimes I do it just to bully mother (Stein, 1952, p. 115).

The stuttering began after the boy was chased by a mad dog (Aikins, 1925, p. 137).

The onset of stuttering in childhood may be precipitated by any experience which, in an emotionally inadequate child, generates anxiety and fear. Such traumatic experiences are fright, accident, illness, operations, forcible conversion from left- to right-handedness or a tense and worrisome environment. The element of fright as a situational traumatic experience plays the most prevalent role. The most common experiences of this type are being frightened by the dark or by lightning; receiving severe punishment at the hands of a domineering and stern parent; being frightened by a dog or some other animal; being chased or mobbed by a gang of "tough boys"; being yelled at by an angered person; being thrown into water for the first time; and being caught in the act of masturbation by a parent (Barbara, 1959, p. 954).

The stress of febrile illness may induce stammering. Stimulating drugs may disorganize the speech function. This is especially true of thyroid substance and ephedrine. Stammering continues during medication; then disappears when the therapy is terminated (Bluemel, 1957, p. 32).

Sixty-two of the mothers were able to describe the manner in which the stammer began. Thirty-five began gradually, 3 began suddenly but were apparently unrelated to any specific disturbance, and 24 were first noticed after a specific incident such as fright or illness (Jameson, 1955, p. 62).

Shock, whether physical or mental, however, can be assigned no role other than that of a precipitating cause, the factor which makes evident a symptom already under preparation. If a boy begins to stammer after a shock (whether called an emotional shock or otherwise) we can be sure that he would have stammered later if the shock had not occurred (Dunlap, 1944, p. 19).

In fact shock, mental or physical, may frequently be said to be the determining cause of a stammer, as the following instances show; Thomas Y., at the age of three, when playing with some older children was locked into a large dark stable as a joke; the key was mislaid, and it was a considerable time before the boy was released. Though he had not stammered before, he was now stammering badly. Albert X. had stammered ever since his father caught him playing with fire and shook him violently. John W. had scarlet fever at the age of four, and was taken to the hospital, where an impatient nurse threatened to "throw him out of the window" if he didn't stop crying. The stammer had definitely developed when John's mother fetched him away (Boome and Richardson, 1932, pp. 25–26).

Only four fathers and five mothers in the experimental group reported anything that could be classified as "complete blocks" and in no case, moreover, did both parents agree in making such a report. According to the parents' descriptions, there was not much effortfulness or tension or emotional distress in the speech behavior originally classified as stuttering (Johnson, 1959, p. 229).

In three of the children the onset appeared to be sudden. One child began to stammer following an attack of measles; another was reported to have stammered severely for two weeks when she hit her head against a door, cried for a long time and "looked very white." A third child was involved in an accident with her mother, and the stammer is reported to have been the sequel to this occurrence (Morley, 1957, p. 41).

Just how being bitten by a dog can produce stuttering in the same fashion in which a habit is acquired is not easy to see; but it is possible that in such a case speech may be regarded as the natural mode of defense through which the nervous shock found expression (Fletcher, 1928, p. 61).

Stuttering may be caused by an injury—such as a fall, blow, or concussion—or a violent fright. Even in cases of injury, fright may have significance for the onset of stuttering. But one may, as Coen has done, overrate the significance of these occasional causes. One must not always take the reports of parents in these cases naively. Many times they assign one of those events as a cause but upon closer examination most of them reveal that the stuttering was present at an earlier age (Treitel, 1894, p. 22).

I have talked with several people from rural North Carolina who are familiar with the local saying, "Don't tickle your child too much or he will stutter" (Orchinik, 1958, p. 38).

Of 1250 patients, 302 were stammerers due to war injuries (Arnold, 1948, p. 72).

Of 144 stutterers at Brooke and MacGuire General Hospitals, 77 were preinduction stutterers and 37 were postinduction cases (Peacher and Harris, 1946, p. 303).

Frequently the immediate effect of the shock is a period of mutism or loss of consciousness; stammering then ensues when the more profound disturbances subside. When stammering results from shock, it is preceded by mutism or unconsciousness in 28 per cent of the cases (Ssikorski, 1891, p. 232).

Cases of postencephalitis have symptoms indistinguishable from those of stuttering (Gerstmann and Schilder, 1921, p. 35).

Two men who suffered from blast concussion and were unconscious for several days began to stutter on recovering consciousness; a third was a soldier who after being wounded in the shoulder developed a variety of psychoneurotic symptoms including stuttering (Van Thal, 1950, p. 166).

Another case was that of a man who as a child had had a very mild stutter which had disappeared. Under fire in a battle he had a complete loss of speech for one day and an acute stutter for four days more (Blanton and Blanton, 1936, p. 78).

. . . parental anxiety, undue attention directed to speech, perfectionistic attitudes, reinforced by the child's own secondary gains, will tend to make a stutterer out of a youngster whose speech apparatus is still immature and who has a low threshold of stability in the language area. In such children careful attention must be paid to their general emotional adjustment. They use their language disability as a psychologic mechanism in the parent-child relationship and at times to oppose a hostile environment (De Hirsch and Langford, 1950, pp. 937–938).

. . . no specific emotional or environmental factor produces stuttering with any significant regularity. This applies to constant and even harsh correction of a child with rapid, repetitive or slovenly speech, as well as to any other type of environmental disturbance. Sibling rivalry, for instance, either in the form of rejection feelings at the birth of a younger sibling or inferiority feelings at inability to compete with an older sibling, is conspicuously present in some stuttering children. Yet 45 per cent of the cases here discussed were only children, whose emotional disturbances arose from totally different causes (Glasner, 1949, p. 136).

BIBLIOGRAPHY

Aikins, A., "Casting Out the Stuttering Devil," *Journal of Abnormal Social Psychology,* XVIII (1925), 137–52.

Ainsworth, S., "Studies in the Psychology of Stuttering XII. Empathic Breathing of Auditors While Listening to Stuttering Speech," *Journal of Speech Disorders,* IV (1939), 149–56.

Ajuriaguerra, J. R. de, Diakine, H. de Gobineau, S. Narlian, and M. Stambak, "Le Bégaiement," *Presse Mèdicale,* LXVI (1958), 953–56.

Andrews, G., "The Nature of Stuttering," *Journal Australian College of Speech Therapists,* XV (1965), 6–15.

Andrews, G., and M. Harris, *The Syndrome of Stuttering.* London: Heinemann, 1964.

Arnold, G. E., *Die traumatischen und konstitutionellen Störungen der Stimme und Sprache.* Vienna: Urban and Schwarzenberg, 1948.

Aron, M. L., "An Investigation of the Nature and Incidence of Stuttering Among a Bantu Group of School Children." Doctoral dissertation, University of Witwatersrand, South Africa, 1958.

———. "Nature and Incidence of Stuttering Among a Bantu Group of School Going Children," *Journal of Speech and Hearing Disorders*, XXVII (1962), 116–28.

Baba, K., "A Cured Case of Infantile Stuttering," *Japanese Journal Otology*, LV (1952), 51–52.

Barbara, D. A., "Stuttering." In S. Arieti (ed.), *American Handbook of Psychiatry*, Vol. I. New York: Basic Books, 1959.

Baurand, G., and L. Striglioni, "Importance du Facteur Parental dans le Symptome Bégaiement," *Journal Française O. R. L.*, XVII (1968), 209–16.

Berry, M. F., "Developmental History of Stuttering Children," *Journal of Pediatrics*, XII (1938), 209–17.

Blanton, S., and M. G. Blanton, *For Stutterers*. New York: Appleton, 1936.

Bloodstein, O., "Development of Stuttering," *Journal of Speech and Hearing Disorders*, XXV (1960), 219–37; 366–76.

Bloodstein, O., J. Alper, and P. Zisk, "Stuttering as an Outgrowth of Normal Disfluency." In D. A. Barbara (ed.) *New Directions in Stuttering: Theory and Practice*. Springfield, Ill.: Thomas, 1965.

Bluemel, C. S., *Stammering and Cognate Defects of Speech*, Vol. I. New York: Stechert, 1913.

———. *The Riddle of Stuttering*. Danville, Ill.: Interstate, 1957.

Boome, E. J., and M. A. Richardson, *The Nature and Treatment of Stuttering*. New York: Dutton, 1932.

Breur, J., and S. Freud, *Studies on Hysteria*. London: Hogarth Press, 1955.

Brodnitz, F. S., "Stuttering of Different Types in Identical Twins," *Journal of Speech and Hearing Disorders*, XVI (1951), 334–36.

Darley, F. L., "The Relationship of Parental Attitudes and Adjustments to the Development of Stuttering." In W. Johnson (ed.), *Stuttering in Children and Adults*. Minneapolis: University of Minnesota Press, 1955.

Darley, F. L., and H. Winitz, "Age of First Word: Review of Research," *Journal of Speech and Hearing Disorders*, XXVI (1961), 272–90.

Daskalov, D. D., ["Basic Principles and Methods of Prevention and Treatment of Stuttering,"] *Nevropatologii i Psikhiatrii imeni S. S. Korsakova*, LXII (1962), 1047–52.

De Hirsch, K., and W. S. Langford, "Clinical Note on Stuttering and Cluttering in Young Children," *Pediatrics*, V (1950), 934–40.

Denhardt, R., *Das Stottern: Eine Psychose*. Leipzig, 1890.

Despert, J. L., "Stuttering in Children," *Nervous Child*, II (1943), 79–207.

Duncan, M. H., "Home Adjustment of Stutterers and Non-Stutterers," *Journal of Speech Disorders*, XIV (1949), 195–98.

Dunlap, K., "Stammering: Its Nature, Etiology and Therapy," *Journal of Comparative Psychology*, XXXVII (1944), 187–202.

———. "The Stuttering Boy," *Journal of Abnormal Psychology*, XII (1917), 44–48.

Eisenson, J., "Aphasics: Observations and Tentative Conclusions," *Journal of Speech Disorders*, XII (1947), 290–92.

Fahy, T. J., M. H. Irving, and P. Millac, "Severe Head Injuries," *Lancet*, CCLXXII (1967), 475–79.

Fletcher, J. M., *The Problem of Stuttering*. New York: Longmans Green, 1928.

Fogerty, E., *Stammering*. New York: Dutton, 1930.

Freund, H., *Psychopathology and the Problems of Stuttering*. Springfield, Ill.: Thomas, 1966.

Fritzell, B., ["On Stuttering and on Studies of Stuttering in Marburg,"] *Svenska Lakartidningen*, LX (1963), 3396–3405.

Froeschels, E., "Die spracharztliche Therapie im Kriege. III. Das Stottern," *Monatsschrift für Ohrenheilkunde*, LIII (1919), 161–90.

——. "Pathology and Therapy of Stuttering," *Nervous Child*, II (1943), 148–61.

——. "The Significance of Symptomatology for the Understanding of the Essence of Stuttering," *Folia Phoniatrica*, IV (1952), 217–30.

——. "Zur Differentialdiagnose zwischen frischem, traumatischem, und veraltetem Stottern," *Med. Klin.*, XII (1916), 694–96.

——. "Zur Frage der Entstehung des tonischen Stotterns und zur Frage der Wirkungslosigkeit der elektrischen Stromes in der meisten Fallen von Stottern," *Med. Klin.*, XIII (1917), 448–50.

Fujita, K., et al., ["The Diagnostic Statistics of 80 Cases of Stutterers,"] *Japanese Journal Otorhinolaryngology*, LXVII (1964), 343. Abstract No. 297 in G. Kamiyama, *Handbook for the Study of Stuttering*. Tokyo: Kongo-Shupan, 1967.

Gertsmann, J., and P. Schilder, "Studien über Bewegungstörungen über die typen-extrapyramidaler pseudobulbar Paralyse," *Zeitschrift für Neurologie und Psychiatrie*, LXXIX (1921), 350–54.

Glaser, E. M., "Possible Relationship Between Stuttering and Endocrine Malfunctioning," *Journal of Speech Disorders*, I (1936), 81–89.

Glasner, P. J., "Personality Characteristics and Emotional Problems in Stutterers under the Age of Five," *Journal of Speech and Hearing Disorders*, XIV (1949), 135–38.

Goda, S., "Stuttering Manifestations Following Spinal Meningitis," *Journal of Speech and Hearing Disorders*, XXVI (1961), 392–93.

Gondaira, T., "A Case Study of a Boy with Stuttering and Physical Malformation," *Japanese Journal of Child Psychology*, I (1960), 340–50.

Graf, O. I., "Incidence of Stuttering Among Twins." In W. Johnson (ed.), *Stuttering in Children and Adults*. Minneapolis: University of Minnesota Press, 1955.

Greene, J. S., "Your Child's Speech," *Hygeia*, II (1924), 11–12.

Guillaume, J., G. Mazars, and Y. Mazars, ["Epileptic Mediation in Certain Types of Stammering,"] *Revue Neurologique*, XCVI (1957), 59–62.

Gutzmann, H., "Erbbiologische, soziologische und organische Faktoren die Sprachstörungen begunstigen," *Archive für Stimmheilkunde*, III (1939), 133–36.

Harle, M., "Dynamic Interpretation and Treatment of Acute Stuttering in a Young Child," *American Journal of Orthopsychiatry*, XV (1946), 156–62.

Hastings, I., "A Case of Stammer and Tongue Thrusting," in *Speech Pathology, Diagnosis, Theory and Practice*. Edinburgh: Livingstone, 1966.

Hirschberg, J., "Stuttering," *Orvosi. Hetilap* CVI (1965), 780–84.

Hoepfner, T., "Stottern als assoziative Aphasie," *Zeitschrift für Pathopsychologie*, I (1911–1912), 448–552.

Irwin, J., and J. K. Duffy, *Speech and Hearing Hurdles*. Columbus, Ohio: School and College Service, 1955.

Jameson, A. M., "Stammering in Children—Some Factors in Prognosis," *Speech* (London), XIX (1955), 60–67.

Johnson, W., "A Study of the Onset and Development of Stuttering." In W. Johnson (ed.), *Stuttering in Children and Adults*. Minneapolis: University of Minnesota Press, 1955.

―――. *The Onset of Stuttering*. Minneapolis: University of Minnesota Press, 1959.

Kamiyama, A., *Handbook for the Study of Stuttering*. Tokyo: Kongo-Shupan, 1967.

Kanner, L., *Child Psychiatry*. Springfield, Ill.: Thomas, 1942.

Kastein, S., "The Chewing Method of Treating Stuttering," *Journal of Speech Disorders*, XII (1947), 195–98.

Katsovskaia, I. I. K., ["The Problem of Children's Stuttering,"] *Deafness, Speech and Hearing Abstracts*, II (1962), 296.

Kingdon-Ward, W., *Stammering*. London: Hamilton, 1941.

Klinger, H., "The Onset of Stuttering in Adults: A Presentation of Three Cases," *Asha*, V (1963), 782 (Abstract).

―――. personal communication, 1966.

Kopp, H., "The Relationship of Stuttering to Motor Disturbance," *Nervous Child*, II (1942–1943), 107–16.

Levina, R. Y., "Study and Treatment of Stammering among Children," *Journal of Learning Disabilities*, I (1968), 24–30.

Luchsinger, R., and G. E. Arnold, *Voice–Speech–Language*. Belmont, Cal.: Wadsworth, 1965.

Makuen, G. H., "A Study of 1000 Cases of Stammering with Special Reference to the Etiology and Treatment," *Therapeutic Gazette*, XXXVIII (1914), 385–90.

Martyn, M. M., and J. Sheehan, "Onset of Stuttering and Recovery," *Behavior Research and Therapy*, VI (1968), 295–307.

Maslow, A. H., and B. Mittelmann, *Principles of Abnormal Psychology: The Dynamics of Psychic Illness*. New York: Harper, 1941.

McCallien, C., "Problems of Speech Defect in the Accra District," *Speech* (London), XX (1956), 15–18.

McAllister, A. H., *Clinical Studies in Speech Therapy*. London: University London Press, 1937.

―――. "The Problem of Stammering," *Speech Pathology and Therapy*, (London), I (1958), 3–8.

McDearmon, J. R., "Primary Stuttering at the Onset of Stuttering: A Re-examination of the Data," *Journal of Speech and Hearing Research*, XI (1968), 631–37.

Mochizuski, S., personal communication, 1962.

Morley, M. E., *Development and Disorders of Speech in Childhood*. Edinburgh: Livingstone, 1957.

Mygind, H., "Über die Ursachen des Stotterns," *Archive für Laryngologie und Rhinologie*, VIII (1898), 294–307.

Nadoleczny, M., (1938), quoted in R. Luchsinger, and G. E. Arnold, *Voice–Speech–Language*. Belmont, Cal.: Wadsworth, 1965.

Nelson, S., N. Hunter, and M. Walter, "Stuttering in Twin Types," *Journal of Speech Disorders*, X (1945), 335–43.

Orchinik, C. W., "On Tickling and Stuttering." *Psychoanalysis and Psychoanalytic Review*, XLIV (1958), 25–29.

Otsuki, H., ["Study on Stuttering: Statistical Observations"], *Otorhinolaryngology Clinic*, V (1958), 1150–51.

Peacher, W. C., and W. E. Harris, "Speech Disorders in World War II: Stuttering," *Journal of Speech Disorders*, XI (1946), 303–8.

Rand, W., M. E. Sweeny, and E. L. Vincent, *Growth and Development of the Young Child,* 3rd Ed., Philadelphia: Sanders, 1962.

Razdol'skii, V. A., ["State of Speech of Stammerers When Alone,"] *Zhurnal Nevropatologii i Psikhiatrii imeni S. S. Korsakova,* LXV (1965), 1717–20.

Schachter, M., "Aphémie Suivie de Bégaiement d'Origine Psychodramatique chez une Fillette de Quatre Ans," *Acta Paedopsychiatrica,* XXXIV (1967), 1–32.

Schmeer, G., "Zur Genese des Stotterns," *Praxis Kinderpsychologie,* XV (1966), 45–50.

Schuell, H., "Working with Parents of Stuttering Children," *Journal of Speech Disorders,* XIV (1949), 251–54.

Scripture, E. W., *Stuttering and Lisping.* New York: Macmillan, 1912.

Seeman, M., *Sprachstörungen bei Kindern.* Marhold: Halle, 1959.

Shames, G., and C. Sherrick, "A Discussion of Nonfluency and Stuttering as Operant Behavior," *Journal of Speech and Hearing Disorders,* XXVIII (1963), 3–18.

Sheehan, J., "Conflict Theory of Stuttering." In J. Eisenson (ed.), *Stuttering: A Symposium.* New York: Harper, 1958.

Shiraiwa, T., "Study of the Cause of Stuttering," (1958) Abstract No. 185. In G. Kamiyama, *Handbook for the Study of Stuttering.* Tokyo: Kongo-Shupan, 1967.

Smith, L. G., "Speech Defect Resulting from Ether Shock," *Pedagogical Seminary,* XXVII (1921), 308–12.

Solomon, M., "Incipient Stuttering in a Preschool Child Aged Two and One Half Years," *Proceedings American Speech Correction Association,* III (1933), 38–44.

Soufi, A., "One Month Stutterer," *Journal of Speech and Hearing Disorders,* XXV (1960), 411.

Ssikorski, I. A., *Über das Stottern.* Berlin: Hirschwald, 1891.

Stein, L., *Speech and Voice.* London: Methuen, 1942.

Takagi, S., et. al., ["The Characteristic of Young Stutterers and Their Follow Up Study"], Abstract No. 272. In G. Kamiyama, *Handbook for the Study of Stuttering.* Japan: Kongo-Shupan, 1962.

Taylor, G. L., "An Observational Study of the Nature of Stuttering at Its Onset." Master's thesis, State University of Iowa, 1937.

Toyoda, B., ["Stuttering of Infants"], *Voice and Language Medicine,* VI (1965), 14–15, Abstract No. 328. In G. Kamiyama, *Handbook for the Study of Stuttering.* Tokyo: Kongo-Shupan, 1967.

Treitel, L., "Störungen der Lautfolge: Stottern," (1894). Excerpts from this work are found in M. V. Jones, "Leonard Treitel on Stuttering," *Journal of Speech and Hearing Disorders,* XIII (1948), 19–22.

Van Riper, C., "The Influence of Empathic Response on Frequency of Stuttering," *Psychological Monographs,* XLIX (1937), 244–46.

Van Thal, J., "The Relationship Between War Conditions and Defects of Voice and Speech," *Folia Phoniatrica,* II (1950), 165–67.

Vlasova, N. A., ["Prevention and Treatment of Children's Stuttering in U.S.S.R."], *Ceskoslovenska Otolaryngologie,* XI (1962), 30–32.

————. ["Late Follow-up Analysis of Some Cases of Recurrent Stuttering,"] *Zhurnal Neuropatologii i Psikiatrii imeni S. S. Korsakova,* LXV (1965), 750–51.

Wallen, V., "Primary Stuttering in a Twenty-Eight-Year-Old Adult," *Journal of Speech and Hearing Disorders,* XXVI (1961), 394.

West, R., "The Pathology of Stuttering," *Nervous Child,* II (1942), 96–106.

West, R., S. Nelson, and M. Berry, "The Heredity of Stuttering," *Quarterly Journal Speech*, XXV (1939), 23–30.

Woolf, M., "Zur Frage der Genese und Entwicklung des Stotterns," *Psychotherapie*, II (1957), 235–41.

Wyatt, G. L., *Language Learning and Communication Disorders in Children*. New York: Free Press, 1969.

five

THE DEVELOPMENT OF
STUTTERING

Most observers agree that stuttering behaviors often change, growing more abnormal with the passage of time. Although a large number of beginning stutterers (perhaps as high as 80 per cent) show the disorder only for a short time and then regain or acquire normal fluency, this chapter is mainly concerned with those who continue to stutter. When it persists, stuttering rarely continues to present the same picture shown at onset, new behaviors replacing or joining the original ones. In the confirmed stutterer there is an incredible variety of contorted, tense struggling and morbid emotional reactions bearing little resemblance to the earlier stuttering. These bizarre new behaviors seem meaningless unless considered in the light of their developmental history. Much of the mystery and confusion that befogs our understanding of stuttering results from our failure to realize how it grows. Stuttering theories often conflict with one another because they have been based on the nature of the disorder after it has already made its morbid growth. Because stuttering develops differently in different people, our research, which has been done mostly with the adult population, has often added to the confusion.

Several of the older writers have commented on the fact that stuttering changes its appearance with the years. The anonymous author of *The Irrationale of Speech,* quoted by Hunt (1861) says:

. . . the stammer may take very different forms from year to year; and the boy who began to stammer with the lip may go on to stammer with the tongue, then with the jaw, and last and worst of all, with the breath; and in after life try to rid himself of one abuse by trying in alternation all the other three (p. 187).

Potter (1882) is more explicit. He writes:

At first there is noticed a halt on some syllable beginning with an explosive consonant, followed by anxiety and a condition of expectancy on the part of the person affected for the next difficult syllable, producing a mental search for a synonym of easier pronunciation, resulting in a halting, irregular hesitation in speech, an outré manner of expressing the ideas. Soon another difficult syllable is encountered, for which a synonym cannot be found, the embarrassment of the sufferer is increased, spasms of the various organs of articulation occur more frequently;—now of the lips, affecting the labial sounds; then of the tongue, affecting the dental consonants; the articulating organs seeming as if temporarily glued together in some cases, in others as though alternately attracted to and repelled from each other. As embarrassment increases, the spasms become more violent, until in severe cases a general spasmodic condition of the muscles of articulation, phonation, and respiration ensues, with even tetanic rigidity of some groups; the patient's voice becomes lost, he gasps for breath with a nearly empty lung, and silence alone brings temporary relief to the general distress of body and mind (p. 81).

In his first book, *Stammering and Cognate Defects of Speech,* Bluemel (1913) recognized these changes. He differentiated between "pure stammering" and "secondary or physical stammering," the latter being characterized by learned fears and learned motor behaviors. In later works (1932; 1935; 1940) he developed further his concept of stuttering as a learned habit based on conditioned inhibition and his terms "primary" and "secondary" stuttering are still used by many to indicate the changing nature of the disorder. In Europe, Hoepfner (1912) sketched the course of stuttering development, but the most detailed exposition of how the disorder grows was provided by Emil Froeschels (1964). He showed, in a series of publications, that stuttering follows a fairly consistent course of development. Here, in outline form, is the first part of Froeschels' sequence:

STEPS IN THE DEVELOPMENT OF STUTTERING
(*After Froeschels*)

I. Syllable and word repetition; normal tempo; no tension. Child's reaction: stops and tries again. II. Syllable and word repetition; normal tempo; no tension. Reaction: child continues until word is uttered. III.

Syllable and word repetition; normal tempo; some tension. Child still stops and begins again. IV. Syllable and word repetition; faster tempo than normal; tension. Reaction: child stops and begins again. V. Syllable and word repetition; faster tempo than normal; increased tension. Child continues until word is uttered. VI. Syllable and word repetition; slower than normal tempo; marked tension. Child now may stop and try again consciously and deliberately or may hurriedly continue until word is uttered. VII. Prolongation of a sound or articulatory posture; slower tempo than normal; marked tension. Child will stop and try again or struggle until word is emitted.

In Froeschels' (1955) own words:

> If the tonic (pressure) component is dominant, abnormal breathing will result, for the openings through which the breath should escape are temporarily blocked. In the state of primary clonus (repetition) no breathing difficulty is present. Another consequence of the tonic component is accompanying movements, such as grimaces, clenched fists, etc. At later stages, and in exceptional cases at an early stage, all sorts of accompanying movements develop, such as stamping of the foot, looking to one side or up and down, as well as the so-called embolophrasias. Embolophrasias are sounds, sound combinations, or words used as starters in moments of speech difficulties (p. 113).

Froeschels says that the overt features of stuttering in this advanced stage are so variable that in 16,000 cases he never found two alike. He also goes on to describe a terminal phase which he calls "concealed stuttering" wherein the stutterer develops various tricks and strategies for hiding his speech difficulty. Concealed stuttering "is almost universal in the development of stuttering in Europe, but relatively rare in the United States" (Froeschels, 1942, p. 86). He believes that all genuine stuttering tends to follow this sequential pattern and, when it does not, he attributes the exceptions to imitation or hysteria or to faulty therapy.

Bloodstein (1960) tried to delineate the developmental course of stuttering. In a series of three articles he summarized his clinical observations of 418 stutterers, aged 2-16 years. His findings were based solely on the first interview of the parent and the first examination of the child. In interpreting his result and conclusions, we must bear in mind that Bloodstein's study was not longitudinal. It does not tell us anything about how the stuttering behaviors changed in an individual child. Instead it was cross-sectional, based on groups at different age levels without regard to the length of time the individuals had had the disorder. Thus, the six-year-old group might include some who had just begun to stutter and some who had been stuttering for several years. At best this is a crude way of gathering developmental data, and the results must be interpreted very cautiously, as the author himself admits. It is surprising, then, that gross developmental trends were indeed revealed. Table 1 shows the data from Blood-stein's study (1960, p. 220).

TABLE 1. PERCENTAGE OF SUBJECTS EXHIBITING EACH OF VARIOUS FEATURES OF STUTTERING BEHAVIOR AT AGE LEVELS FROM 2 TO 16. NUMBERS IN PARENTHESES INDICATE THE NUMBER OF SUBJECTS ON WHICH THE PERCENTAGE WAS BASED WHERE THIS DIFFERS FROM THE TOTAL NUMBER (N) IN THE AGE GROUP.

	Age Level						
	2–3	*4–5*	*6–7*	*8–9*	*10–11*	*12–13*	*14–15–16*
	N-30	*N-74*	*N-79*	*N-60*	*N-79*	*N-47*	*N-49*
	%	%	%	%	%	%	%
Slow, easy repetitions ...	30	34	28	37	30	9	8
Easy repetition or prolongation as sole symptoms of stuttering	43	32	18	18	11	4	4
Hard contacts	40	32	44	45	53	51	53
Associated symptoms	33	39	57	58	57	64	65
Fluent periods	47	45	27	10	10	9	00
Difficult situations			27 (15)	67 (27)	71 (56)	75 (40)	72 (39)
Difficult words or sounds				82 (17)	62 (45)	72 (32)	73 (33)
Anticipation				38 (26)	45 (51)	62 (37)	71 (41)
Word substitution				48 (23)	65 (48)	66 (32)	83 (36)
Avoidance of speech	00	5	11	17	28	40	45

Bloodstein's findings are difficult to interpret. If we assume that most of his subjects had begun to stutter at two to five years of age (which is what our review of the onset research seems to indicate), then certainly gross changes in stuttering behaviors have occurred. The stuttering patterns change from simple to complex and grow in severity in each consecutive age group. Making the same assumption, it appears that hard contacts and struggle and avoidance reactions gradually increase as children continue to stutter, and that their fluent periods diminish. (Bloodstein's anticipation data is especially suspect since his criterion for anticipation was the consistency effect, and later research has shown that the same consistency of hesitations and nonfluencies occurs in normal speakers who certainly are not afraid of stuttering.) What Bloodstein really found is that stuttering does not remain static, that it changes with time. On the basis of these data, Bloodstein also discerns four phases of stuttering development, and he gives profiles of each. In illustrating the profile of a Phase III stutterer Bloodstein cites the following case:

P.M., aged 10–3, exhibits severe hard contacts, preformations, long pauses, frowning, and sharp exhalations. He has more difficulty at school than in any other situation. He reports some anticipations and difficult words and sounds, but no substitutions. He does not avoid speaking, frequently volunteers to recite in class and is a "talker" by reputation (p. 374).

STAGES OF STUTTERING

In the foregoing discussion we have indicated that there may be something wrong with the whole concept of stages of stuttering. Are there really any Phase I, II, III, or IV stutterers? Or for that matter, what validity is there in Bluemel's primary and secondary kinds of stuttering or in Van Riper's (1963) primary, transitional, and secondary stages, or any of the other developmental categories which have been spread over so many pages of print? We must confess that we have never been very comfortable with the criteria for our own developmental stages. Too many of our cases resisted placement in any of them. In preparing this book, the miserable task of going through 30 years of case folders and a mountain of clinical notes to see what developmental data we could uncover has at least opened our eyes to our error. Seduced by Bluemel's concepts of primary and secondary stuttering, which were attractive because they described the marked differences between beginning and advanced stutterers, we first accepted these two kinds of stuttering, then added a third, called transitional stuttering, to accomodate those who fit neither category. Finally, in 1963, we added a fourth stage between primary and transitional. It was sheer folly. Carried to the extreme, we could have had an infinite number of minimally differentiated categories. In clinical practice, we had often found the distinctions difficult to use. Some children never showed any primary stuttering; some never became secondary. Also, a child could be a secondary stutterer one day, a transitional stutterer the next, and within a week be a primary stutterer or even a normal speaker. Or he could run the gamut back and forth within a single day. Bloodstein's four developmental phases of stuttering (based on averaging behaviors in terms of chronological age), suffer from the same limitations.

The inadequacy of all this sectioning and categorizing now seems quite clear, and when adequate longitudinal data are available the concept of phases or stages will probably be completely discarded. This does not mean that the beginning stutterer should be treated in the same way we would treat him after he has learned to struggle or avoid. It means that our treatment should fit his needs as shown by his current behaviors, including their history; it should not be a prescribed treatment appropriate only to the child's classification in a developmental category. Human beings have a way of slipping through the meshes of all categories. We are tired of wielding empty nets.

THE NEED FOR LONGITUDINAL STUDIES

Andrews and Harris (1964) and Morley (1957) failed to investigate in any systematic way the changes in stuttering that occur as the child grows older. Their observations indicate, however, that the disorder becomes more severe with time. We urgently need longitudinal research. It is difficult research to do, and the money and time needed seem almost prohibitive. It will require a team of dedicated investigators working for years to assemble the information.

The next sections of this chapter contain our observations of individual cases in a longitudinal way. These findings do not fulfill the requirements of objective research. We could not see all of the subjects routinely at specified intervals. The number of contacts, though they were many, varied from stutterer to stutterer. At times our clinical notes were too sketchy. The early observations were made before tapes were available, and even afterward we found that recordings have a astonishing ability to disappear from the files. How much contamination was produced by therapy we do not know, but certainly it had some influence. We tried to help all the subjects. We counselled their parents, and we worked directly or indirectly with all of them. The 44 stutterers whom we were able to follow from onset to adolescence or adulthood thus represent clinical failures, and it is on this small population that the conclusions are mainly based. It is our impression, however, that many other stutterers, for whom we succeeded in arresting the development of the disorder, or who did so themselves, showed similar developmental patterns. Maybe we have again deluded ourselves in thinking that we have found some common paths down which children stumble to lose themselves in the dark swamp of stuttering. In essence, we think the course of stuttering is often oscillatory, and there are at least four tracks the stutterers may follow in development.

THE OSCILLATORY COURSE
OF DEVELOPMENT

One of the weaknesses in the concept of progressive stages of development is that it implies that the course of the disorder is linear, that it moves consistently forward toward greater severity and morbidity. Many authors have noted the prevalence of remissions in young stutterers. For a week or months or even longer the stuttering disappears, only to return again at a later time. An examination of our records, not only of the 44 stutterers we were able to follow from onset to maturity, but also of several hundred others with whom we had contact for only three or four years, demonstrated to our satisfaction that the development of stuttering is usually oscillatory. Only when it reached its final form did we find any stability of behavior.

In most instances, the younger the stutterer, the more he tended to oscillate from one level of severity to another. Periods characterized by many syllabic repetitions on many words alternated with other periods as long as a week or month when only two or three such repetitions occured per day. Later in development, when frustration reactions with facial contortions and struggle appeared, they would persist for weeks and then give way to the earlier, simpler stuttering pattern. (Developmentally the severity of stuttering seems to see-saw back and forth.) Sometimes on the backswing, the stutterer may become completely fluent for days. We have watched children develop situation fears and avoidances, then lose them in succeeding weeks. Vivid awareness of their speech difficulties will be followed by long periods when no sign of awareness can be detected.

These swings are very important to the diagnostician. He must make sure that what he is observing in the examination situation is a representative sample for the period. He must also try to get an idea of the *range* of stuttering behaviors. We always try to assess not only the average or most characteristic kinds of behavior shown by the child, but also (through parental interview or repeated examinations) the extremes of greatest and least severity, its furthest and nearest points on the developmental schedule. We want to know, for example, if the child has any extended periods when the stuttering appears only as unforced, normally timed syllabic repetitions of if he is ever fluent for sustained periods.

It has been our clinical observation that these extreme points on the range of stuttering behaviors can provide very important information in terms of both diagnosis and prognosis, as will become evident in the following sections.

DIFFERENT TRACKS OF DEVELOPMENT

An examination of 300 case folders of stutterers we first saw in childhood (including the 44 on whom we had sufficient longitudinal observations) revealed certain common patterns of progressive change. Despite the oscillation, the general course of the disorder in those who continued to stutter for some years showed a series of features that seemed to follow each other in a definite sequence. In this search we were not looking for types of stutterers or etiological factors—we were trying to find out how stuttering changed with the passage of time. At first, we found the same sequence occurring so often we thought there was only one track, but as we hunted for exceptions it became fairly clear that there were instead several tracks. All but 3 of our 44 cases and all but 69 of the 300 fell into four major courses of development. Not all of the individuals in any one track followed its sequence exactly in every detail, and of course the sample may not be representative. So, it is only our opinion that in general the disorder developed with fair consistency according to one of four major sequential patterns. Despite initial doubt and continued skepticism we became convinced that the course of stuttering was not after all a random wandering in the wasteland. Selah!

TRACK I

Track I was by far the most common. Of the 44 stutterers in our best sample, 21 showed this developmental sequence and 141 of the other children followed it at least part of the way. It went like this. Stuttering first appeared, after a period of normally fluent speech, between 30 and 50 months, though actual age of onset was difficult to establish since it began gradually. Several remissions occurred for periods of a week or longer within the first two years after onset. In fact, Track One stutterers showed the greatest amount of oscillation in development. Their swings are more frequent and more extensive than those of the children on the other tracks. They are less consistent, sometimes showing a behavior characteristic of the most advanced forms of stuttering, then in a day or two returning to the simplest of syllabic repetitions or even quite normal speech. Track One stutterers have more complete remissions and for longer periods of time than those of the other groups. Also most of the stutterers who spontaneously recover or who profit most swiftly from therapy have shown this course of development.

The behaviors of Track I stutterers consisted of frequent syllabic repetitions (without the schwa), uttered at the same tempo as the normally spoken syllables. They were multiple repetitions, averaging about three per word and rarely exceeding five per word. They were effortless, and so far as we could tell the child showed no signs of awareness. They occurred most frequently on the first word spoken after a pause or on the most meaningful word of the sentence. The single-syllabled words were repeated as wholes but polysyllabic words were not. Often the repetitions occurred in volleys or clusters which in turn were followed by considerable normal fluency. The stutterings constituted only a small but very noticeable fraction of the total speech output. When the children were fluent, they were very fluent. Luper and Mulder (1964) give their version of these features as follows:

> Incipient stuttering fluctuates considerably. Periods of days, weeks, and months may go by without the appearance of an unusual amount of stuttering. Sometimes the stuttering is reported to disappear completely before reappearing. More rarely, instances of periods of a year or more of fluency

may be reported. Gradually (and the periods of time necessary for these changes to occur varies considerably) the periods of fluency become shorter and shorter and the presence of stuttering is noted more than its absence. It is noteworthy that at the onset of stuttering the disorder is essentially episodic—shifting to essentially chronic and finally to chronic insofar as observable periods of fluency are concerned (p. 21).

Next the tempo changes as the disorder develops. The repetitive syllables become irregular and are often spoken more rapidly than other fluent syllables. An occasional schwa is heard. The number of repetitions per syllable increases, first in terms of their range and then in terms of their average. The percentage, or number of stutterings per 100 or 1000 words, increases. To the listener they seem compulsive. Freund (1966) expresses the latter impression well:

> The repetitions here are not used for the purpose of filling in a gap but for the purpose of overcoming a hindrance which, as it were, towers within the syllable itself, between its articulatory closure phase and phonation. These forms of intrasyllabic, struggling repetitions become quickly compulsive, fixed and conditioned (p. 72).*

Further development is marked by an occasional prolongation of a voiced continuant sound. At first they appear largely at the conclusion of the repetitions and upon the first sound of the word that is then spoken, but later they may be heard earlier in the stream of repetitions. Following this, some children demonstrate prolongations of the vowels within the syllables. We hate to see any of this development, and we regard these vowel prolongations as a definite danger signal. We have seen too many children react to them with awareness and frustration which often leads them to produce a rise in pitch resembling a fire siren on the prolonged vowel.

In most of these children, as the disorder grows, the prolongations move forward, from the final repeated syllable of a series to the initial syllable. Very soon thereafter prolongations tend to become increasingly predominant behaviors (though syllabic repetitions may occur sporadically throughout life in a confirmed stutterer.) Tension and forcings then make their appearance, first on the voiced and then on the silent prolongations of an articulatory posture during these prolongations, and we find the stuttering tremor showing itself for the first time. It is in this phase that many of the children begin to show concern. The frustrating awareness manifests itself initially as surprise, almost shock. The child may stop talking abruptly, look at his listener helplessly or angrily or even say, "I can't talk." They may cry or strike out at their listener.

As we have also discovered, Bloodstein (1960) found that these behaviors can occur very early in life:

* From *Psychopathology and the Problems of Stuttering*, by Henry Freund. Charles C Thomas, Publisher, Springfield, Ill. Copyright © 1966 by Henry Freund. Reprinted by permission of the author.

Of the nine two-year-old subjects, four were said to have reacted to repetitions or other types of blockage by exclaiming, "I can't talk," by crying, or by looking down and blushing. In one case, seen three weeks after reported onset, the child was said to have become "so annoyed" by his repetitions that he hit himself on the mouth and stopped talking for three days (p. 233).

Despite these comments and reactions, this awareness seldom lasts very long. In a few days the disorder has again reversed its course and no signs of frustration can be detected. The stuttering is still very intermittent with remarkably long periods of completely fluent speech, but when the volleys occur they last longer. One can also witness the growth of these prolongations in time. At first very short, their durations increase depending upon the communicative stress and other factors to be described later.

Next, surges of tension appear and with them signs of obvious struggle as the child seeks to interrupt his closures and fixations. Facial contortions, jaw jerks, co-movements of the limbs are seen in various combinations, much of the behavior almost appearing random and unstereotyped. The tension, first located in the lips or jaws, overflows to adjacent structures. The child is now highly aware of his difficulty, greatly frustrated by it, and doing his utmost to interrupt it so that he can continue to communicate. Stein (1942) puts it this way:

> His deliberate efforts have brought the stammerer "out of the frying pan into the fire." He is now quite convinced that speaking is hard work, and is puzzled about how other people are able to master it. He now follows the rule which we all follow when our motor attempts are not successful: we think we have not made enough effort (p. 121).

As the child makes an effort to overcome what he senses as the obstacles in his speaking, he shows various kinds of struggle behavior. Some of them are signals to himself, devices to aid in timing the next attempt or to help force out the word. But they are often simply the result of spreading tension. When these behaviors appear, the parents react with surprise and horror, reactions which the child notices soon enough, and which in turn create even greater struggling or lead, as we shall see, to anticipation, expectancy, and fear. Remember the oscillatory course of the disorder. We have seen extreme behaviors of this sort disappear a few days later so that the child is stuttering effortlessly again. We recognize their danger of course. As the swings move further forward, the chances are less that the back swings will return within the range of normal fluency. But our concern deepens when we see signs of fear.

In quicksand, the more you struggle the deeper you sink, and the child soon finds himself in a quagmire of fear. Fear is the anticipation of unpleasantness, and once the child has repeatedly experienced the frustrations of interrupted communication, he comes to expect it when certain stimuli that were associated with the experience earlier now present themselves again. Most of the young stutterers we have studied show their first fears on words rather than situations—but this may be due to our active intervention to keep the child's associates from penalizing him for the stuttering. In all the children who showed situation fears before word fears, the child's associates, parents or siblings, had somehow called the stuttering to his attention, had shown their anxiety and concern, or had mocked or punished him. Where we were able to prevent this, the word fears came first.

What are these fears and what are their nuclei? It is always difficult to determine. In their play-talk commentary, one of the older children told us of invisible little green men who squirted glue in his mouth; another said that something squeezed in his tongue tight when he wasn't looking; still others, simply that some words were just too hard to say and that they could see them coming. One little girl would whisper something with her mouth onto a piece of paper and then erase it hard. She said it was a "trouble word." One boy insisted that some words wanted to go down when they should come up, and he often squatted when struggling with his stuttering. Most of the children cannot tell you. The clinician, however, will not find it difficult to identify the signs of fear. There are pauses before the utterance or before the word. The rate of speech suddenly slows, becomes hesitant. Words are tackled gingerly, almost pre-tasted for danger. The breathing is altered with jerky over-inhalations, it is held before vocalization, or it becomes very shallow. The voice loses its flexibility of intonation. And you can see the fear on the child's face and in the sudden immobility of his body posture.

Once fear arises, avoidance follows. Synonyms are used and stallers, rituals of timing, or disguise behaviors. The loci of stuttering become more consistent. We have watched the spread of these fears in many children. The earliest gradient of generalization seems to be phonemic rather than semantic. The fear of /p/ words spreads to /b/ words, then to the other bilabials, then to labiodentals. Even advanced stutterers are often able to use synonyms with some success, which probably reflects this same observation. Other verbal features are scanned for danger signals: the length of the word, its familiarity, its position, its propositionality. All or any of these can become cues.

Situation fears show a similar pattern of growth by generalization. When a given listener, whether it be parent or playmate, reacts to the child's stutterings punishingly, other listeners become able to generate fear depending on how much they resemble the punisher. We have watched fear spread from its origin in reaction to the impatient mother of a favorite playmate to other older women, and then to the child's own mother. We have seen the stuttering child who formerly played freely with all the children in the block gradually restrict his play space and partners until finally he would play only with a little sister in his own yard. The first situational fears tend to be fears of people rather than of the conditions of communiction. Later we find them precipitated by cues associated with communicative experiences such as talking at the dinner table, answering questions, making requests. One child showed his first situational fear in the family car after having been shouted at by his father for an especially severe moment of stuttering. Afterward, he was not afraid of speaking to his father in any situation other than while being transported, even when his mother did the driving. We have been unable to discern any common patterns in the growth of these sound, word, and situation fears except that the process of stimulus generatization makes itself evident, and that avoidance increases their intensity. The fears grow and the fears spread, but each child develops his own unique constellation depending on the specific circumstances under which he has experienced communicative frustration or punishment.

In the final phases of the disorder's development, which we shall describe with more detail in a succeeding chapter, a series of important changes occur. Patterns of stuttering behavior, both overt and covert, become stabilized and stereotyped. The stuttering child acquires the self-concept and role of a "stutterer" with all the evil these entail. Personality changes may occur; defenses are set up. The disorder becomes an integral part of his existence.

TRACK II

The analysis of our records also revealed another fairly common developmental route. Of the 44 stutterers whom we were able to study until they reached maturity, 11 showed Track II development as did 31 others on whom we have less complete records. One of the marked differences between these children and those of Track I is that the fluency disruptions began much earlier in speech development. Most, though not all, of these children also showed retarded speech development and did not use phrases or sentences until they were from three to six years of age. What is distinctive is that the disorder appeared when they began to talk consecutively. In those whom we observed, and from the parental reports of those we did not, it seems clear that these children had no previous history of sustained normal fluency. The onset of stuttering came with the onset of connected speech. We are pretty sure of this since six of the 11 persons mentioned above began to stutter (or clutter?) while they were receiving help for delayed speech and language in our own clinic, and we have had more than a few reports from other speech therapists who saw "stuttering" develop before their eyes in the children they were trying to teach to talk.

These then are the children who have been able to comprehend the long involved sentences of others for some time before they themselves could communicate verbally. For some time, even years, they have used gestures, a few single words, or jargon to make their wants known. As they break free from their shackles, their urge to communicate creates an exorbitant demand on their small store of available expressive symbols. The speech is very unorganized. Arranging, sorting, sequencing according to dimly perceived, standard syntactical patterns, these children need more than the usual amount of time and do not usually get it. They need simple models and much patience from their listeners and when these are not forthcoming, breaks in fluency appear. We find some of the same picture in aphasics as they began to regain their speech.

The literature has many accounts of this sort of onset. In Hungary, Hirschberg (1965) writes:

> In our own series of patients, we found in 48 cases, i.e., in nearly one third of all the patients examined, a delayed speech development. This agrees with the figures reported by Borel-Maisonny, who found late development of speech in 58 per cent of her stutterers (p. 783).

Andrews and Harris (1964) noted that the children who were severely delayed in speech at the age of three and four began to stutter as they became intelligible. Dostalova and Dosuzkov (1965) classified them as belonging to a group they called "Balbuties Tarda" and stated that they had the poorest prognosis. De Parrel (1965) echoes a long French tradition of ascribing stuttering onset to the delayed beginning of true speech. Some children do seem to start stuttering in this way.

The early behaviors in Track II are not exactly the same as those of Track I. There are the same syllabic repetitions, but from the beginning they are hurried and irregular, and whole words of one syllable constitute the greater proportion of these early repetitions. Later on this changes. There are more silent gaps, more hesitations, than in Track I. More stumbling occurs, more abortive beginnings, more revisions, more interjections. Before they speak these children often hold their breath, then blurt. They seem to be searching for words. There are more back-ups, more retrials, more changes in direction. Articulation errors are prevalent. This is the unorganized speech described so clearly by Bluemel (1957); it is the early cluttering-like speech delineated by Weiss (1964).

The children on this track seem relatively free from frustration. Their tolerance of fluency breaks seems to be very great, perhaps because so many of them have never known what it feels like to talk without stuttering. Moreover, awareness, fear, struggle, and avoidance develop much more slowly than in Track I. Track II children do not seem to listen to themselves. It is conceivable that this auditory imperceptiveness to their own speech was one of the factors which produced the original delay. They may have skipped the stage of self-listening which most children go through before they learn to monitor their utterance primarily by proprioception. Perhaps their inattention to their own fluency breaks results from the fact that they often have many other problems too, problems of coordination, musicality, articulation, language, and general organization. We have followed some of these children from onset to adulthood and marvelled to see how they filter out the junk in their speech.

This track also differs from Track I in that these children rarely show prolongations and fixations. They repeat long strings of syllables or words, often very swiftly and compulsively, but they rarely hold a sound or articulatory posture during the early development of the disorder. Occasionally on the first word of a sentence or phrase (especially if it begins with a vowel) they silently preform the vowel, holding back in preparation for the verbal rush to follow, but this seems different from the tremor-infused prolongations of Track One. These children are often tremor-free for a long time. They also have fewer complete blockings of the airway at the lips or palate or in the larynx than other stutterers in the later stages of development.

There are also characteristic differences in the development of fears in these children. Situation fears come first, and for many they remain the only ones. Phonemic fears are at best vague and unreliable. They are not intense, not phobic. The children on Track II do not show the complexity, the spread, or the intensity of logophobia so characteristic of other stutterers. When they have word fears, the cues that precipitate them are word length or unfamiliarity rather than particular sounds associated with frustration or penalty.

Track II children seldom exhibit grotesque facial or body movements, even late in the disorder's development, perhaps because they have so few prolongations or fixations. Since Track II children rarely have complete blockage, they have little need for the timing or releasing jerks or associated movements which create so much abnormality in others. What they do show, in the more severe cases, are long series of repetitions of syllables and whole words, often produced so compulsively as to render their speech completely unintelligible. These "runaway" behaviors (so labelled by older members of Track II) are difficult to describe in words. The person begins a syllable, and it seems to recycle preservatively like some normal speakers on the delayed feedback apparatus. The syllabic repetitions are very fast, often accelerating throughout their duration, and arhythmic. They are also often accompanied by a rise in pitch. Once caught in these oscillations, the Track II stutterer seems unable to terminate them until the exhalation is finished. We have seen some even yelp or shout in the effort to interrupt the compulsive oscillatory yapping. During these spasmodic experiences, the eyes of these stutterers often seem fixed and glazed, but they are highly aware that something devastating is happening to them. Older ones have told us that when they get started on one of these "runaways," they can't stop. Interestingly enough, for those in the terminal phase of Track II, even after many of these experiences, although they have a few word or sound fears, it is the experience itself or the situation in which it occurred which is most dreaded. Only a very few of the children of Track II, however, reach this traumatic destination; most of them terminate in speech that is mildly stuttered but mainly cluttered.

It might be objected that what we have been describing is not stuttering but cluttering. The early patterns shown by these children could certainly be viewed as cluttering, but later on they certainly show all the characteristics of true stuttering. The problems of differential diagnosis are difficult, and almost all authorities agree that stuttering may emerge from cluttering and that both disorders may coexist in the same individual. The individuals in Track II end up as stutterers. They do not become fluent when they try to talk slowly and carefully. They eventually become aware of their disordered speech (especially on the "runaway" repetitions) and they develop some rare but real situation and phonemic fears. They talk in torrents. They use avoidance tricks and consider themselves stutterers. Some cluttering component is probably present since, when their stuttering decreases as a result of therapy, they speak more clutteringly than before. Without arguing the diagnosis, we can say that some stutterers show this pattern of disorder development. De Hirsch and Langford (1950) make the following comment on the Track II type:

> There is another smaller group who have similar symptoms but at a later age. Many of these children start talking late. . . . Frequently their motor speech patterns are so poor that their speech is practically unintelligible. . . . Investigation of the family background of these children frequently reveals a history of language difficulty. . . . The speech of these children closely resembles a type of disturbance seen at all ages and known as cluttering (p. 936).

TRACK III

We would like to illustrate the third route of stuttering development with a brief case presentation.

> B.J., a boy of five years, was walking with his father down a residential street one evening when a dog rushed out from a yard and bit him so severely he had to be hospitalized for two weeks and given the painful series of rabies shots. He had been speaking at the time he was bitten. Until this incident, the boy had been very fluent, but in the hospital and thereafter his speech was marked by spasmodic inhalations prior to all utterance.

Laryngeal closures with marked tension initiated all speech attempts after all pauses. We had known the child before the trauma and visited him while still in the hospital. Despite all we could do, this child developed a very severe stuttering problem, and it has persisted now for over 20 years. Its symptomatology has changed little, though the laryngeal blockings with their preceding inhalations do not occur after *every* pause as formerly. They show themselves only under various kinds of communicative stress, in reciting, in talking to authority figures, etc. The normal speech is completely fluent. B.J. has word and phonemic fears, the vowels being especially dreaded. He has developed a variety of avoidance behaviors, primarily of postponement, but they fail him more often than they help. The stuttering behavior is remarkably consistent and stereotyped and monosymptomatic. He has had psychotherapy and speech therapy for years and still stutters in the same way he began.

Only 5 of the 44 persons we studied longitudinally and on whom we had sufficient data fit the pattern of this track, but we were able to discern the same patterning in 13 other cases whom we were able to treat successfully before they reached the terminal behaviors. Few of the stutterers in Track III provide as clear a history of the circumstances surrounding onset as that of B. J. Usually all we know is that the disorder started very suddenly and that it began with an apparent inability to speak or to continue speaking. Most parents cannot account for this sudden appearance of what they call "blocking," but some attribute it to frightening experiences, shocks, sudden changes in environment, and a host of other causes most of which when investigated appear to have little pertinence. Since this section is not concerned with etiology but only with how stuttering develops, we want to stress the initial behavior rather than the presumed conditions under which it arose. Vague as these parents often are about the "causes," they are very specific about what made them aware that the child was having trouble. "He opened his mouth and tried to talk but nothing came out." "It was like he couldn't get any sound out." "She would try and try again to get started but wasn't able to." "It really wasn't like stuttering. She didn't repeat over and over; she just tried to talk and couldn't. Now she repeats, but not at first. She was stuck that's all."

All of the children in this group had spoken quite fluently for some years, and the age of onset is usually later than in Track I. Most of them begin stuttering during the years from five to nine, although we have found the same patern occasionally in a child as young as two years and also in adults. The stuttering is at first consistently confined to the beginning of an utterance after a pause, and once the sentence or phrase is under way no further difficulty is experienced until another and different utterance is begun. The basic initial behavior is fixation not oscillation; it is tonic, not clonic. The first articulatory posture is held and prolonged. It is accompanied by tension and struggle almost from the first. The closure is primarily at the level of the larynx. Breathing abnormalties appear very soon and often become stereotyped rituals of attack. An intermittent vocal fry can be heard during the struggle for phonation.

These children develop awareness and frustration almost immediately. Struggling and forcing also appear very soon. Tremors show up in the tensed musculature. Often the child will cry helplessly or attack the listener or stop talking for long periods. Regressions in social behavior patterns ensue: enuresis, thumb-sucking, other long-outgrown forms of infantile behavior. We have seen the eyes cross during the struggle. An overflow of tension results in facial contortions and associated limb movements. The child may finally shout the word with which he has attempted to begin his utterance. All of this behavior develops very suddenly and swiftly although it may completely and dramatically disappear for a considerable period only to show up again in a slightly different form. But in far too many, the disorder grows like a brushfire. From the frustration and the struggle and the great concern shown by the child's associates—a concern that is most difficult to conceal since it seems so merited—the fears and avoidance arise. No one who has witnessed the malignant growth of this behavior can doubt the traumatic experience felt by the child.

As the child progresses along Track III the silent fixations at the level of the larynx spread to the lips and the tongue. We have noticed in the few of these children with whom we could work directly that multiple occlusions of the airway occurred. First, after a quick intake of breath, the larynx was raised up under the hyoid, and the vocal folds were tightly adducted as in startle. Then abdominal pressure was suddenly increased in an effort to break the blockade. This was the elementary pattern of behavior that took place during the abortive attempt to speak. Next we noticed that other structures were also beginning to occlude the airways. First the lips were closed, then the tongue was pressed against the palate. In the longest moments of this kind of stuttering, all three closures occurred simultaneously. Most of the children showed only one closure during any one moment of stuttering. We found generally, however, that within a few weeks prolongations of vowels and the continuant consonants would make their appearance and that then there was a sudden decrease in the number of the old silent laryngeal closures. It seemed almost as though the child was able to substitute this other type of prolonged fixation. As proportionately more prolonged /s/, /f/, /m/, /n/, and other phonemes appeared, the pronounced struggle behaviors also decreased and the child seemed less frustrated. He began to talk more again.

Next in the development of stuttering in this group of children, syllabic repetitions appear for the first time in substantial quantity. There is some repetitive behavior in the early behavior, but it is more retrial than clonic repetition. In other words, the child would get so stuck, he had to stop completely and then try again. This is quite different from the automatic syllabic bouncing of the Track I children. In the Track III children, the repetitions follow the prolongations, and often each repetition begins with a slight prolongation of the first sound (tonoclonus). It seems as if the child is trying to find the proper integration of the initial syllable of the word. One of the characteristic features distinguishing this group is the relative rareness of their stuttering on the later syllables of a polysyllabic word, even upon a syllable carrying the primary accent. They simply have trouble getting started! Evidently this phase presents a favorable opportunity for the reacquisition of fluency since we have noted that a good many of the children who do recover, do so at this stage of development.

Those who do not are swept over the falls of fear and into the whirlpool of chronic stuttering. They present the most morbid picture of any of the three groups of children we have described. Their fears are stronger; their patterns of stuttering behavior more complex. Avoidance is very marked. They scan approaching situations and prospective utterances with greater anxiety. They become very severe stutterers, often of the interiorized type described by Freund (1934) and by Douglass and Quarrington (1952).

TRACK IV

The onset of the disorder in these children is usually later than for those of the other tracks. As in the children of Track III, stuttering begins suddenly and after several years of fluency. The initial behavior, however, is different. From the first it seems highly stereotyped, almost deliberate and contrived. The child seems very aware of it from the first and even more aware of its impact on the listener, whom he watches carefully. He is testing, testing, testing. Often he may smile slightly.

In some of these children the first behaviors are repetitions of whole words or phrases rather than syllables, although they soon change to include the latter. The initial word or phrase is repeated many more times than is usual in normal nonfluency. The inflection and intonation patterns are demanding, insisting. The child begins a sentence with "I-YI-YI-YI-YI-I-I-I" or "Mommy-mommy-mommy-mommy-mommy" or "When can, when can, when can, when can, when can, when can I go?" A bit later that same child will be saying, "Whe-whe-when-when-wh-wh-when-when can I go?" The lengthy repetition of words already spoken normally is a continuously characteristic feature of this group. Even in the advanced stages these children sometimes say a word or phrase correctly, then stop and say it again with pronounced nonfluency. They return to the utterance to stutter upon it.

There are some, who seem to belong to this group, who show no repetitions at all. The first behaviors are gaps and pauses accompanied by stereotyped postures and activities such as sobbing, grunting, biting, or tongue or lip protrusions. The jaws may be opened widely and retching noises made. Whimpering sounds accompanied by tremulous movements of the lower lip may fill the pauses.

One of the children we studied intensively was brought to us by his anxious mother because he had suddenly begun to interrupt his fluency with successive inhalations until his chest was greatly distended. He would hold this thoracic posture for some moments, sometimes until he staggered. We learned that early in infancy the boy had done a lot of breath-holding in moments of frustration. It was plainly evident that he was using the behavior to control his mother and we did what we could through referral to a child psychiatrist to solve the problem, but in vain. We have watched the disorder develop over the years and at present this person, now an adult, would be classified as a severe stutterer by anyone. Other reactions have joined the initial respiratory behavior, but the latter still dominates the symptom picture. He is infantile, neurotic, controlling still.

One of the major distinguishing characteristics of Track IV is that the behavior changes very little over the years. The frequency of stutterings may increase, but the basic patterns seem very stable. Most of the other stutterers we have described pass through many phases and finally develop a repertoire of different avoidance or release reactions. Those on this track, however, tend to be monosymptomatic. Moreover, they develop few avoidance tricks; the disguise and masking behaviors are conspicuous by their absence. Interruptor behaviors are few. These children offer you their stuttering openly. They watch you as you react to it. And they are rarely emotional about it. As adults, they talk a lot about their tragic speech handicap, but somatic evidence of stress is not impressive. GSR recordings show little disturbance even when pronounced speech interference is demonstrated. When they are fluent, they are very, very fluent. When they are not, their behavior is stereotyped, almost symbolic, and there is that small, brave smile. These stutterers suffer less than their listeners. One can sense the controlling, punishing, wheedling, exploitative urges behind the behavior. Only four of our 44 children fit the pattern we have outlined as characteristic of this track and only five others of our larger population seemed to show the described onset and development. It is our impression that those who begin to stutter in adulthood are more likely to portray these behaviors than children. And the adults show very few changes once they begin to stutter this way. They continue to stutter much the same way they began.

We have described four of the common courses of stuttering development, and the first two are by far the most common. Some stutterers we have studied do not follow any of these tracks; some shift intermittently from one to another at different times. We could not fit three of our smaller group and 69 of our larger group into any track. Remember also that these are just observations, the gleanings of 35 hectic years. Until we have careful longitudinal studies of large groups of stutterers, studies which present very great difficulties in design and administration, we must rely on such clinical observations or on the information we get from cross-sectional studies. The following chart summarizes these four courses of development.

AT ONSET

Track I	*Track II*
Begins 2½ to 4 years.	Often late. At time of first sentences.
Previously fluent.	Never very fluent.
Gradual onset.	Gradual onset.
Cyclic.	Steady.
Long remissions.	No remissions.
Good articulations.	Poor articulation.
Normal rate.	Fast; spurts.
Syllabic repetitions.	Gaps, revisions, syllable, and word repetitions.
No tension; unforced.	No tension.
No tremors.	No tremors.
Loci: First words, function words.	Loci: First words; long words; scattered throughout sentence; content words.
Variable pattern.	Variable pattern.
Normal speech is well integrated.	Broken speech with hesitation and gaps even when no disfluency.
No awareness.	No awareness.
No frustration.	No frustration.
No fears; willing to talk.	No fears; willing to talk.

Track III	*Track IV*
Any age after child has consecutive speech.	Late, usually after four years.
Previously fluent.	Previously fluent.
Sudden onset, often after trauma.	Sudden onset.
Steady.	Erratic.
Few short remissions.	No remissions.
Normal articulation.	Normal articulation.
Slow, careful rate.	Normal rate.
Unvoiced prolongations.	Unusual behaviors (see text).
Laryngeal blockings.	
Much tension.	Variable tension.
Tremors.	Few tremors.
Beginning of utterance after pauses primary.	First words; rarely on function words; content words especially.
Consistent pattern.	Consistent pattern.
Normal speech is very fluent.	Normal speech is very fluent.
Highly aware.	Highly aware.
Much frustration.	No frustration.
Fears speaking; situation and word fears.	No evidence of fear; willing to talk.

DEVELOPMENTAL CHARACTERISTICS

Track I

Repetitions of syllables increase in frequency and speed and become irregular.

Then:

Repetition of syllables begin to end in prolongations.

Then:

Prolongations show increased tension, tremors, struggle. Evidence of frustration.

Then:

Overflow of tension; facial contortions; retrials; speech output decreases; signs of concern.

Then:

Situation fears join other behaviors and avoidance behaviors. Then word fears, and fears of certain sounds arise. Child uses tricks to disguise and cover up. Speech attempts often hesitant. Poor eye contact. Output of speech decreases. Both repetitions and prolongations as core behavior.

Track II

Behaviors remain the same but the speed increases; their number also increases.

Then:

Little change in form.

Then:

Little change; little awareness; little frustration.

Then:

Duration of nonfluencies increases; more syllabic repetitions; little awareness.

Then:

Occasional fears of situations, not of words or sounds. Long strings of syllabic repetitions at fast speed are added to other behaviors. Some fears of situations. Good eye contact. No disguise. Output of speech increases. Little avoidance. Primarily repetitive. Unorganized.

Track III

An increase in the frequency but the behavior at first changes little. Signs of frustration.

Then:

More retrials are seen; lip protrusions, and tongue fixations appear; prolongations of initial sounds.

Then:

Tremors; struggling; facial contortions; jaw jerks, gasping; marked frustration.

Then:

Interruptor devices become prominent; rate slows; more hesitancy; more refusals to talk.

Then:

Intense fears of words and sounds; many avoidances; patterns change in form and grow more bizarre; much overflow; output of speech decreases; will cease trying to talk. Poor eye contact; the normal speech becomes hesitant. Nonvocalized blockings are frequent. Primary tonic blocks with multiple closures.

Track IV

The number of instances increases, and they are shown in more situations.

Then:

Little change in form; monosymptomatic and symbolic.

Then:

Little change.

Then:

Little change in type but duration and visibility increase; no interruptors or new forcings; increased output of speech.

Then:

Very few avoidance or release behaviors. Not much evidence of word fears. Few consistent loci. Very aware of stuttering. Stutters very openly. Good eye contact. Little variability in the stuttering behavior. Normal speech very fluent. Talks a lot. Consistent pattern; few silent blockings. Either tonic or clonic.

COMMENTARY

From observations on more than 3000 children treated at our institute we conclude that the disturbance in breathing and voice is secondary. In the beginning, when the first signs appear, these disturbances are found only rarely. More usually, they appear somewhat later, when the stuttering, becoming more severe, begins to make the child uneasy (Vlasova, 1962, p. 32).

In the vast majority of cases the development of genuine stuttering proceeds in the following way: First, iterations occur; in other words, a child occasionally repeats a word, a syllable or a sound. It must be stressed that such iterations are a physiologic feature in children from three to five years of age. Several pediatricians and the writer found that these iterations occur in the speech of about 80 per cent of all children (Froeschels, 1964, p. 80).

Whatever may be its source, stuttering seldom remains static. It grows. And as it grows, it tends to change in form as well as in severity. Early patterns are replaced, obscured, or supplemented by more pronounced and abnormal behavior. Repetitions or prolongations become troublesome "blocks." Tremors may appear in certain oral structures. Word attempts may be interrupted and replaced with synonyms. Reattempts on words may be prefaced by noticeable pauses during which a child can appear to be experiencing some sort of internal struggle. Some children become less talkative and occasionally may refuse to speak (Robinson, 1964, p. 47).

Above all, the development of stuttering is actually a continual and gradual process to which any sharp division into phases does some violence. There is little use to a ruler without markings, however (Bloodstein, 1960, p. 366).

These children were referred to the author for diagnosis and treatment because of abnormal speech. In most cases the repetitions, prolongations, or blocking of sounds were in various ways different from the familiar repetitions and stumblings of children. Their speech was characterized by a change in muscle tonus, pitch, speed, and rhythm. This difference, in most cases, was observed by the physicians, usually pediatricians. One mother, who had been a nursery school teacher, said of her two-year, ten-month-old child, "All children repeat at times in their speech, but hers is different from any I've ever heard. She is so tense when she speaks." As a rule, there was an element of tension and compulsion in their speech which distinguished them from other children (Glasner, 1949, p. 135).

The stuttering continued into the second week. Signs were beginning to develop suggesting that Sandy was reacting at times to broken fluency. He would start a questioning sentence, then interrupt it with, "Oh, never mind" (Robinson, 1964, p. 106).

It is conceivable, nevertheless, that a speaker, even a young child, might feel frustrated by his nonfluency, particularly if it is extreme, and in reacting to the frustration speak still more hesitantly and even tensely. Through this experience he might also become increasingly attentive to his non-fluencies and more apprehensive of them, evaluating them as unacceptable or as "stuttering," and reacting accordingly with avoidant tensions. In some such way a speaker might conceivably create the problem of stuttering for himself by virtue of his intolerance of the nonfluencies in his own speech—and it is an incidental rather than a fundamental observation that any such onset of stuttering seems to be extraordinarily rare (Johnson, 1959, pp. 258–259).

In about an equal number of Phase 4 stutterers there appears to be no past history of repetitions at all.

J.R., aged 4–5, protrudes her tongue rapidly and attacks some words with her mouth wide open. No other symptoms are apparent. The earliest stut-terings, noticed at age three and a half, are said to have been forcings.

R.W., aged 5–7, has a stuttering pattern which contains some repetition of monosyllabic words, but is made up chiefly of somewhat tense prolonga-tions. The symptoms were noticed initially at age three years. At that time, it is said, he would flush, and his whole body would become tense as he exhausted his breath.

The severity of stuttering in some of the illustrations of Case 4 just pre-sented is noteworthy. The concept of a "primary" stage of stuttering has fostered the assumption that the stuttering of early childhood is simple and innocuous. While this is true in many instances, there are actually many more severe cases than some of those found in the first phase of stuttering (Bloodstein, 1960, p. 370).

When encountered in the adult, stuttering has accumulated so great an emotional overlay that the problem of its genesis and treatment is much confused. This is a natural result of the experience of the individual who had been blocked, by reason of his impediment, from free social intercourse and who has very often indeed accumulated a heavy load of inferiority and a fear of speaking. In by far the great majority of stutterers, however, the difficulty with their speech began in childhood, and at the time of onset of stuttering, the picture is very different from that seen in the adult. The emo-tional and personality factors which are so striking later and which have led many observers to classify all stutterers as neurotics, are notably absent in childhood. Many early stutterers when seen within the first year of their difficulty show no demonstrable deviation in the emotional sphere and present no history of environmental or psychological difficulties which seem at all adequate to explain the disorder (Orton, 1937, p. 122).

Some of these children, whose attention had apparently not been directed to their speech, after a prolonged repetition or block would blurt out or whisper, "I can't talk." Some showed their frustration by crying, others by stamping their feet or walking away without completing their sentence. Some placed their hands over their mouths whenever they were about to stutter. Two had been known to avoid speech for a period of two days. Obviously, many of these children were disturbed or anxious while stuttering, but whether this is the cause or the effect of the stuttering cannot readily be determined. The only thing that can be said with certainty is that many children under five when stuttering *do not* exhibit the same calm, totally unconcerned attitude characteristic of normal children when they speak with usual childhood repetitions and speech inaccuracies (Glasner, 1949, pp. 135–36).

L.B., age 4–6, began to stutter at two and a half years of age with "easy interruptions" which disappeared after six to eight months. After that, stuttering "came and went" until several months before the interview when it became more chronic with severe forcing and "contortions" (Bloodstein, 1960, p. 225).

Another step "forward" is the replacement of more conspicuous symptoms by less conspicuous ones. For instance, a patient who is used to stamping his foot, making all kinds of grimaces, etc., will then perhaps only clench his fist in his pocket and/or stare at an object. This state is called *concealed stuttering* (Froeschels, 1964, p. 86).

He had stammered in the usual manner up to age of about 15, but at that period of life he began to make great efforts to overcome his impediment and found that, when in difficulty, he could always pronounce the word by having recourse to this "drawback method" of phonation. Practicing this method voluntarily at first, he soon found that it became involuntary and habitual with him (Wyllie, 1894, pp. 18–19).

When I did screw up courage to try, the words came with so many contortions and such overwhelming self-consciousness, that I could not be understood. I would be wet with perspiration (Pellman, 1947, p. 31).

The child, believing in speech difficulties, and perhaps asked not to iterate, will try to overcome the "difficulty" by using more muscular energy. In this way the iterations will be spoken with strongly contracted muscles, and the single iterations will thereby proceed more slowly than the iterations without pressure. The writer has proposed calling the combinations of iterations and pressure *clonotonus* or *tonoclonus* depending on which of the two symptoms, iterations or pressure predominates (Froeschels, 1964, p. 113).

Cluttering is "the mother lode of stuttering" (Weiss, 1960, p. 217).

In young children, the symptoms of cluttering are less clearcut; the main characteristic—drivenness—does not show up because difficulties in word-findings, grossly incorrect spelling, vague sound images, poor motor innervation, impede that kind of onrush (Roman, 1959, p. 37).

In brain-damaged children, the speech interruptions date from the trauma or from the first onset of speech and are accompanied by omission of words or whole syllables, by peculiar syntax, perseverations, and often by the hyperactivity termed "drivenness." The latter is often reflected in the excessively rapid rates of utterance and confusions in thinking these children show. Here we could talk about an organic form of cluttering which is, unfortunately, very difficult to influence therapeutically (Freund, 1966, p. 145).

The following is a sequential account of the development of stuttering and its remission by the late Rigmor Knudsen (1948), an outstanding pioneer Danish therapist:

> This is the case history of a speech-retarded boy who developed stuttering and lost it again. Niels Ole was born 20/2 1938. Has an older brother and a little sister. Teething began with 1 year, cleanliness also. He walked at 18 months and began to talk when 2 years old. Came to the Institute for treatment on the 1st of September 1944 (6 years old). Is quite a big boy for his age, a little pale. Very quiet but stubborn. Is apt to say "I can't." and hates the fact that he speaks badly. Gets on fine with the other children. Is eager to come and practises at home by himself. When he came he lacked the following consonants: /p, f, h, s, t, l, k, r, n/; in the middle or at the end of a word the /s/ is replaced by /d/; /l/ by /ŋ/; /f/ by /b/; /p/ by /b/. All double consonants are missing (for "fly" he says "by" etc.). He does say /m, b, v, d, j, g, ŋ, or n/ in initial position. His speech is completely unintelligible. Some paragrammatism ("him" and "her" for "he" and "she." Conjugation and declination uncertain). In a week he had learned /p, f, s, h, l/. He quickly became very lively, wants to learn everything (i.e., tie a bow, wind the clock etc.). Tells a lot of fibs. After having learned the /s/, he puts it everywhere.
>
> On Sept. 27th I noticed primary cloni for the first time. On October 2d the mother tells me "He stutters a lot." I instruct her carefully how to react to this. By the 2d of November he can say all /l/-blends and all single consonants. On November 15th I notice the first tonus. Niels Ole has begun to talk very fast. I have stopped teaching him sounds and stopped correcting him altogether, I just let him repeat little stories slowly when he likes to. December 18th; stutters with both toni and cloni and tono-cloni. January 19th 1945 has stopped stuttering. January 22d 1945 stutters again but only in clonic form. March 16th 1945 does not stutter at all. Speaks correctly but a little agrammatically. (I cannot translate all the examples. They are something like "Iseed" for "I saw" etc.). Treatment discontinued on March 28th 1945. Came to see me on the 9th of April. No stuttering. Came to see me on the 19th of June. Speaks normally in every respect. Came to see me on the 17th of August. Goes to school. Is much more "grown up". Wants me to teach him to say "religion" (he says "regilion"). Does not stutter in the least.
>
> I have talked to the boy or his mother with regular intervals during these years and they seem to have forgotten that he ever stuttered (Knudsen, 1948).

There is yet another group of children, in which no family history of language difficulty is present nor is there any confusion in motor leads.

Many children in this group talk early and fluently. They begin stuttering, seemingly out of the blue, at any age, as early as 3 and as late as 14 years of age. The stuttering sometimes follows an emotionally traumatic incident which seems to serve as a precipitating factor. These children most often give a long story of emotional disturbance prior to the onset of the stuttering, manifesting symptoms of personality disorder such as recurrent vomiting, fears, sleep disturbances, feeding problems, enuresis, or persistent thumb-sucking. In these cases pronounced tonic elements and accompanying muscular movements, generally a feature of the individual who has been stuttering for some time, appear very early. In this group stuttering definitely seems but a symptom of an emotional disturbance involving the total personality, the expression of severe underlying anxiety which appears to disrupt cortical integrative functions with the result that speech reverts to an earlier and disorganized pattern.

Mark B., is five years, seven months old: He is the younger of two children; his older brother, Simon, is eight and a half years of age. Family history is free of language disturbance. The mother, who herself is a tense and anxious person with high blood pressure, describes her husband as "very nervous." As an infant Mark suffered from severe colic and cried continuously. From the time he was 17 months old he vomited after most meals, especially on occasions when his mother forced him to eat things he did not like. "He was a difficult child," Mrs. B. says, "and I used to hit him a lot." Mark produced his first words at 16 months and his first short sentence came through when he was not quite two years old. By the time he was three years, the boy talked fluently and easily, showing only a few sound substitutions normal for his age. At the time Mark was four and a half years old, his brother was kept home from school for several months recovering from rheumatic fever. The children fought a great deal, and it seems that one night Simon had pretended to choke the younger boy. Shortly afterwards Mark started to stutter and continued stuttering even after his brother went back to school. On examination the stuttering pattern was seen to consist of severe tonic blocks, many of them at the level of the larynx so that at times the child could not get a word out. Blocking was accompanied by various muscular movements, above all by jerking up of the head.

"My——brother won't let me——play. If——I go downstairs in the m—orn ing he could k—kill me cause, cause he is jealous. If——I go with Daddy he makes a picnic—no.——I'm——m-mean a racket." At times Mark is practically free from blocks: "I can't sleep at night times." At other times blocking is so severe that he flushes with the effort to bring a word out. "Mummy has too——m-much trouble, must——force——Simon to eat————I eat too much. I f—f—fight too much." In this example, note should be taken that blocking is most severe on emotionally laden terms (De Hirsch and Langford, 1950, p. 938).

BIBLIOGRAPHY

Andrews, G., and M. Harris, *The Syndrome of Stuttering*. London: Heinemann, 1964.

Bloodstein, O., "Development of Stuttering," *Journal of Speech and Hearing Disorders,* XXV (1960), 219–37; 366–76; XXVI (1961), 67–82.

Bluemel, C. S., "Primary and Secondary Stammering," *Quarterly Journal of Speech,* XVIII (1932), 187–200.

———. "Stammering and Inhibition," *Journal of Speech Disorders,* V (1940), 305–8.

———. *The Riddle of Stuttering.* Danvill, Ill.: Interstate, 1957.

———. *Stammering and Allied Disorders.* New York: Macmillan, 1935.

———. *Stammering and Cognate Defects of Speech,* Vol. I. New York: Stecher, 1913.

De Hirsch, K., and W. S. Langford, "Clinical Note on Stuttering and Cluttering in Young Children," *Pediatrics,* V (1950), 934–40.

De Parrel, S., *Speech Disorders.* Oxford: Pergamon, 1965.

Dostalova, N., and T. Dosukov, Uber die drei Hauptformen des neurotische Stotterns," *De Therapia Vocis et Loquellae,* I (1965), 273–76.

Douglass, E., and B. Quarrington, "Differentiation of Interiorized and Exteriorized Secondary Stuttering," *Journal of Speech and Hearing Disorders,* XVII (1952), 377–85.

Freund, H., *Psychopathology and the Problems of Stuttering.* Springfield, Ill.: Thomas, 1966.

Froeschels, E., "Core of Stuttering," *Acta Otolaryngologica,* XLV (1955), 115–19.

———. "Pathology and Therapy of Stuttering," *Nervous Child,* II (1942), 146–61.

———. *Selected Papers (1940–1964).* Amsterdam: North-Holland, 1964.

———. "Survey of the Early Literature on Stuttering, Chiefly European," *Nervous Child,* 2, (1943), 86–95.

———. "The Significance of Symptomatology for the Understanding of the Essence of Stuttering," *Folia Phoniatrica,* IV (1952), 217–30.

Glasner, P. J., "Personality Characteristics and Emotional Problems of Stutterers Under the Age of Five," *Journal of Speech and Hearing Disorders,* XIV (1949), 135–38.

Hirschberg, J., ["Stuttering,"] (Hungarian text) *Orvosi Hetilap,* CVI (1965), 780–84.

Hoepfner, T., "Stottern-als assoziative Aphasie," *Zeitschrift für Pathopsychologie,* I (1912), 448–553.

Hunt, J., *Stammering and Stuttering, Their Nature and Treatment* (original Edition, 1861). Reprinted New York: Hafner, 1967.

Johnson, W., *The Onset of Stuttering.* Minneapolis: University of Minnesota Press, 1959.

Knudsen, R., personal communication, 1948.

Luper, H. L., and R. L. Mulder, *Stuttering Therapy for Children.* Englewood Cliffs, N.J.: Prentice-Hall, 1964.

Morley, M., *The Development and Disorders of Speech in Childhood.* Edinburgh: Livingstone, 1957.

Orton, S. T., *Reading, Writing and Speech Problems in Childhood.* New York: Norton, 1937.

Pellman, C., *Overcoming Stammering.* New York: Beechhurst, 1947.

Potter, S. O. L., *Speech and Its Defects.* Philadelphia: Blakeston, 1882.

Robinson, F. B., *An Introduction to Stuttering.* Englewood Cliffs, N.J.: Prentice-Hall, 1964.

Roman, K. G., "Handwriting and Speech," *Logos,* II (1959), 29–39.

Stein, L., *Speech and Voice.* London: Methuen, 1942.

Van Riper, C., *Speech Correction: Principles and Methods* (4th Ed.). Englewood Cliffs, N.J.: Prentice-Hall, 1963.

Vlasova, N. A., ["Prevention and Treatment of Stuttering in Children in the U.S.S.R.,"] *Ceskoslovenska Otolaryngologie,* XI (1962), 30–32.

Weiss, D. A., *Cluttering.* Englewood Cliffs, N.J.: Prentice-Hall, 1964.

———. "Therapy for Cluttering," *Folia Phoniatrica,* XII (1960), 216–28.

Wyllie, J., *The Disorders of Speech.* Edinburgh: Oliver and Boyd, 1894.

six

PHENOMENOLOGY:
OVERT FEATURES

This chapter describes the features of stuttering in its full fledged form. Having discarded the phrase "secondary stuttering" for reasons mentioned earlier, adjectives such as "advanced" or "confirmed" will be used to refer to fully developed stuttering. Wyllie (1894) gives a vivid description of stuttering in its morbid maturity.

> He (the stutterer) closes the oral canal at one or other of the closing points, according to the nature of the letter to be articulated, and this he does as well as a man who possesses the faculty of speech could do it; instead, however, of allowing the vowel to follow without delay, he presses his lips, or his tongue and teeth, or his tongue and palate, more firmly together than is necessary; the explosive escape of the air does not take place, the other muscles of the face and those of the glottis and even the muscles of the neck become spasmodically affected like those of articulation; gesticulatory movements are made, the abdomen is retracted, the head is drawn backward, and the larynx is drawn forcibly upward, until finally he works himself into a state of frightful agitation; his heart beats forcibly, his face becomes red and blue, his body is bedewed with perspiration, and he may present the appearance of a complete maniac * (pp. 21–22).

---

* Wyllie evidently translated this from an earlier article by Kussmaul in Ziemssen's Medical Encyclopedia (1877). We are glad to help the old German's words reverberate a little longer.

VARIABILITY

Not all confirmed stutterers show so severe a disorder, but anyone who has worked with more than a few adult cases will recognize the picture as a familiar one. And this is only one of many such portraits in the rogue's gallery of stuttering. The newcomer to this gallery is often both appalled and bewildered by the variegated display. How can all these behaviors constitute one disorder? Why does the stutterer do what he does when trying to talk? One young man stopped suddenly in the middle of one of his contorted struggles, grinned at us, and then blurted with complete fluency, "The trouble with stuttering is that it just doesn't make any sense." We hope this chapter will help make overt stuttering behaviors more comprehensible.

In most stutterers, the early behavior is primarily syllabic repetitions and prolongations of a sound or articulatory posture (see Chapter 5). But people react to the frustration and penalties that follow these behaviors in many different ways. There are literally thousands of possible reactions that can be used to escape, avoid, or disguise the inability to say a word. We have reports of identical twins who stuttered differently. Most adult stutterers pass through a whole series of different reaction patterns before they develop the final set which is as unique as their fingerprints. At four years of age, the stutterer may have only syllabic repetitions; at five, postural fixations. By his 11th birthday he could be retching and gasping; by his 16th, his speech may also be punctuated by long pauses. When he is 30, all of these behaviors may be in his stuttering repertoire, and there may also be some head-jerks. But some of these behaviors may also be suddenly discarded or replaced by others less abnormal. We knew one man, at the age of 70, who stopped the struggling and avoiding of many years and began to stutter easily and with the syllabic repetition of his childhood. He told us he was too tired and too old to stutter so hard any longer.

At any age, a stutterer shows some variety. Those who are monosypmtomatic are very rare, and they are the kind Freund (1966) calls hysterical. Most advanced stutterers have more than one behavior in their repertoire, and some have so many that at times of great stress they hardly know which one to use. Different kinds of behaviors may be used when stuttering on words beginning with vowel sounds than when stuttering on words beginning with stop consonants. A stutterer who used a nasal snorting noise to interrupt a long tremorous fixation on the first sound of the word "take" never showed this behavior when stuttering on the word "ache." Instead he had an intermittent vocal fry or a rise in pitch. One stutterer used a quick inhalatory vocalization to release himself from hypertensed laryngeal closures on voiced cv or vc syllables, but never used it on syllables beginning with an unvoiced consonant. These different responses seem to have no reason for existing until we note that the nasal snort may at least initiate airflow, that vocal fry cannot be produced with true or ventricular vocal fold occlusion and so on. Many of the strange behaviors shown by stutterers seem to have some method in their madness when they are viewed as attempts to search for the integrations that will make the utterance of the word possible. If we look only at the variability itself, the picture is indeed confusing.

HIERARCHIES OF
STUTTERING BEHAVIORS

When the advanced stutterer's overt behaviors are closely scrutinized, it becomes apparent that they are arranged in a sort of hierarchy. Some of the responses in the stutterer's armamentarium (as Robert West might have called it) are fairly inconspicuous. Saying "ah" to postpone the speech attempt, or to interrupt a prolongation, belongs in this category. So might a single licking of the lips or a sudden inhalation. If the fear is weak, these inconspicuous reactions are the only ones used, but, as the fear or frustration become more intense, more conspicuous behaviors are called into play. The stutterer now struggles more visibly; his gasping, grunting, and other sounds (such as the vocal fry) become more audible. The tongue now comes out all the way. Stutterers in an extreme panic of helplessness sometimes run through their entire repertoire several times, finally ending with large trunk movements almost seizure-like in their severity. Bluemel (1957) gives an example:

> When asked a direct question such as his age, the young man sniffs loudly several times through his nose, then he sucks in his cheeks and exhausts the breath from his lungs. Meanwhile his face becomes suffused. He bends his head forward and blinks his eyelids vigorously. He opens his mouth, whereupon the jaw and facial muscles engage in violent "spasm." His head pulls over to the left; and the entire body, especially the left side of the body, becomes rigid. Finally, after violent and prolonged effort, the patient suddenly speaks rapidly and fluently on almost exhausted breath (pp. 47–48).

Why does the stutterer use one behavior first or second or third? How does the sequence develop? We have been able to watch this aspect of the disorder develop in only a few cases, but it is our impression that there are two factors determining the sequence of the various behaviors. First, the final hierarchy often reflects the order in which the coping behaviors were acquired. Those the stutterer adopted first are those that occur first in the sequence; those developed last are the final ones to be tried out as he struggles to utter the word. Second, the behaviors may occur in the order of their social visibility or listener wince-value. Thus the stutterer may use the least conspicuous coping behavior first. If this fails, he uses one that is just a bit more visible or abnormal, and so on until finally he gives up trying to hide his difficulty. It is then that he shows his most bizarre struggle. Gottlober (1953) gives this description:

> [The substitution of synonymns] works but soon he fears the word he is using for substitution, and it is not long before he runs out of synonyms. Then the "starters" begin, sounds or acts which he thinks will help him begin talking. He snaps his fingers, stamps his feet, clenches his fists, screws up his face or whistles. Each trick has its few moments of effectiveness and then helps no more. But he continues to use them just the same and the ritual that precedes even a single word may take from a few moments to more than a minute to complete (p. 87).

STUTTERING AS INTEGRATED BEHAVIOR

To the naive observer, this incredible variety of stuttering behaviors appears chaotic, spasmodic, and random. When a stutterer's abnormal behaviors are scrutinized carefully, however, they are found to be highly organized, well integrated, almost stereotyped patterns. The breathing abnormalties of such a stutterer as he stutters *on the same word* at different times are remarkably similar (Van Riper, 1936,). Sonographic, electromyographic, and sound pressure recordings also show highly consistent features. Each confirmed stutterer acquires his own unique *set* of stuttering behaviors. The superficial impression of randomness is not justified. Perhaps the casual observer thinks these behaviors are random because they are so inappropriate. For example:

> An adult of our acquaintance suddenly would look as though she were about to pray as she talked. Both palms would be placed together in front of her, pressed together tightly, then a word or phrase would be produced as she suddenly pulled them apart. . . . Another moved her feet around as she talked. If she were standing, it would at times look like she were about to perform a soft-shoe routine (Robinson, 1964, p. 6–7).

> . . . Some patients for example, will repeatedly jerk the head backwards or forwards; others will preface speech with violent movements of the arms or legs; others again will exhibit facial twitchings, eye-blinking, or clenching of the jaw (Boome and Richardson, 1932, p. 42).

> The act of stuttering is often accompanied by various associated movements. Most commonly involved are: wrinkling of the forehead, frowning, blinking, pressing the eyelids together tightly, and many other forms of grimacing appear as soon as the child makes an effort to speak. The head may be thrown backwards. Swallowing movements may occur. The patient

may jerk the extremities, or clench his fists or stamp his feet (Kanner, 1942, p. 314).

As one stutterer said, these behaviors seem to make no sense. They are completely unadaptive. Why should anyone close his lips tightly in order to say a word beginning with a vowel? Or open his jaws for one beginning with an /m/? Why should anyone gasp and jump and jerk trying to say "Good morning?" Why interject a prolonged *zzzzz* or squeeze one's eyes shut? Surely all this is not only maladaptive behavior; it must also be random. But it is not. The patterns occur too consistently. They are not a complete breakdown; they do not have the chaotic characteristics of panic behavior. Instead they are highly integrated responses, and when their history of development is examined, they appear to be the habituated descendants of instrumental acts that were once highly meaningful. Most of these responses, as Van Riper (1937) pointed out long ago, were originally used to postpone, avoid, or time the dreaded speech attempt, or to disguise, interrupt, or escape from the stuttering so as to avoid penalty. As such, they did make sense.

Not all of the contortions, grimaces, retrials, rituals, and forcings of the developed stutterer have their origins in conscious and deliberate attempts

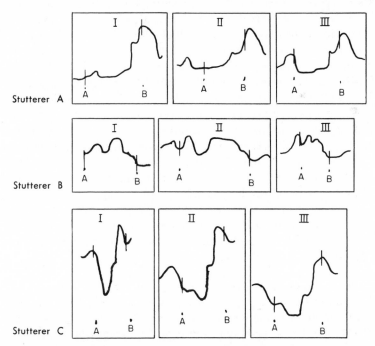

Figure 5. Consistency of breathing abnormalities in three productions of the word "stutterer" by three different stutterers. A. Beginning of stuttering; B. End of stuttering. Roman numerals indicate the three attempts by the same speaker.

to cope with the core behavior. Some of them are learned almost by chance. They may have coincided with release from tremor or with utterance. If, for example, a stutterer jerked his head, and if, just as he did so, he also said the word on which he had been stuttering, the utterance itself would reinforce the head-jerk. At that moment, there would be some relief from specific anxiety or least from frustration. What is more important, the head-jerk would be followed by communication. He could continue. The head-jerk also terminates any phonemic, word, or situation fear. All these events are powerfully rewarding. A pigeon can be taught to continuously rotate clockwise by shaping its movements with reinforcement. The stutterer may also find himself doing some oddball things that seem unrelated to speech. In acquiring many motor skills, learning to play golf for example, certain inappropriate movements or limb or head postures may become fixed because they occasionally preceded a fair wallop of the ball. These behaviors are difficult to unlearn and become more so as they are practiced.

THE STUTTERING TREMOR

One of the most prominent features of severe stuttering is tremor of the muscles of speech. Tremors are so prominent that it is difficult to understand why they have largely escaped investigation. They often form the basic behavioral substructure upon which the clonic repetitions are superimposed. The lips, jaws, tongue, and the extrinsic muscles of the larynx are thrown into rhythmic vibration at rates ranging from 7 to 9 per second. These oscillations are usually small in amplitude, depending on the structure involved. Their regularity resembles that of the physiological tremors, but they are often interrupted by larger jerking movements, apparently attempts made by the stutterer to interrupt the perseverating tremor. The tremor affects the stutterer strongly. He feels seized by it; he does not understand how it begins or is maintained. A normal speaker can perhaps get some understanding of the experience by recalling times when he felt a spasmodic facial twitching or a chattering of the teeth when very cold. Or perhaps he can imagine what it would be like to suddenly find an arm or leg vibrating in a sustained tremor. These tremors violate the integrity of the self. They are highly unpleasant and frustrating. They contain the seeds of panic. As Robinson (1964) says:

> The tremors cause a child to feel literally blocked in his efforts to talk. Feelings of frustration change to fear. Fear may change to panic. Escape is sought in any possible way. Unfortunately, the very devices that release the tremor and free the child to talk serve only to complicate his problem (p. 62).

Some of the interruptor devices do terminate the tremor, and they may occur just before the word is finally uttered, but at other times the larger

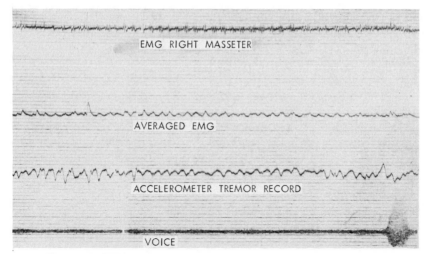

Figure 6. EMG and accelerometer recording of silent tremor on the word "start."

jerking movements fail to interrupt, and then the stutterer returns again to the tremoring. Our electromyographic recordings indicate that when the sudden movement (e.g., a jaw jerk imposed upon a lip tremor) is out of phase with the tremor, release occurs, but if the larger movement is in phase, the tremor resumes and the stutterer remains blocked. Generally, just prior to the moment of release and utterance, the tremor slows down in frequency and smooths out in amplitude. Most of the longer fixations (toni, prolongations) are accompanied by these tremors, and many of the repetitions (cloni) are either superimposed upon them or the final syllabic repetition shows a tremor of short duration. In severe stutterers a tremor may be set off in a group of oral muscles even before they begin to be used for speech. Our polygraphic recordings of breathing show them appearing in this area prior to utterance as well as during the blockings. As such they are probably conditioned to feared phonemic cues.

We find three conditions necessary for the initiation of these stuttering tremors: (1) a localized area of hypertension, (2) a postural fixation of the muscle groups involved, a posture different from that normally used for the sound, and (3) a sudden ballistic movement, or a surge of tension or air pressure. All three of these factors seem to be required before the tremor can be started, and the omission of any one seems able to prevent tremor. Though usually localized in a single area, stuttering tremors can spread to other structures. Some of these structures are those involved in speech, but we have seen tremors in the eyelids and legs accompanying those of the lips, tongue, jaw, or laryngeal areas. Usually, the tremor has its locus first in the speech muscles and then overflows to other structures.

Without trying to explain tremors, we will say only that they seem to arise as the result of the stutterer's struggle to release himself from speech arrest or from repetitive movements which have persisted too long. Only occasionally do they occur in very young stutterers shortly after onset. Generally they appear much later in the developmental sequence of the disorder. Again we turn to Wyllie (1894) for a description of this behavior:

> The lagging of the voice and the misdirection of energy already explained, cause the stammerer to surcharge his oral mechanism with energy, so that he sticks or stutters at his explosives, and prolongs his fricatives and nasal resonants, producing those of the latter voicelessly or with feeble vocalization. He sticks and stutters very specially upon his explosives, both voiceless and voiced.
>
> From the nerve centers of oral articulation thus surcharged, an overflow, in many cases, occurs; so that spasmodic and involuntary movements may be excited, both within the organs of articulation, and in other parts of the face, or even the body. Among the spasmodic movements thus produced, may be enumerated *trembling movements* and spasmodic twitchings of the lips and cheeks, working of the jaw, forcible winking of the eyes, twitching or tonic contraction of the sternomastoid on one or both sides, and sometimes spasmodic working of the arms.
>
> There may be drawback phonation. This is the production of speech during inspiratory effort; the vocal cords being approximated, and made to vibrate, when air is being drawn in between them.
>
> During phonation, this part of the larynx (the false cords and the ventricles of Morgagni) remains unclosed, while the true cords below are in apposition. What would happen if, during phonation, the false cords closed over the true, and by their valvular action, shut off the passage of air? Exactly that does happen in a variety of stammering (Wyllie, 1894, p. 19).

BLOCKAGES AND CLOSURES

Very severe stutterers often feel that blockages are the heart of the problem. In the midst of a tremor, the stutterer feels helpless. Something has happened to him that he cannot control. He tells us he feels "stuck" and "blocked." It is our considered opinion that many of the bizarre avoidance and struggle reactions shown by stutterers are coping devices, instrumental acts used to free themselves from these tremors or to prevent their occurrence.

Stutterers who are highly aware of their problem describe the core experience of stuttering as a "blocking" or "spasm," although the latter term is not used as frequently today as formerly. The term "blocking" or "stuttering blocks" refer to the momentary occlusion of the airway, a closure which is very real and evident in the advanced stutterer. This closing may occur at the level of the larynx when the true or false vocal folds or both are tightly approximated. Then the stutterer contracts his thorax and compresses his abdomen to emit the air forcefully to overcome the blockade. Or the closure may take place within the mouth, the rear or the front of the tongue creating a tight seal and a barrier to airflow and sound. The blocking of the airway may also occur at the lips. Of course it is the stutterer who is erecting these blockades, but they seem involuntary to him. At times there are multiple occlusions of the airway, and it is fascinating to observe, during a prolonged moment of stuttering in a severe case, that as one of these stoppages is released, another is activated in a different place. We have tried to determine whether, in these multiple blockades, certain of the areas are released before the other, and it is our impression that the closure at the laryngeal level is the last to be released in most stutterers. Kenyon (1943) and others always held that the vocal fold fixation was the primary and basic stoppage, but we have seen many stutterers whose closures were never laryngeal.

These blockings or closures are some of the most important phenomena in the multifaceted disorder of advanced stuttering. The stutterer senses such a closure very vividly. For a moment he feels impotent, out of control. The normal speaker may be able to share the experience by imagining a sudden inability to lift his hand or move a finger on command, Stutterers speak of having their lips glued together, of the tongue being cemented to the roof of the mouth. They say that something seems stuck in their throat. It is a deeply threatening experience, and the stutterer reacts to it with panic and frustration, with struggle and forcing, or by recoil and reattempt. Over 50 years ago Makuen (1914) said it this way: "To be suddenly stricken dumb when one is in full possession of his faculties is an alarming predica-

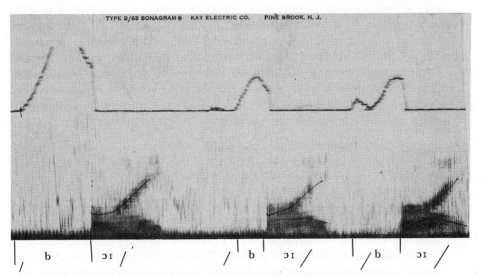

Figure 7. Intra-oral air pressure and sonographic recordings of complete blockages in the adaptation production of the word "boy." (*Courtesy of Dr. Joseph Agnello.*)

ment, and even a few repetitions of this will very naturally arouse an over-powering fear in the afflicted individual" (p. 386).

INTERRUPTOR DEVICES

Many of the most bizarre behaviors found in severe stutterers are those we have chosen to call interruptor devices. They are attempts to overcome blockings. Most of them are sudden—head and body jerks, foot or hand movements, inhalations, facial grimaces, nasal snorts. There is an incredible variety of interruptors, but most stutterers use only a few, trying first one then another, or repeatedly using the same one in the hope that finally the closure will be broken.

We cannot stress too strongly the importance of closures and interruptor devices because far too much has been written about avoidance as the dominant characteristic of stuttering. Stuttering often includes avoidance as a response to anticipated unpleasantness, but escape responses are a much more important feature. When the stutterer's forward progress is blocked by a closure, the unpleasantness is already under way, and he needs to escape from it as quickly as possible. It is both psychologically and semantically unwise to stretch the term avoidance to include these escape reactions. Wendell Johnson loved a paradox, and when he defined stuttering as the stutterer's attempts to avoid stuttering or disfluency, he beclouded the issue. A closure is a closure is a closure! Closures are devastatingly unpleasant, and most stutterers want to get out of them as quickly as possible. The ways they learn to do so contribute much to the abnormality of the problem. More practically, the therapist will find that escape behaviors are much more easily extinguished than avoidance reactions but that they demand different therapeutic procedures, an observation which may throw some light on the curious finding that many of the most grotesque and severe stutterers respond more favorably and quickly to therapy than milder stutterers who have fewer actual stutterings but more avoidance.

POSTURAL FIXATIONS

Closely related to closures of the airway, but differing in that the blockage is not complete, are the postural fixations of advanced stuttering. Although complete closures can occur on any phoneme, they are most pronounced on the plosives, as one might expect. The postural fixations in which the airway is abnormally constricted, but not completely blocked, occur primarily on the continuant sounds. Airflow or voice may be maintained, though often the voiced continuants show no phonation. The $/z/$ for example emerges as a prolonged /s/, and the /m/ or /n/ show silent nasal emission. The articulators are held in a highly tensed and fixed position, thus producing the prolongation. Tremors of the tongue, lips, and jaw may accompany these fixations though usually they are of slower rate and larger amplitude than those accompanying complete closures.

VOCAL FRY

As the unvoiced prolongation of a sonant proceeds in time, intermittent brief bits of weak phonation or vocal fry can be heard, and the word is uttered when these become stronger or persist longer than 0.3 seconds, according to our sonographic studies. We suspect some feedback mechanism may be operating here, but another explanation for the eventual release from fixation may lie in the characteristics of the phonation itself. Most of the little bits of intermittent phonation that occur during stuttering show the brief aperiodic waveforms of vocal fry, the harsh ticker-like sounds which according to Moser (1942), who gave it the name, resemble the sound of bacon frying in the pan. At the moment of release they become more regular and longer and finally the rhythmical waveforms of true phonation appear just before the word is finally spoken.

We have come to view vocal fry as another searching behavior. Somehow the stutterer has discovered that it is incompatible with tight laryngeal closure, that when he uses vocal fry his tight laryngeal closures are loosened. Rarely is he consciously aware of the mechanism involved or how it facilitates phonation. All he really knows is that somehow the airflow and sound have begun to emerge. Vocal fry is found very frequently in severe stutterers. In a long moment of stuttering on vowels or voiced sounds, the stutterer may first show complete laryngeal closure involving both true and false vocal folds; then, as he strains and struggles, little snatches of vocal fry appear between the surges of tension. They are irregular and initially very brief, but toward the end of the stuttering the vocal fry becomes sustained and smooth, and as this happens true phonation is superimposed upon it. Then release occurs and the syllable is uttered. This is how many stutterers finally manage to integrate the basic synergies involved in sound production. Tragically, they do not know how they accomplish the integration or how they use the vocal fry to help create the necessary conditions for phonation. Instead they often attribute the release from laryngeal closure to their struggling.

Not all stuttering on vowels or voiced continuants is marked by vocal fry. Some stutterers show abortive and weak but true phonation. We were puzzled by this until sonographic recordings showed that these prolonged or repeated segments did not have the transition components that are shown in the normal utterance of the desired sound. Normally, the production of

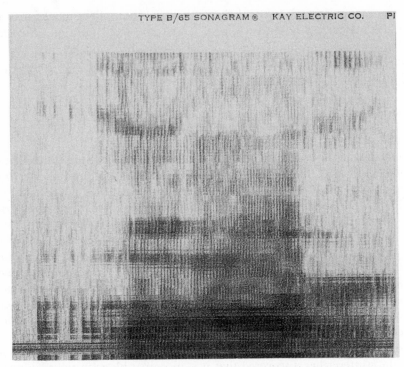

TYPE B/65 SONAGRAM® KAY ELECTRIC CO. PI

Figure 8. Vocal fry in the initiation of the stuttered word "are."

an *isolated* voiced sound such as /n/ or /v/, or a vowel such as /i/, gives a different sonogram than the same sound used in a syllable or word. In the latter, transitional formant patterns appear which are determined by the sounds that precede and follow the sound in question. These transitional formant patterns are lacking in the stutterer's prolongations until just before the release takes place. The same absence of coarticulation may even be observed visually at times. During prolongation of the /s/ in the words "see" or "Sue" the stutterer may not show the usual preparatory lip postures of the vowels that follow the /s/, as he does when speaking these words normally. Instead he uses the lip posture for the schwa vowel. He produces the neutral, isolated /s/, not the allophone for the word he is trying to say. This is doubtless due to the manner in which he perceives the feared word. He may be fearing its initial sound, the isolated /s/, the "suh" or "ssss" sound. Or some of his difficulty may occur because he begins his utterance with a totally inappropriate sound. The prevalence of the schwa vowel in the repetitive abortive releases is another indication of this behavior. The advanced stutterer seldom says "mmmmo . . . mmmo . . . motor." He says "mmmmuh . . . mmmmuh . . ." And when he says "vvvvvvvvvery" or "aaaaaaaapple" the /v/ or the /æ/ are produced differently and have a different spectrographic pattern than when he says the /v/ or /æ/ of "very" or "apple" normally. He seems to be searching and hunting for the appropriate transitions he needs.

REPETITIVE STUTTERING

In the last paragraph we discussed what happens when the stutterer has difficulty uttering syllables beginning with a voiced sound. In repetitive stuttering, for example, something quite similar also occurs when the syllable begins with an unvoiced consonant. Instead of finding serial short bursts of vocal fry or weak phonation, we notice brief pulses of airflow. Observing the airflow pulses closely, even without instrumentation, it seems that here also the stutterer is searching for the basic timing he needs if he is to integrate the complex pattern of simultaneous and successive muscular contractions that are required. He is trying to get airflow going, trying to integrate the basic synergy of utterance. Stetson (1951) maintained that the breath pulse was the basic integrator of the syllable. The stutterer tries and tries again, sometimes almost achieving the necessary timing of his breath pulse, then losing it, then finally finding it. He seems to be searching, to be hunting cybernetically for the target pattern, overshooting, undershooting, and finally at long last finding the bull's-eye. The same searching behavior appears in the successive articulatory postures found in the repetitive type of stuttering. Superficially, it looks as if the stutterer is only saying the same syllable over and over again. On close examination, however, there are some intriguing variations in these syllables. On the first repetition highly inappropriate articulatory postures may be used; on the second, some revision takes place; on the third, the posture may be almost appropriate; on the fourth and final syllabic repetition the stutterer has found the posture he needs, the one with coarticulatory features, and then the word is spoken. Sometimes the stutterer, in this searching behavior, almost gets his fix on the target only to lose it completely so that he has to begin hunting all over again.

SPEAKING ON COMPLEMENTAL AIR

In effecting the release from closures or prolonged syllabic repetition, many stutterers begin the actual speech attempt on complemental air, on the air that is left in the lungs after a normal exhalation. They squeak out their words at the very end of their breath, and sometimes several attempts must be made even then before the word is finally uttered. It may be significant that this behavior occurs rarely on sounds other than continuants.

Strong contractions of the muscles responsible for collapsing the thoracic cage accompany speech on the end of the breath. Some stutterers use this behavior as a last resort when all other ways of terminating the stutter-

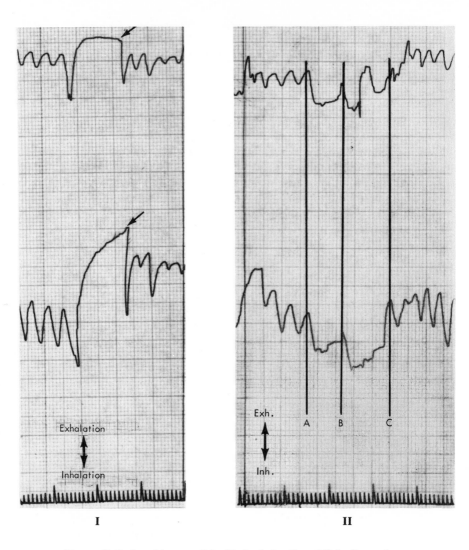

Figure 9. I. Speaking on "the End of the Breath" in Stuttering. II. Covert Rehearsal of Breathing Abnormality Prior to Overt Stuttering. A. Presentation of Stimulus Word; B. Signal to Speak; A-B Rehearsal; B-C Overt Stuttering.

ing have failed. In a few cases, however, it and vocal fry are the only behaviors shown. Why does this use of complemental air seem to facilitate speech for the stutterer? None of the explanations seem satisfactory. One stutterer said,

> By waiting until almost all my air is gone and then starting to say the word, I commit myself. I can postpone no longer. It's then or never, or rather, if I fail to say the word at that last moment, I'll have to take a new breath and begin all over again.

Another stutterer said, "At the end of my breath my vocal cords relax because they know they'll have to open soon or I die." We wish we could fit this little piece of the puzzle into the larger pattern. Perhaps someone else can. Why do so many advanced stutterers use this device? Why does it apparently enable them finally to begin an integrated syllable or word?

TRIGGER POSTURES

The articulatory postures used by stutterers on both voiced and unvoiced sounds are often wholly inappropriate, even grotesque. One of our cases habitually used an extremely unilateral /f/ and /v/ posture when prolonging these sounds. He said them out of the side of his mouth. Another, in trying to say words beginning with /f/ and /v/, thrust his tongue upward into the position normally used for /1/—as we discovered by palpating the cheeks. There are many other variations of inappropriate and even antagonistic postures. When the first sound of a syllable or word is distorted in this way, the utterance will obviously be impeded. What is not so apparent is the function these abnormal postures perform in triggering tremors. When stutterers try to throw themselves into "real" stuttering, they immediately assume such characteristically abnormal postures, then suddenly tense the structures and then go into a tremor. This they sense as being involuntary and real stuttering, quite different from the experience they have when doing pseudostuttering or faking.

We have been able to precipitate such "real" blocks, or alternately to produce normal speech, on a word beginning with /b/, by inserting a swab stick between the lips at different places and asking the stutterer to press it before attempting speech. In one of our young stutterers, the crucial pressure point was located with precision at a point one third of the distance from the corner of the lips to the midline of the vermillion border on the right side. This pressure point produced the longest blocks. By moving the probe away from this spot on either side, a definite gradient was seen in which the *duration* of the stuttering moment varied directly with the distance from the crucial spot. Moreover, when the swab stick was placed on the midline or anywhere along the left side of the tensed lips no stuttering occurred and the boy could not throw himself into real blocks when he focussed the pressure there. These trigger contacts and trigger postures play an important part in stuttering, and their modification is important in therapy.

RECOIL BEHAVIOR

For some stutterers the experience of what is felt to be involuntary closure is so traumatic, especially when the occlusion is accompanied by tremors, that an instantaneous recoil occurs. The behavior seems as involuntary as the recoil from touching a hot stove. Since the drive to speak is strong, the stutterer immediately makes a new attempt, and again, sensing the first feeling of closure or tremor, again recoils. The stutterer repeats the syllable, but the new attempt does not resemble either a deliberate retrial or a repetition since a very sudden arrest occurs before the syllable is automatically recycled. The recoils seem almost cybernetic. They are usually accompanied by surges of tension and are irregular. Schwa vowels predominate at first in the abortive attempts, but as the successive recoil-repetitions take place, revisions of these vowels occur until finally the appropriate one appears and then the word is spoken. To the stutterer the whole process seems to be automatic and involuntary. It is a very unpleasant experience. One of our girl stutterers who showed many of them said,

> It's devastating! I start to open my mouth to say a word and suddenly it starts jumping and bouncing as though it had a life and will of its own. Oh, I can stop it, but when I begin to say that word again, the same thing happens. It feels as though I'm not doing it.

Recoils are the essence of the behaviors stutterers call "runaway blockings." Electromyographically, they begin when both antagonistic muscle groups show strong action currents to produce a tremor and then one of them makes a sudden contraction *in phase* with the tremor's oscillation.

DISGUISE REACTIONS

We have been attempting to show that stuttering behaviors, despite their variability and inappropriateness, do make some sense if they are viewed as habituated attempts to cope with and escape from fixations and oscillations. There are certain reactions, however, that cannot be explained in this way. Why does one stutterer cover his mouth with his hand compulsively every time he stutters? Why does another laugh almost hysterically every time he stutters? Or a third turn his head far to the left? The answers are often in the histories of these behaviors. Initially they were adopted quite deliberately to hide or disguise the stuttering and then became automatized through the powerful force of intermittent reinforcement. One of our stutterers consistently cocked his head upward and to one side, wrinkled his brow, pursed his lips, and closed one eye whenever he had a severe blockage. The pattern was highly stereotyped and was very difficult to modify in therapy until we found that it had originally been a trick of pretending to think which he had often used in the past to disguise the fact that he was stuttering. Stutterers develop many ingenious ways of hiding their disorder. Some of these unfortunately become incorporated into it.

AVOIDANCE BEHAVIOR

No description of stuttering behavior would be complete without a discussion of the behaviors stutterers use to avoid the experience of fractured fluency. After a long history of communicative frustration and social penalty most confirmed stutterers will try almost anything that will prevent stuttering from occurring. They scan approaching speech situations and certain words with an alertness almost inconceivable to the normal speaker. Their radars are constantly revolving. They devise and revise strategies; they marshall alternative modes of avoidance to be used if the one selected fails; they assess the probability of unpleasant listener response; they estimate their own tendency to block. In their heads, the computers of probability whirr.

The most successful avoider, however, eventually finds this incredible burden of vigilant scanning so unbearable that the volleys of stuttering that occur sooner or later (even despite all his stratagems) are almost a relief. When the stutterer has successfully used some device or reaction which enables him to speak with no apparent difficulty, his fears do not subside. Indeed they are increased, for he reasons that this time he was not only alert but lucky. He knows that the avoidance tricks or rituals have not always "worked." Just because he has escaped the experience or revelation of his abnormality doesn't mean he can decrease his alertness.. He walks a jungle path of communication where many enemies and hazards lurk. If this description seems unbelievable to the normal speakers who read it, we doubt that it will to the stutterer who is a chronic avoider.

As one stutterer said, "Stuttering is like the mythical hoop snake. If you run after it, it flees; but if you run away it chases you." The tragedy of chronic avoidance is that it causes the situational and phonemic fears to spiral. Flight from stuttering makes it all the more frightful. It provides no opportunity to test reality. The expectation of approaching misery often is exaggerated, and successful avoidance corroborates the exaggeration. Perhaps it is for this reason that avoidance conditioned responses are so difficult to extinguish.

It is interesting that the more severely a person stutters, the less he resorts to avoidances. This happens because the severe stutterer soon discovers that he is stuttering even on the stallers, postponement tricks, starting phrases, synonyms, or circumlocutions that he uses to avoid feared words. Milder stutterers have more avoidances because they have more fluency and a better chance to hide their abnormality. Often, however, they have more intense word fears than the severe stutterer, probably because of their chronic avoidance. We worked for a year with one woman of 35 who claimed that she had really stuttered only once, and that at the age of 17.

We never heard her actually stutter in all that time, but we have never known a case to have such tortured, almost unintelligible speech because of her panicky substitutions and circumlocutions. We have never seen word phobias of such intensity. She carried a heavy burden.

Types of avoidance behavior. Since the basic purpose of avoidance behavior is to prevent stuttering from occurring there are several behaviors that are fairly common. First there is *refusal behavior.* The stutterer refuses to enter communicative situations in which he expects to stutter, or he refuses to attempt certain feared words. Here too there is alert scanning, a frantic estimation of probabilities, a search for ways to prevent stuttering from happening. In our intensive work with thousands of stutterers we have been continually amazed at the lengths to which these people will go to avoid exposing their abnormality or experiencing frustration. They have had the telephones removed from their houses; they have sold their homes and changed their addresses; one even legally changed his name. Many stutterers feign stupidity in school to avoid reciting; others feign deafness so they can write out what they have to say. A few stutterers simply stop speaking when they sense a feared word coming, leaving the sentence unfinished, thus inviting other listener penalty. Bluemel (1957) has a good passage:

> The chronic stage of stammering is usually marked by speech avoidance and aversion. The stammerer avoids difficult words, and he attempts to escape menacing situations. He is obsessed in his attitude toward his speech difficulties, and he lives his anxieties in retrospect and in anticipation.
>
> The stammerer dodges not only words; he dodges people and situations. He will cross the street or turn the corner rather than face the necessity for conversation. In scanning a menu he will look for words that he can say, and when he gives his order it represents a choice of words and not a choice of foods. Often the stammerer maneuvers a conversation so that difficult words will fall to his partner's questions instead of his own statements, and not infrequently the stammerer remains silent rather than face the struggle with speech (p. 59).

Most frequent of all the refusal behaviors are those involving substitution and circumlocution, the use of synonyms, or alternative coding of the thought. Some stutterers develop very large vocabularies as a result of habitual substitution, and their speech is so tortuous and strangely imprecise that a listener must work hard to comprehend its meaning. One of our cases told us of a telegram he had to send by phone. He wanted to say "Returning noon Friday by plane. Please meet me." This is what the wire finally read: "I'll be on airplane coming home day after tomorrow about lunchtime. Hope you will be able to have car for me there." The message cost him three times as much, and despite all this avoidance he said he stuttered on more words and more severely than he would have if he had kept to the essential information. Despite this insight no real learning occurred, for as he told of the experience he was constantly revising, substituting, and garbling his account of what had happened. In contrast, other stutterers, especially those for whom the frequency of stuttering is very high, develop a sort of telegraphic speech. Talking is such hard work that they speak as tersely as possible. We have seen a stutterer so fatigued by the terrific struggle accompanying each word of a sentence that at the end of it he was on the verge of physical collapse. We have watched little children stop talking and cry helplessly and, oddly, silently. Several of our cases of voluntary mutism and spastic dysphonia began with refusal behavior related to stuttering.

POSTPONEMENT

Refusal behavior is often accompanied by postponement. Most confirmed stutterers learn that the probability of abnormality or frustration can occasionally be lessened by delaying the speech attempt. There are several possible explanations for this, the most plausible being that fear seldom has a steady state. It fluctuates in time, rising and falling in intensity, flaring suddenly, then subsiding a bit. Stutterers tell us that if they can time the speech attempt at the very instant that the fear is decreasing—in the trough of the wave, so to speak—they can sometimes say the word normally or at least better than they had originally anticipated.

We have done some unpublished research in which we made polygraphic recordings of the respiration of stutterers attempting single words following a signal by the experimenter. When the signal to speak was given at the moment when the anticipated stuttering had come to the end of its rehearsal, as indicated by the polygraph, fewer moments of overt stuttering occurred and they were of shorter duration than when the signal to speak was given at the beginning of the rehearsal behavior. It may be that stutterers use postponement reactions because they try to time the moment of speech attempt to coincide with the moment of maximum reactive inhibition. It is very difficult to do, but even if it succeeds only once in a while it may provide the intermittent reinforcement necessary for maintenance. Wendell Johnson (1930) describes his own early stuttering in these words:

> . . . words imbedded in a sentence sometimes offer less difficulty than words, even the same words, at the beginning of a sentence. Knowing this, I frequently back up, so to speak, and take a running start at sounds on which I expect to encounter difficulty in order to permit the articulatory and vocal momentum to carry me over (pp. 115–116).

Stutterers use many different strategies to gain time without being conspicuous. Many postponements resemble the same behaviors used by normal speakers when confronted by uncertainty in formulation, or listener loss.

All of us filibuster at times, using "ahs," "ums," "ers," facial and hand gestures, repeating previously spoken phrases or words, inserting communication-holding phrases such as "What I mean is . . .", "Let me see . . .", "and uh, and uh," or other interjections whose major function is to maintain verbal momentum and to prevent silent gaps. We use them to ward off interruption by others, to maintain our hold on the listener's ear. They are signals that we have not finished sending our message.

By deliberately using postponement mechanisms that closely resemble those used by nonstutterers, the stutterer gains more time to wait for the fear to ebb or for the covert rehearsal behavior to be completed than he could get by using silence alone. Filled time, as many experiments have shown, is perceived as shorter than empty time by both the speaker and the listener. In addition, silence, as Sheehan (1958) and others have made clear, is often threatening, especially in our highly garrulous and swift-paced culture. Silence may even hint of impotence or death for the more morbid souls. Some stutterers postpone silently without moving a muscle for interminable lengths of time, then suddenly blurt out the word. These interiorized nonvocalized stutterers are as hard on the therapist as they are on their other listeners. One of ours resembled the peasant mentioned by the Latin poet Horace who came to the bank of a river and waited for it to run by. Most stutterers are not so interiorized nor so tolerant of silence. They fill their communicative gaps with some sort of overt audible or visible behavior.

Occasionally we find postponement behaviors that are extremely complex. One of our stutterers had developed a stereotyped hierarchy of postponement reactions to the anticipation of stuttering on a feared word which ran as follows. First, he licked his lips; then he said "ah;" then he said, "Well . . ."; then he looked upward with furrowed brow as if thinking; then he coughed; finally he yawned. If the fear was intense all six behaviors occurred, and always in that order. If it were mild, perhaps only the first, or the first and second of these reactions would precede the speech attempt. Van Riper and Milisen (1939) found that stutterers can successfully predict the crude duration of their stuttering. This stutterer was so good at it that he seldom showed any overt blocking. He only postponed, apparently using the ritualistic disguise behavior as a stuttering equivalent. After each component of the sequence he made a sort of predictive assessment of the probability of stuttering were he to make the speech attempt at that instant. He said he never gave himself the benefit of the doubt; he tried to say the word only when he was certain he wouldn't stutter. We asked him what happened when he had exhausted his repertoire but still felt uncertain, and he answered that he went back to the first item of his postponement hierarchy, licking his lips, and started over. His behavior corroborated this account.

Not all stutterers are as fortunate, if that is the appropriate term, in using postponement to prevent overt stuttering. Despite their tricks, the inevitable moment comes when speech is mandatory, when they can postpone no longer. The stuttering that then occurs is often more severe than if the postponement had not been used. Why then does the stutterer continue to use his stallers? There may be many reasons. Careful observation and interview will reveal what reasons motivate a particular stutterer. Here are a few reasons, listed in random order. The stutterer postpones:

1. To give him time to scan the listener's tolerance of speech interruption.

2. To torture the listener, to make him wriggle with impatience, to make him reject. This occurs especially in hostile, neurotic stutterers.

3. Because he is caught midway in an approach-avoidance conflict. He wants to speak, but he fears the exposure of abnormality. These are usually silent postponements.

4. To permit the fear or tension to ebb. To help him relax, to build up his courage. To combat time pressure.

5. To take advantage of reactive inhibition in his rehearsal behavior.

6. To revise the anticipatory behaviors, to modify the tremors and false postures which he feels will almost ensure stuttering.

7. To regain some sense of self-contact and self-control. These are usually vocalized postponements or gestural rituals, coughs, yawns, etc. Feeling unable to utter the feared word, the stutterer does something else voluntarily to reassure himself.

8. To bypass the moment of spasmodic breakdown if such moments exist.

9. To plan a revised attempt to time the sound, syllable, or word and thus to reduce the probability of severe stuttering.

10. As an equivalent of expected overt stuttering.

The automatization of postponement behaviors. Some very odd behaviors develop as postponement behaviors become automatic. (See also Chapter 5.) One of our cases used a most peculiar vocalization of something like [l:m:si] prior to speech attempt on feared words. Often he would repeat this bit of jargon many times if he expected great difficulty. His parents said it was a contraction of "Let me see," a postponing phrase he had used very frequently and often inappropriately during his adolescence. Another stutterer showed no behavior other than the compulsive repetition of "Andodododoh . . . andoh . . . andoh . . . andodoh . . ." His wife said that this behavior had begun only recently and that formerly he had used the phrase "And don't you know" in the "oddest places when he was talking." We have seen the decayed residue of the swallowing reflex similarly truncated and persisting in a stutterer who had formerly pursed his lips and swallowed to gain time. This behavior was socially acceptable, but he had overused it, and finally, like many anticipatory behaviors that become habitual and automatized, it had become compressed into a pursing of the lips and the elevation of the hyoid, though with no resulting completion of the swallow. We have watched the development of such post-ponement mechanisms in several cases, seen them originate in deliberate behavior, become stimulus-tied or bound, and finally observed them end in responses which were the bare skeletons, almost caricatures, of the former instrumental response. The key features of the original postponement are retained; the rest drop out. Many of the bizarre and strange behaviors of the stutterer are explained in such histories of habituated compression.

TIMING DEVICES

Much has been written about the perseverating nature of the stuttering response. Repetitions and prolongations are by definition perseverations. Postponements also persist in time, but the time always comes when a stutterer must either give up communication altogether or finally make the speech attempt. The time pressure of the approach gradient increases with every instant and finally the stutterer dare not postpone any longer. What does he do then?

The answer is of course that he stops postponing and tries to say the word. It is at this point, however, that a new state of behaviors appears, instrumental responses designed to compel utterance at a specific moment in time. Otherwise, postponement would go on and on. It is difficult to stop postponing once you have started it, especially when its termination may be very unpleasant. Accordingly, certain timing devices or rituals are used to make the attempt mandatory. Anyone who has ever had to jump over a ditch or a stream that seemed wide can understand why the stutterer be-haves this way. The variety of timing devices is endless. Some are quite socially acceptable. Many stutterers repeat words they have already spoken normally in order to get a running start so that the feared word is part of the total sequence. Others are very odd: head nods, foot twitches, sudden gestures, a facial grimace, a quick inhalation. Often the timing device used to end postponement is the same one that is used to interrupt a closure or postural fixation or a perseverative repetition. The stutterer may reason that if the interruptor trick occasionally works to get him out of the un-pleasantness it may also aid him as a "starter," a term stutterers commonly use among themselves for this behavior. Sometimes starters may occur in organized sequences as ritualistic behavior, each component of which must be used before its successor is employed:

> In opposing his impediment, the stammerer has frequent recourse to starters and wedges. He may begin his sentences with such words as *Oh* or *listen,* or *well,* or *now;* he may use such phrases as *I say* or *let's see;* or he may use irrelevant sounds such as *ha-ha*—or *he-he*—or *uh-uh-uh-uh-uh.* One young man began his sentence with *it-tay-yer,* which he sing-songed, and repeated with rising pitch and increasing intensity (Bluemel, 1957, p. 48).
>
> Many who stutter work out "starters" for themselves. Some pound with

their foot, some make a certain grimace, some have trick sounds, or voice pitch. All of them deplore this and feel it to be unfortunate; but such things, which are considered voluntary, are often compulsive and are a part of the stutter (Blanton and Blanton, 1936, p. 77).

We know one stutterer who used an old nursery rhyme spoken in pantomime and accompanied by different gestures: "One for the money (head nod); two for the show (squeezing the lips); three to get ready (slow inhalation); and four to go! suddenly hitting himself on the side)." The speech attempt was made always in unison with the last of these. Occasionally, after a long postponement in which he was usually completely silent and immobile, this stutterer would run through the sequence several times, and then the performance would be far more abnormal than if he had merely struggled through the utterance to begin with. No one who saw this behavior would ever think it was disorganized or breakdown behavior. It was highly integrated and stereotyped, although it was certainly difficult to believe it was useful. Nevertheless, this stutterer said, "it worked" (i.e., he felt it prevented the more devastating experience of closure and tremor often enough so that he continued to use the routine.) Many stutterers continue to use starters that seldom "start," and much of their abnormality can be traced to these behaviors.

ABULIA

This term refers to the inability to make decisions or to act or perform certain voluntary movements. It is a sort of psychosomatic dyspraxia. It is the ultimate of procrastination and is well known in psychopathology. The stutterer, caught midway between two alternatives, both full of misery, just stays put. Abulia always represents a very advanced stage of the disorder and is a most difficult problem for the therapist to treat. The mand * type of self-talk seems to be lacking. We have seen stutterers almost in a trance, almost cataleptic, their postures frozen and rigid. They tell us that in these states, their consciousness of self is very low and that often they do not even see or hear their listeners. Fortunately, most stutterers do not reach this stage. It is found more frequently in those who use silent postponements than in those who use vocalized ones.

THE HISTORY OF ACCESSORY REACTIONS

In several cases we have been able to study the development of these instrumental responses. Most stutterers start off using behaviors that are socially acceptable and quite normal: the pauses, the use of "ah" or "um," the repetition of words previously spoken. Next appear the timing devices

* See Skinner (1957).

to terminate the postponement. Then these reactions change and become foreshortened, retaining only their dominant features in skeletal form, e.g. the pursing of the lips and elevation of the larynx as the residue of a former swallowing reaction. As this compression of the response takes place, the reaction becomes more and more automatic and stereotyped. It becomes tied to word fear. It becomes habitual, even compulsive in response to the phonetic, durational, or semantic cues of a feared word, a part of the stuttering language he speaks. At this stage the stutterer feels unable to inhibit or even to vary the postponement behavior. The duration and form of the postponement reactions vary directly and automatically with the amount of the fear.

It is at this point that something new is added. The tremors, the closures, the postural fixations, and recoils that formerly had their locus in the actual speech attempt now move forward in time to invade the postponement behavior that was originally used to avoid them. When this happens, the stuttering, as may be imagined, increases greatly in severity. Now the postponement behaviors do not postpone but instead precipitate. The distraction devices no longer distract or prevent the occurrence of abnormality but rather contribute to it. The stutterer's starters do not start. His timing tricks no longer facilitate utterance but only complicate it by their compulsivity.

We have watched stutterers go up these steps, sometimes skipping one or two of them in the process, but the disorder always spirals in severity as the automaticity increases. In the most severe stutterers there is a final stage in which the stutterer either becomes interiorized and abulic or gives up all avoidance and resorts to intense struggle and interruptor devices. Some stutterers just stop talking. Of course not all stutterers run the entire gamut. Most in fact stop short of these final behaviors, but every therapist should be highly aware of the dangers involved in any therapeutic method that may enhance the natural tendency of stutterers to avoid or postpone their speech attempts.

THE RESEARCH ON OVERT BEHAVIOR

Clinical descriptions of stutterers' behavior are found throughout the literature, but actual research on this aspect of the disorder is scanty. Van Riper (1937) analyzed the behaviors of severe stutterers and found that many of them were learned reactions to the anticipation or experience of being blocked. He analyzed these into five categories: avoidance, postponement, starters, antiexpectancy devices, and release reactions. He found that although the patterning of these learned responses showed much variability from stutterer to stutterer, it was very consistent for the individual stutterer.

Sheehan (1946) made phonetic transcriptions of the speech of 20 stutterers who had not had therapy. The only common features were repetitions of syllables or prolongations of sounds. There was a wide variability of other reactions, but for each subject, stuttering behaviors aligned themselves into a definite sequence or pattern. Most stutterers showed several of these characteristic patterns, depending on the phonetic properties of the word or sound involved.

Barr (1940) found that all her stutterers showed repetitions of syllables and prolongations of sounds. Nine specific phenomena accounted for more than 25 per cent of all stuttering behaviors. They were: repetition, prolongation, silent gap, lip tremor, extraneous sounds, eye-blinking, breath-holding, jaw tremor, and movements of the forehead or eyebrow. She also mentions marked intersubject variability but consistent patterns for the individual stutterer. Black (1957) investigated this consistency in two readings of the same material. She found a mean rho of .64 for sequences of stuttering behaviors; specific behaviors were even more consistent from reading to reading. Bloodstein (1960) in his cross-sectional developmental study of stuttering behaviors found that repetitions and prolongations occur at all ages and that hard contacts, struggle, and associated movements as well as avoidance behaviors increase with age. This was corroborated by Andrews and Harris (1964). Many studies, notably those by Fossler (1930), Henrickson (1936), Van Riper (1936), and Brankel (1961) have displayed the many breathing abnormalities shown by stutterers. Schilling (1960) reported tremors and irregular clonic movements of the diaphragm during both speech and silence.

Stutenroth (1937) analyzed autobiographical material for the presence of avoidance behaviors and found that they clustered around vocational, heterosexual, and status relationships. Kimmel (1938) repeated the study more carefully and found similar results. Douglass and Quarrington (1952) showed that much of the behavior of so-called interiorized stutterers was the result of avoidance. Quarrington and Douglass (1960) compared groups of stutterers in whom stuttering was predominantly vocalized with another group in whom it was not, and discovered that the nonvocalized group had less stuttering in a situation where the stuttering was not heard by a listener than in a situation where it was.

Snidecor (1955) studied the tension patterns reported by stutterers and found the chief locus of tension in the speech muscles, although spreading to other areas often occurred. An earlier study by Draseke (1921), based on snapshots, showed a similar overflow of struggle from a central locus in the mouth outward even to the limbs. Sheehan and Voas (1954) found that electromyographic recordings of a small number of subjects demonstrated a peak of tension just before the release from blocking. This peaking of tension at this point in the stuttering sequence was not observed, however, by Schrum (1967). Also using electromyography, Schrum found that stutterers showed more tensions, and that the tension lasted longer in the jaw, neck, and chest areas on stuttered as compared with nonstuttered words. Gertner and Luper (1967) found that stutterers as compared had longer linguoalveolar contacts than nonstutterers as observed with cine-fluorography. Chevrie-Miller (1963), employing glottography, studied the action of the larynx in stuttering. She found many anomalies of laryngeal function including breaks in the rhythm of vocal fold vibration and a clonic fluttering of the folds in some but not all of her stutterers. Lohr (1969) made a frame-by-frame analysis of motion pictures of stutterers and found marked variability from subject to subject and a lack of consistency in behaviors even for the same individual. Unfortunately she did not investigate the consistency of stuttering patterns on the same words or words beginning with the same sound, and it is in this context that consistency is most apparent. One very interesting finding was that unilateral deviations of the lips and jaws to the left side were twice as frequent as deviations to the right. Eye closing and blinking, and suspension of lip and jaw activity were characteristic of the stuttering of all subjects. These subjects were confirmed stutterers receiving therapy in a summer camp and had a mean age of 17 years.

COMMENTARY

Most stutterers strive for fluency, but their devices usually result in increased abnormality. When the speech blockage occurs, they attempt to force their way through the spasm and may succeed in uttering the word fluently. The amount of effort to achieve this, however, results in abnormal and bizarre bodily struggle phenomena. For a few seconds, usually not more than fifteen seconds, the stutterer struggles and displays facial grimaces, with contortive movements of all or any part of the body. For this period, not only is phonation arrested, but respiration too is suspended. Eventually the word or syllable is emitted (Douglass, 1954, p. 366).

Blocks have a great variety of forms. Some are very conspicuous with many audible and visible characteristics such as tremors, grimaces, irrelevant sounds, and great struggles which sometimes resemble epileptic seizures (Lennon, 1962, p. 1).

It was terrible at times when he tried to talk. He'd squeeze his eyes and grit his teeth and sometimes he hit his fist against his leg (Robinson, 1964, p. 6).

What he does when he stutters is similarly a series of movements of which he is largely unaware, though they may include a number of extraneous movements that are, from the viewpoint of an observer with some awareness of how the vocal mechanism operates, sometimes superfluous and sometimes directly contradictory to the movements that are needed. For example, a stutterer who blocks on the first sound of "mother" may, at the moment of blocking, have his mouth open, although the normal production of the first sound in *mother* requires that the mouth be closed. Or he may have his mouth closed as he attempts to initiate the word *uncle* whose first sound requires that the mouth be open (Villareal, 1962, p. 108).

One capable young man, a pupil of ours, would always go through this complex form of response on the approach of a /c/ word. His tongue would always take the /t/ position first, and then the last acquired /c/ position, saying the word as t-t-t-c-come. Three times on the /t/ position, then two attempts on /c/ and a complex "come" was produced (Young, 1928, p. 86).

Another kind of symptom occurs in the "er," "well," etc., that the stutterer used to get started. Sometimes this "starter" is an inarticulate but complicated grunt. Often the patient has to make severe contortions of the face or the head or the body before he can begin. A frequent phenomenon is the expulsion of the breath just before speaking. It is not unusual to find a patient who never has any symptom of stuttering in the presence of the physician except the monotonous laryngeal tone. I have never seen a stutterer without this symptom (Scripture, 1923, p. 13).

It is suggested by the present writer that one reason why the stutterer's motor plan breaks down is that he puts his articulators into an unnatural position as part of getting ready for the point in the sequence which is perceived to be difficult. As a result of being in this unnatural position, he literally does not know how to get out of it—because he has departed so far from the correct and unconscious sequence of overlapping movements that he cannot get back into the right sequence. It seems not at all unlikely that the reason why many stutterers go back and repeat several words which preceded the word on which the block is taking place is that they are attempting to start over again in the right sequence in its entirety without interruption. This type of behavior on the part of the stutterer seems quite analogous to what the musician will do when he has played a note incorrectly. The probability is that the musician will return to the beginning of the passage and play that entire passage again. This he will do in contrast to any attempt to stop immediately after playing the given note incorrectly, play that note again correctly and then continue from that point to finish the rest of the passage (Frick, 1965, p. 6).

It is readily apparent that stuttering patterns vary from one stutterer to another, and that for an individual stutterer the pattern may change with time. The basis for this variation, it is believed, is to be found in a learning process. Those symptoms are acquired which are accompanied by reinforcement. Clinical observation indicates that stutterers may consciously utilize certain movements, facial and bodily, because as they say "they feel it helps them to get the word out." Such movements ultimately become integrated through continual reinforcement into the total stuttering pattern (Wischner, 1950, p. 333).

Respiratory disturbances are common in this secondary phase of stammering. The stammerer holds his breath, then gasps as though in distress.

He may exhaust the breath, then attempt to talk on empty lungs. He may open his mouth and gasp loudly before beginning to talk. He may gasp for breath between words and even in the middle of words. He may make little gasping sounds which give an aspirate quality to his consonants; his words may sound as though they were full of h's (Bluemel, 1957, p. 46).

Tremor is a biologically preformed component of the anxiety reaction. When stress is past, it subsides and disappears. Many men emerged from acute war trauma trembling violently all over, but in most cases the tremor gradually subsides. In certain cases, however, the tremor did not subside, it lasted and became a permanent hysterical symptom.

The tremor patients, therefore, could be considered as quite involuntarily sustaining their reflex tremor by keeping up a slight hypertonicity of musculature (Brown and Menninger, 1940, p. 286).

Hard contacts and prolongations are the characteristic symptoms of stuttering. They appeared, associated with considerable strain, in even the youngest children. In a few cases it seemed that they were the first symptoms of stuttering, although it was possible that the repetitions had been overlooked and the stutter diagnosed only when the more markedly abnormal symptoms became prominent (Andrews and Harris, 1964, p. 10).

When needle electrodes were placed in the stutterers' lingual muscles for taking electrocardiograms, it was found that the stutterers became fluent. It is usually observed that stuttering tremors are inhibited when the stutterer bites his tongue or pinches his tongue by paper clip, or pinches the lips or when pressure is given to any musculature which is directly related to speech production. The investigator explains this phenomena in terms of its resemblance to the tremors of Parkinsons and paralysis agitans, which can be stopped by pressing the affected areas by a hand. This inhibitory mechanism is explained in terms of the neurological function of the extrapyramidal system (Fujita, 1954, p. 290).

Each stutterer fears certain sounds. In order to avoid them, he continually attempts new *alternations of sentence construction*. From these efforts result stereotyped but meaningless clichés of speech with dysgrammatic or syntactical disturbances of sentence structure. When the stutterer decides to avoid the cliffs of his verbal obstacles after he has begun his utterance, he may even end up saying the opposite of what he had planned to say (Luchsinger and Arnold, 1965, p. 751).

Exactly as might be expected, the first devices to develop are those which arise in response to the feeling of being blocked; those which represent reactions to the anticipation of stuttering come afterward (Bloodstein, 1960, p. 224).

The stronger the closure the stronger is the explosion after such a blockage. The amount of closure force and the intensity of the burst of sound are correlated in their intensity (Grewel, 1960, p. 116).

Here's the way one seventh grade boy told us about his difficulty: "I just s-s-s-s-seem to get s-s-s-s-s (here he stopped, inhaled, and started over) s-s-s-stuck on that——s-s-sound." He often expelled practically all the air from his lungs before completing troublesome words, and at times, as on *stuck*, he would interrupt the prolongation to take in more air. This boy had similar though less pronounced trouble on the /f/ and /sh/ sounds as well as tonic-type blocks on plosive consonants (Robinson, 1964, p. 7).

Constant preparedness, constant vigilance to guard against revelation of his stutter, complete avoidance of possible situations anticipated as threatening, are all evidenced. Every eventuality must be anticipated so that he can either avoid the danger entirely or meet it fully prepared. To be caught unprepared would be a tragedy. When stuttering cannot be warded off entirely, he then utilizes rather specific devices like coughing, blowing his nose, hand gestures, standing up and sitting down just at the "right" moment. These and many other "natural" movements used by normal speakers are adopted and adapted by the interiorized stutterer to disguise his stuttering moments. Indeed, with enough dodges, he succeeds in achieving his goal of avoiding overt stuttering.

The typical exteriorized stutterer fears moments of stuttering, also, and does his best to minimize the abnormality. The adoption of stuttering devices, when originally adopted, did, in fact, serve the intended purpose; that is, they facilitated oral expression. Constant exaggeration of the device, however, became necessary (Douglass and Quarrington, 1952, p. 379).

Other patients paroxysmally press nearly all air out of their lungs, and when almost completely exhausted, succeed in uttering one or two words (Stein, 1942, p. 109).

By far the most frequent breathing abnormality at every age is the habit of terminating a stuttering block with a sudden, sharp exhalation that results in the remainder of the word being spoken on residual air. This single mannerism perhaps occurs more often than most other associated symptoms put together (Bloodstein, 1960, p. 233).

The thing that discouraged me most of all was the realization that I could no longer detour around a difficult bugaboo word with the substitution of a clever synonym, a ruse which I had developed very successfully in high school. Much of my study time was spent in searching for synonyms which might be used in place of words that begin with hard, explosive consonants. I never found a synonym for the word *trapezoid*. I remember standing before a class in mathematics, trying to explain something about a lopsided figure on the blackboard. It wasn't a parallelogram or a trapezium—words which I could say because the accent did not fall upon the first syllable—but for this professor it had to be called a trapezoid. I got as far as the word trapezoid in my explanation when my tongue froze to the roof of my mouth. Some kind student in the front row relieved me by saying the word. "Yes," I agreed, "this t-t-t" and again my tongue stuck, tighter than ever, to my palate. One of the campus wits called me "trapezoid" that afternoon and I carried the name for many weeks. Every time I heard the word my conscience burned with self reproach and made me wish I had never attempted college. I developed a keen word consciousness that doubled the severity of my affliction (Wedberg, 1937, pp. 24–25).*

The accessory movements and avoidances "are not merely chance products of random instrumental learning but necessarily reflect the dynamics of the stutterer and the pattern of instrumental relations from which they emerged. The stutterer's pattern is not a superficial symptom but a significant and revealing part of the stutterer's personality (Sheehan, 1958, pp. 129–130).

BIBLIOGRAPHY

Andrews, G., and M. Harris, *The Syndrome of Stuttering.* London: Heinemann, 1964.

Barr, H., "A Quantitative Study of Specific Phenomena Observed in Stuttering," *Journal of Speech Disorders,* V (1940), 277–80.

Black, P. C., "A Study of the Consistency of Sequences of Stuttering Behavior." Master's thesis, University of Pittsburg, 1957.

Blanton, S., and M. G. Blanton, *For Stutterers.* New York: Appleton, 1936.

Bloodstein, O., "The Development of Stuttering," *Journal of Speech and Hearing Disorders,* XXV (1960), 219–37; 366–76; XXVI (1961), 67–82.

Bluemel, C. S., *The Riddle of Stuttering.* Danville, Ill.: Interstate, 1957.

Boome, E. J., and M. A. Richardson, *The Nature and Treatment of Stammering.* London: Methuen, 1932.

Brankel, O., ["Pneumotachographic Studies in Stutterers,"] *Folia Phoniatrica,* XIII (1961), 136–43.

Chevrie-Muller, C., ["A Study of Laryngeal Function in Stutterers by the Glotto-Graphic Method"] *Proceedings, VIIᵉ Congrès de la Société Française de Médecine de la Voix et de la Parole,* Paris, 1963.

Douglass, E., and B. Quarrington, "The Differentiation of Interiorized and Exteriorized Secondary Stuttering," *Journal of Speech Disorders,* XVII (1952), 372–88.

Douglass, E., "Development of Stuttering and its Diagnosis," *Canadian Medical Association Journal,* LXXI (1954), 366–71.

Draseke, J., "Über Mitbewegungen bei Gesunden," *Deutsche Zeitschrift für Nervenheilkunde,* LXIV (1921), 340–46.

Fossler, H., "Disturbances in Breathing During Stuttering," *Psychological Monographs,* I (1930), 1–32.

Freund, H., *Psychopathology and the Problem of Stuttering.* Springfield, Ill.: Thomas, 1966.

Frick, J. V., *Evaluation of Motor Planning Techniques for the Treatment of Stuttering.* Final Report, Grant No. 32-48-0720-5003. U. S. Department Health, Education and Welfare, Office of Education, 1965.

---

* From *The Stutterer Speaks* by Conrad Wedberg. Reprinted by permission of Expression Company, Publishers, Magnolia, Mass.

Fujita, K., ["Tremor Control as a Factor in Stuttering,"] *Japanese Journal of Otology,* LVII (1955), 287–91.

Gertner, L. L., and H. L. Luper, "A Cinefluorographic Study of the Duration and Number of Lingual-Alveolar Articulatory Contacts and Reading Time of Stutterers and Nonstutterers," convention address, A.S.H.A., 1967.

Grewel, F., "Balbuties (Stotteren)" *Logopaedie et Foniatrie,* XXXII (1960), 109–15; 125–28; 145–52; 165–68.

Gottlober, A. B., *Understanding Stuttering.* New York: Grune and Stratton, 1953.

Henrickson, E. H., "Simultaneously Recorded Breathing and Vocal Disturbances of Stutterers," *Archives of Speech,* I (1936), 133–49.

Johnson, W., *Because I Stutter.* New York: Appleton, 1930.

Kanner, L., *Child Psychiatry.* Springfield, Ill.: Thomas, 1942.

Kenyon, E. L., "The Etiology of Stammering: The Psychophysiologic Facts which Concern the Production of Speech Sounds and of Stammering," *Journal of Speech Disorders,* VIII (1943), 337–48.

Kimmell, W., "The Nature and Effect of Stutterers' Avoidance Reactions," *Journal of Speech Disorders,* III (1938), 95–100.

Kussmaul, A., "Die Störungen der Sprache," in H. V. Ziemssen (ed.), *Cyclopaedia Medica* (1877).

Lennon, E. J., *Le Begaiement: Thérapeutiques Modernes.* Paris: G. Doin, 1962.

Lohr, F., "Visible Manifestations of Stuttered Speech," convention address, A.S.H.A., 1969.

Luchsinger, R., and G. E. Arnold, *Voice—Speech—Language.* Belmont, Cal.: Wadsworth, 1965.

Makuen, G. H., "A Study of 1000 Cases of Stammering with Special Reference to the Etiology and Treatment of the Affection," *Therapeutical Gazette,* XXXVIII (1914), 385–90.

Moser, H. M., "Symposium on Unique Cases of Speech Disorders: Presentation of a Case," *Journal of Speech Disorders,* VII (1942), 173–74.

Quarrington, B., and E. Douglass, "Audibility Avoidance in Nonvocalized Stutterers," *Journal of Speech and Hearing Disorders,* XXV (1960), 358–65.

Robinson, F. B., *Introduction to Stuttering.* Englewood Cliffs, N.J.: Prentice-Hall, 1964.

Rotter, J. B., "A Working Hypothesis as to the Nature and Treatment of Stuttering," *Journal of Speech Disorders,* VII (1942), 263–88.

Schilling, A., ["Diaphragmatic Radiokymograms in Stuttering,"] *Folia Phoniatrica,* XII (1960), 145–53.

Schrum, W. F., "A Study of the Speaking Behavior of Stutterers and Non-Stutterers by Means of Multichannel Electromyography," convention address, A.S.H.A., 1967.

Scripture, E. W., *Stuttering and Lisping,* (2nd Ed.). New York: Macmillan, 1923.

Sheehan, J., "A Study of the Phenomena of Stuttering," Master's thesis, University of Michigan, 1946.

———. "Modification of Stuttering Through Non-reinforcement," *Journal of Abnormal and Social Psychology,* XLVI (1951), 51–63.

———. "Projective Studies of Stuttering," *Journal of Speech and Hearing Disorders,* XXIII (1958), 18–25.

———. "Conflict Theory of Stuttering," J. Eisenson (ed.), *Stuttering: A Symposium.* New York: Harper, 1958.

Sheehan, J. G., and R. B. Voas, "Tension Patterns During Stuttering in Relation to Conflict, Anxiety Binding and Reinforcement," *Speech Monographs,* XXI (1954), 272–79.

Skinner, B. F., *Verbal Behavior.* New York: Appleton, 1957.

Snidecor, J. C., "Tension and Facial Appearance in Stuttering," W. Johnson (ed.), *Stuttering in Children and Adults.* Minneapolis: University of Minnesota Press, 1955, 377–80.

Stein, L., *Speech and Voice.* London: Methuen, 1942.

Stetson, R. H., *Motor Phonetics.* Amsterdam: North-Holland, 1951.

Stutenroth, R. I., "Specific Reactions by which Stutterers Attempt to Avoid Stuttering." Master's thesis, State University of Iowa, 1937.

Van Riper, C., "A Study of the Stutterer's Ability to Interrupt Stuttering Spasms," *Journal of Speech Disorders,* I (1936), 61–72.

———. "Effect of Devices for Minimizing Stuttering on the Creation of Symptoms," *Journal of Abnormal and Social Psychology,* XXXII (1937), 63–65.

———. "The Growth of the Stuttering Spasm," *Quarterly Journal of Speech,* XXIII (1937), 70–73.

———. "The Preparatory Set in Stuttering," *Journal of Speech Disorders,* II (1937), 149–54.

———. "Study of the Thoracic Breathing of Stutterers During Expectancy of Occurrence of Stuttering," *Journal of Speech Disorders,* I (1936), 61–72.

Van Riper, C., and R. Milisen, "A Study of the Predicted Duration of the Stutterer's Blocks as Related to Their Actual Duration," *Journal of Speech Disorders,* IV (1939), 339–45.

Villareal, J. J., "The Role of the Speech Pathologist in Psychotherapy," in D. A. Barbara (ed.), *The Psychotherapy of Stuttering.* Springfield, Ill.: Thomas, 1962.

Young, E. H., *Help For You Who Stutter.* Minneapolis: Hill-Young School, 1928.

Wedberg, C. F., *The Stutterer Speaks.* Magnolia, Mass.: Expression Company, 1937.

Wischner, G. J., "Stuttering Behavior and Learning," *Journal of Speech Disorders,* XV (1950), 324–35.

Wyllie, J., *The Disorders of Speech.* Edinburgh: Oliver and Boyd, 1894.

seven

PHENOMENOLOGY:
COVERT REACTIONS AND LOCI

This chapter describes the feelings, reactions, and attitudes of those who stutter. It is a difficult task, almost an impossible one. There is an immense array of these responses to the fear and experience of stuttering. Moreover, their precise definition and measurement would require an objectivity that is impossible because they are covert and hidden. Research deals with them obliquely since the instruments for measuring emotional states are far from satisfactory. Much of our knowledge is based only on verbal testimony, on introspective accounts which themselves leave much to be desired. Those of us who have been stutterers may read our own experiences into these clinical accounts and distort them. It is very hard to find words that fit the squirting of our glands. Only poets have those words. Over a hundred years ago one of these poets wrote the following:

Come, I will show thee an affliction unnumbered among the world's
    sorrows,
Yet real and wearisome and constant, embittering the cup of life.
There be who can think within themselves, and the fires burneth at
    their heart,
And eloquence waiteth at their lips, yet they speak not with their
    tongue;
There be those whom zeal quickeneth, or slander stirreth to reply,
Or need constraineth to ask, or pity sendeth as her messengers,

But nervous dread and sensitive shame freeze the current of their speech:
The mouth is sealed as with lead, a cold weight presseth on the heart,
The mocking promise of power is once more broken in performance,
And they stand impotent of words, travailing with unborn thoughts,
Courage is cowed at the portal, wisdom is widowed of utterance:
He that went to comfort is pitied, he that should rebuke is silent,
And fools who might listen and learn, stand by to look and laugh:
While friends, with kinder eyes, wound deeper by compassion:
And thought, finding not a vent, smouldereth gnawing at the heart,
And the man sinketh in his sphere for lack of empty sounds.
There may be cares and sorrows thou hast not yet considered,
And well may thy soul rejoice in the fair privilege of speech:
For at every turn to want a word—thou canst not guess that want;
It is as lack of breath or bread; life hath no grief more galling (Tupper, 1861).

Nevertheless, enough students of the disorder have been able to record their impressions of the stutterer's covert behavior with enough similarity so that it can be described with some confidence. These cautions, however, should be borne in mind.

FEARS

Perhaps the most common of the advanced stutterer's feelings is fear. Fear is the expectation of unpleasantness. This expectation ranges from vague doubt to complete certainty. The expected unpleasantness itself is also highly variable. The stutterer may be afraid of social penalty and stigma; he may dread listener loss or some other kind of rejection. Nonstuttering therapists often think these are the only things feared, but most of the stutterers with whom we have worked have told us that there is another more basic fear—the expectation of communicative inability and verbal impotence. What they fear most is the momentary loss of self-control. They dread the moment of muteness, of spasmodic contortion; they anticipate with foreboding the repetitions or fixations that seem both mysterious and involuntary. One stutterer called the moment of blockage the *petit mort*, the moment of the little death. The inability to move a muscle when you want to move it, a muscle that you can normally move with ease, is traumatic to the basic integrity of the self. Equally devastating is the experience of being unable to stop doing something that you don't want to do. As one of our stutterers said,

> What really scares me is when I start to say a word and find myself saying the same syllable over and over again and I can't stop, or when I find myself making a yard of an *s* sound when I only want a quarter inch of it. I get petrified when I fear this sort of thing is going to happen. I feel as helpless

as a ventriloquist's dummy. Something, somebody else is in charge of my mouth and I can't do anything about it.

This seems to be a very common and basic experience. We have seen little children stop suddenly after a perseverative repetition, cry uncontrollably, and run to their mothers for comfort. Their eyes, at least to us, seemed full of fear. In our opinion, this core experience is not simply frustration at stymied communication. That is present, of course, but something more traumatic is also occurring. It is the sudden loss of the ability to command oneself.

There are other unpleasant events to anticipate. Chief among these are the various punishing listener reactions. Few stutterers are able to run the verbal gauntlet of their days and years without receiving some hard blows from someone with whom they talk. Pity, rudeness, and rejection are commonly experienced. Most of our cases report having had listeners mock or humiliate them. Most have met at least a few vivid reactions of impatience and irritation. They remember the occasional cruel comment of a stranger, teacher, parent, or playmate. They have watched their friends be amused by some stuttering character on television and many came to think these reactions were universal, although perhaps kept hidden out of politeness. They have winced when, as children, they read about P-p-p-porky the p-pig in the comic strips. There are many jokes about stutterers, some of them very funny too—except to the stutterer. In short, most stutterers have been badly hurt by society's reaction to their disability. Most of them sense their deviance keenly. From India comes this account:

> The patients feel more unhappy by the treatment they meet at the hands of their fellow beings than by the ailment itself. Of course, the ailment itself is a great handicap to make them unhappy but the unsympathetic treatment adds to the misery of the patients. It is the sneering, zeering, and snubbing of the fellow beings . . . that make them feel the burden all the more heavy. And there is no dearth of persons who even take delight in copying a stammerer. The treatment . . . mentioned above creates an emotional mood in the patients. They become suspicious and quarrelsome or timid and shy (Mathur, 1960, p. 58).

But the stutterer often also finds rejection when it is not really there. Because he has difficulty communicating and is reluctant to reveal his sensitivity, he has few opportunities to test the reality of his suspicions. Most normal speakers find it frustrating to listen to a stutterer, but only a few ever show the marked rejection the stutterer attributes to them, simply because they are more concerned with other things. Nevertheless, imagined or real, social penalties are certainly important in the genesis and the maintenance of the stutterer's fears.

One of the more unpleasant aspects of stuttering is the ever present threat of exposure. Until he stutters, the stutterer looks and sounds quite normal. Since stuttering is intermittent and since there are many ways of hiding it, the mild stutterer always lives under the sword of Damocles, never knowing with certainty when the hair that holds it will break. Using his entire repertoire of avoidance and disguise reactions, he may be able to hide his impediment from many of his casual acquaintances or the strangers to whom he must talk briefly. But he always feels the threat of exposure. These stutterers live constantly in verbal jeopardy.

Although social penalties are unpleasant in themselves, the emotional reactions they generate in the stutterer are even more disagreeable. Feelings of unworthiness, embarrassment, shame, and guilt are common. Sometimes these feelings reverberate as the stutterer relives a traumatic experience over and over again, nursing his misery to keep it warm. Old wounds ache most when the wind blows cold. And when the stutterer feels moody or depressed for other reasons his stuttering curse seems intolerable. Some stutterers react to listener penalties with anger and hate. There are some very hostile stutterers, whose rage, bred of frustration and penalty, constantly seethes beneath the surface, occasionally breaking out in asocial attacks with a suddenness and vehemence incomprehensible to the listener. Other stutterers, less able to release their hostility outwardly, turn it upon themselves. Even little children sometimes slap their own faces or pinch themselves viciously after a volley of stuttering. Scripture gives a vivid picture:

> Few persons realize how terrible life becomes to a stutterer. One religious but stuttering lady finally demanded to be "cured or chloroformed." One boy often threw himself on the floor, begging his mother to tell him how to die. Many stutterers become so sensitive that they imagine everybody is constantly making fun of them. The stutterer prefers to be thought lazy or stupid rather than reveal the true nature of his trouble. A condition of mental flurry is usually present. When the patient starts to speak, he becomes partly dazed by his emotion and does not know exactly what he wants to say. This condition may be present even when he does not stutter; in trying to answer a question, for example, he cannot make up his mind just what he wishes to say. The embarrassment and sad experiences of the stutterer often lead to an abnormal mental condition. The patient is nervous, shy, easily embarrassed, retiring, odd in his ways, sad, etc. In some cases the change does not go beyond an increased sensitiveness. Many stutterers, especially young women and schoolboys, acquire a permanent facial expression that is typical of the profoundest sadness. The thought of suicide is frequent. It may be suggested that stuttering is a defect which tends to exclude the person from the society of his fellows, and that persons who already have this unconscious tendency instinctively seize upon such a means of encouraging it (1923, p. 3).

These emotional upheavals can be anticipated by the stutterer, and since they are not pleasant experiences, they are dreaded, whether the anticipation is one of hostility or shame or anxiety. Even fear can be feared.

THE PRECIPITANTS OF FEAR

Stuttering fears first begin as the consequences of these various unpleasant experiences. The context in which the unpleasant experience occurs determines the stimuli that will later precipitate fear. These stimuli fall into several categories: (1) characteristics of the listeners, (2) the content or implications of the message, (3) the words and their position in the utterance, and (4) the acoustic and motoric features of the sounds on which the stuttering occurs. Any of these, and any combination of them can serve as stimuli that will precipitate stuttering fears. It all depends on how the stutterer perceives them. Each stutterer develops his own particular pattern of fear-invested cues based on his perceptions, and these fears can generalize to other cues, following the laws of classical conditioning.

Much has been made of the role of the listener in stuttering since Wendell Johnson suggested that it began in the listener's ear rather than in the stutterer's mouth. Stuttering is apparently as much a disorder of communication as it is of speech; the receiver is at least as important as the sender in the interchange. There is a wealth of testimony from cases and research findings confirming the importance of the listener as a precipitator of stuttering fears. Stutterers scan their listeners with the intensity and care of a robber casing a bank. Again there are many individual differences. One stutterer's computer is programmed to read out FEAR if his prospective listener is of the opposite sex, is voluble, and older; another's so that the facial expression of the listener, his size, and probable vocation are inspected and responded to in that order. One of our stutterers found it impossible to speak to children without immediate fear. "I've had too many mothers who dragged their frightened children away from me," he said. One stutterer even found it easier to talk to listeners who interrupted him because, as he remarked, "I can sneak in what I have to say under the cover of their talking." Another told us that the one situation in which he *always* felt fear was when talking to school teachers. "Old or young, male or female, elementary, secondary, or college, whatever they are, teachers always petrify me."

It is difficult to generalize, considering the wide variety of conditionings, but it seems apparent that listeners whose rejection would have truly unpleasant consequences precipitate more fear than those whose opinion is less important. Accordingly, most stutterers are afraid of speaking to people in authority, prospective employers, parents, teachers or prospective sexual mates. This generalization is also true for normal-speaking trainees in speech pathology who, as part of their practicum, are assigned to fake stuttering for a variety of listeners. One stutterer analyzed the content of 721 consecutive situation fears over a period of one month at the beginning of his therapy. These fears are given below, ranked in order of their frequency:

> 1. Fear of being ridiculed, smiled at, laughed at, viewed as being funny; 2. Fear of being exposed and classed as a stutterer, a deviant, an inferior, abnormal person, a speech defective; 3. Fear of being unable to communicate my message effectively in the allotted time; time pressure; frustration fear; 4. Fear of embarrassing my listener; 5. Fear of rebuke or impatience or rejection, either open or hidden, by my listener; 6. Fear that my listener will pity me; 7. Other (fear that I am not making progress; fear of relapse; fear that I will lose hope again, etc.)

The same stutterer rechecked his situation fears three months later, finding only 104 of them in the same period, and, although they were the same ones, the rank order had changed to 7, 3, 2, 5, 4, 6, 1. Much of the change resulted from reality-testing and the realization that most listeners are more curious than punitive. For example, his fear of mockery had been greatly exaggerated, and when a few listeners seemed to parrot him by opening their mouths when he gaped, or holding their breath when he did, it was more empathy than ridicule.

Many stutterers dread speaking to groups more than to individuals, probably because in a group there is a greater chance of at least one listener rejecting the stutterer. Even here, however, there are stutterers who react the opposite way, especially in situations where the stutterer is making a speech and possesses a captive audience. If he is especially vulnerable to listener loss, then he speaks better before a group. His listeners can't get away. To the beginning therapist in this field, who may feel overwhelmed by the diversity of stimuli that can precipitate the fear of stuttering, we can only say that each stutterer's phobic phenomena are unique because of his past conditioning and the particular patterns of generalization that have taken place. If we are to decondition and extinguish these fears, they must be identified for each individual. There are few rules and many exceptions. Yet these fears make sense. They have a history.

THE COMMUNICATIVE MILIEU: SITUATION FEARS

Stuttering does not occur in a vacuum but in an environment. This environment or milieu possesses distinctive features on which the stutterer may hang his dread. The telephone can become a frightening bugaboo if sufficient misery has been connected with its use. A doctor's office, a beauty parlor, a certain store can become dreaded places. The author of this text, long fluent, still feels fear when he sits in a certain chair of his old family home. For some children the schoolroom is colored with stuttering apprehension; others fear the playground. The bus station or airport, the employer's waiting room, even the church can be feared places. Again the patterns differ with different stutterers.

THE CONDITIONS
OF COMMUNICATION

Stutterers also scan the conditions under which communication will occur for signs that mean approaching stuttering. Chief among these is temporal urgency, the time factor. When the stutterer knows in advance that he must finish his communication in a hurry, the red flare of fear arises. One of our stutterers, a soldier in combat, said that when going out on night patrol his major fear was not of the enemy but of being challenged to give the password on his return. Part of the fear of the telephone is due to the knowledge that the stutterer must begin to speak within a relatively short time or hear the click of a hung-up receiver at the other end of the line.

Since stuttering is a disorder of time, and the communication of messages is impeded by repetitions, prolongations, or any of the coping behaviors, most stutterers seem especially vulnerable to this time pressure. Under such stress, they usually stutter more, and longer, and with greater abnormality. The apochryphal story is told of the stuttering king of England who, while a young man and an officer on board ship, was marching his marines on the foredeck. When the front ranks had their forelegs about to step over the ship's side, and he was still completely blocked from all utterance, one of his fellow officers is reputed to have queried, "Gad, sir, aren't you even going to bid them goodbye?" Once again, however, some stutterers have surprised themselves and their listeners by being able to speak completely fluently under great urgency. One of our patients was a member of a submarine crew who discovered a malfunctioning of some of the controls and was able to give a series of directions and reports under great time pressure without a trace of his usual stuttering, though he claimed his hair began to turn grey as the result of the experience. We asked him how he could explain his fluency under such stress. "I'm not sure," he replied. "I guess I had no time even to think of stuttering, or what I was going to say. I just had to say it and did." Others in similar emergencies have testified that great fears or great necessities have wiped out the specific fears or rehearsal behaviors that trigger the stuttering response, and so for a moment they are able to be fluent.

Usually, the amount of stuttering varies with the meaningfulness of the message to be communicated. The greater the propositionality or meaningfulness, the more stuttering. Stutterers can often repeat what someone else has already said. "Small talk" in conversation provides little difficulty. Stutterers can often interject the little "asides," the bits of commentary on what they have said, with little stuttering.

For some stutterers the presence of certain types of masking noise arouses fear. One stutterer claimed that every time he rode in the back seat of a car he knew he would stutter and that he had the same apprehension in the hubbub of a cocktail party. "It's hard to make yourself understood in these situations," he said, "and if I stutter I know I'll have to say the whole thing over again which means more trouble. That's why I fear noise." Other stutterers, usually the milder ones with few silent closures, find that such situations are much easier than those in which silence must be broken.

Some stutterers fear oral reading or recitation of memorized material because there is little opportunity for avoidance or disguise. The words cannot be dodged; all pauses will be apparent. Other stutterers find the same activities much easier because no burden of responsibility for message formulation is required, and a certain amount of distraction from the stuttering is produced by the necessity for reading or remembering. Again, in all of these, we find the loci of the stutterer's fears determined by individual past experience.

The frequency, duration, and abnormality of stuttering varies with the listener's reaction as the stutterer perceives it, a perception which may not be realistic. In general, stutterers have more difficulty speaking to rejecting listeners, or to those who show impatience, irritation, pity, or embarrassment. The *threat* of possible punishment for stuttering seems to evoke more of it. Thus, speaking to a listener of higher status, or who has the power to facilitate or negate the stutterer's desires, ordinarily produces more stuttering. Nevertheless, some stutterers speak much better when confronted with a hostile, rejecting listener. As one of them said,

> I won't let that bastard hear me stutter! Somehow, for a short time, I can rise to the occasion and summon up my energies and just refuse to stutter. I won't let him get the best of me. Of course, I couldn't keep it up very long, but I'd never put myself in a situation so I'd always have to be with a person like that.

A nice little old grey haired lady once put her arm around the author when he had been stuttering badly to a store clerk, and said to him, "My son, oh you poor boy, do you always have to stutter like that, you poor thing." To his surprise, if not to his credit, he answered, and with complete fluency for once, "No, Madame, only when I talk!" Although many stutterers have more difficulty speaking to strangers, others have none in this situation. One of the latter said:

> When I speak to a total stranger, one I have never seen before or expect to see again, I can talk perfectly, though I stutter badly to all the people who know me. I figure that the reason for this is that the stranger doesn't expect

to hear me stutter—there's no reminder. For a short time I can pass as normal as I look.

Again, the variability seems due to different learning experiences.

THE COMMUNICATIVE CONTENT

There are also certain semantic variables that precipitate the fear of stuttering. We have much research which indicates that propositionality (the amount of meaning) in a word or utterance produces more stuttering. The stutterer knows this well, and so he scans his anticipated communication for signals of this sort. Nouns, verbs, and adjectives generate more fear than do articles or conjunctions. The key word or phrase of a joke is approached with more trepidation than other words. Vital utterances are more dreaded than casual ones. The words of a given sentence do not all carry the same load of meaningfulness, and the stutterer knows that more communicative disruption will occur when he stutters on an important word than on an unimportant one. A common trick used by some stutterers to defeat the expectancy of stuttering is to lead up to the main message with a few sentences of casual, meaningless conversation. Small talk is less to be feared than big talk. Indeed, many stutterers employ such meaningless gambit phrases or words ("Well," "You know," "What I mean is . . .") as devices to get started. Perhaps the reason most stutterers sing without trouble is that the content of the message sung is so low in information value, though there are other explanations too. The adaptation effect—the reduction in stuttering with repeated utterances of the same material—has been attributed variously to anxiety reduction, or to reactive inhibition, but also to the inevitable reduction in the meaningfulness of the material being spoken over and over again. Even the most frantic adolescent would find it difficult to maintain the same meaningfulness in the phrase "I love you" were he to say it sequentially one hundred times. Nevertheless, there are stutterers who find small talk very difficult, and most stutterers, when they are compelled to repeat what they have already said fluently, will show more stuttering. There are also stutterers who do not show the usual adaptation effect, and there are those who speak much better when they are especially concerned with the content of their communication. One of them told us, "When I can just quit thinking about stuttering and think about what I'm trying to tell the other person, I'm very fluent."

The emotional content of the message may also serve as a precipitant of stuttering fear. Bardrick and Sheehan (1956) and others have shown that emotionally loaded words produce more stuttering than either ordinary communication or nonsense material. Stutterers say they fear these emotional utterances. In part this fear may arise from anticipated listener rejection. One of our stutterers left the Catholic church because of his stuttering experiences during confession. "It was not, alas, that I had many sins to confess but the tremendous fear of having to suffer so much stuttering over and over again every time I went to confession." Almost all ordinary speech has some emotional content, but some utterances are filled with it, and on these the stutterer anticipates unpleasantness, not only because listeners may react unfavorably, but also because of the inevitable confrontation of his own miserable feelings. Unpleasant speech doesn't taste good. It is interesting and understandable that expressions of anxiety and guilt seem to be more feared than those of anger.

LINGUISTIC PRECIPITANTS

One of the most prominent features of the confirmed stutterer is his intense scanning of a prospective utterance for linguistic cues associated with stuttering. We should not be surprised to find this since, after all, stuttering does occur on sounds, syllables and words. Furthermore, no one stutters on every word or sound, so one would expect the stutterer to scrutinize his sounds and words and their placement for danger signals if only to avoid the consequences. We have said that this scanning is intense. It is very difficult for the normal speaker to comprehend the vigilance, the alertness, the complex pre-testing of stuttering probabilities that goes on in the mind of the stutterer. It is one of his greatest burdens. Kazin (1951) gives this autobiographical account:

> The word was my agony. The word that for others was so effortless and so neutral, so unburdened, so simple, so exact, I had first to meditate in advance, to see if I could make it like a plumber, fitting together odd lengths and shapes of pipe. I was always preparing words I could speak, storing them away, choosing between them. And often, when the word did come from my mouth in its great and terrible birth, quailing and bleeding as if forced through a thornbush, I would not be able to look the others in the face, and would walk out in silence, the infinitely echoing silence behind my back, to say it all cleanly back to myself as I walked in the streets . . . only then was it possible for me to speak without the infinite premeditations and strangled silences I toiled through whenever I got up in school to respond with the expected, the exact answer (p. 67).

PHONEME FEARS

Of all the verbal stimuli that precipitate stuttering fears, phonemes and their distinctive features are probably the most vital. When stutterers remember their past experiences, the initial sounds of words stand out most clearly. "Words beginning with /b/, /p/, and /t/ consonants give me more trouble," one stutterer will tell you. Another may have a totally different set of feared phonemes. Again the past conditioning accounts for the variation. We even find stutterers claiming that 'h' words such as 'hour' are feared (although that word really begins with a vowel), thus indicating that the visual aspect of the spelling has come to be a stimulus. Stutterers may say that they fear the "s" sound when actually they produce that sound fluently far more often than they stutter on it. Some will inform you that vowel sounds are their "Jonah" or unlucky sounds but only when they occur in the initial position of a word. Others have generalized their feared stimuli to include all lip sounds or all tongue-tip sounds. The important thing to remember is that these stimuli are not distributed at random in any given stutterer; they have loci and foci; they have been conditioned.

Stutterers rarely fear the final sounds of words or syllables. Spencer Brown (1938) says:

> The beginning of a word has for the stutterer a far greater importance than the rest of the word. This is shown by the fact that of the spasms recorded in the data studied, 92 per cent were in relation to the initial sound of the words with only 8 per cent occurring at all other points. Other evidence showing this primacy for the stutterer of the initial part of the word is found in the introspections of stutterers. They report that they think of "s-words" or "k-words" and fear stuttering with relation to the initial sound of the word. Several stutterers who reported that they feared s-words such as *see, seven, side,* etc., did not report such fears with relation to the *s* sound when it occurred at the beginning of the second or third syllable of a word, and questioned on the point said they did not fear the *s* in such words as *inside, consent, Robertson,* etc. Furthermore, many stutterers insist that they never stutter except at the beginning of a word (p. 113).

However they do have occasional fears of the sounds beginning accented syllables of longer words, especially on the sounds also feared in the initial position. Perceptually, each word presents to the stutterer a configuration of features any one of which may have been associated with unpleasant past experiences. The phoneme with which the word begins, the length of the word, the way it is spelled, its relative familiarity, its dominant syllable—any of these may signal danger quite apart from the word's propositionality or emotional loading. After a stutterer has fallen into the stuttering booby-trap repeatedly and has been hurt, he scrutinizes his verbal terrain with great care lest unsuspectingly he fall into it again.

WORD FEARS

Stutterers develop fears of words as well as sounds. He fears the word as a whole because in the past his communication has been impaired by its utterance. For example, stutterers are often afraid to speak their own names or addresses, because on former occasions their inability to say these partic-

ular words provoked penalty and embarrassment. Some stutterers can recall
very vividly the original experience that led to word fear. For most, however, the origin of the fear has been forgotten, and fear is magnified by
mysteriousness.

Other word fears have their origin in the ambivalence of uncertain pronunciation as in foreign or unfamiliar words. Because of their need for
synonyms, some stutterers have developed supervocabularies, many words
of which they know only by sight but not sound. When they try to say them,
mispronunciations add to the difficulty. Other words, such as the name of
the disorder itself—stuttering—are feared because they are emotionally loaded.
Some words seem to signal approaching stuttering merely because they are
used so frequently in important communication. Child stutterers often show
a word fear of "Mother" and adults of the pronoun "I" for this reason.
These words have been used so often to initiate sentences concerned with
emotional upheaval that the sand burrs of fear stick to them. Interrogatives
such as "Where? Why? When? How?" are also often used under the same
circumstances and become feared words. There are few valid generaliza-
tions about the type of words that stutterers fear but we can be sure that
some words are feared as wholes and that stutterers scan them as such.

As though all this scanning were not burden enough, stutterers also
search for and find danger signals in the *arrangement* or positioning of the
words within the prospective sentence. "It's the starting word that I fear,"
they tell us, and they mean not only the first word of a sentence but any
word that follows a pause such as that used for verbal punctuation. The
stutterer often responds to these perceptions of positional fear by rearrang-
ing the sequencing of his speech. He may attempt to bury the word that has
evoked fear in the middle of the sentence instead of using it in the beginning as he originaly intended, or he may preface it with some starting
phrase such as, *"I believe that"* and thus reduces the positional cue on the
feared first word. Words of high propositional value or emotional content
are similarly shuffled about in the silent rehearsals that precede the speech
attempt to lessen the certainty or expected severity of the anticipated stuttering. Sentences consist of configurations just as single words do. Certain
features loom large: the starting word, the key word. The fear of stuttering
lurks among these prominences.

RELATIONSHIP OF SITUATIONAL
TO WORD FEARS

Situational fears are fears that have become conditioned to features of interpersonal communicative relationship. Situational fears are energizers of
word fears. They create the fund of fear that drains into and finds its focus
in the word fears. Typically, the situation fears in the adult usually come
first. The stutterer, confronted with an approaching speech situation, scans

it for danger signals. "Oh, oh," he says to himself. "I'm going to have trouble. I'm going to stutter." At this point he anticipates his distress, the probable punitive audience reactions and the communicative frustration. But these fears are often vague and without focus. It is only when the stutterer begins to formulate what he will say (and sometimes only as his speech unfolds) that the scanning for difficult words, sounds, and positional cues takes place. When these are identified, the fear gets suddenly stronger. It finds its focus. Tentative rehearsal behaviors then arise during which the stutterer rehearses his expected abnormality. He silently samples the approaching tremors and struggle reactions. He runs through his repertoire of possible avoidance strategies, selecting and discarding as time ticks on. Then finally he tries the first word of his utterance.

This relationship between word and situation fears may be seen when a stutterer is asked to say a sentence repeatedly in a given communicative situation. Because of the adaptation effect, first one word, then another will be spoken fluently on successive readings. Then, if situational stress is increased by bringing in new listeners, the sequence will reverse itself. The word most feared will usually be the last to become fluent during adaptation and the first to be stuttered upon as the stress is increased. Moreover, the relative severity of the stuttering on a given word, as measured by its duration or struggle or avoidance reactions, remains roughly constant. This is shown in Figure 10 where the verticals *above the adaptation reading baselines* represent the severity of stuttering on the word, and the horizontal lines the consecutive speaking or reading trials.

Ignoring for the moment the labeling on the right side of the diagram which we shall discuss later, note that the length of the vertical above the lowest baseline for the word "Smith" is the longest for any of the four words spoken. This means that the hypothetical stutterer had the most severe stuttering on this word as compared with the others. The vertical for "stutterer" is not as tall, which means that the severity of the stuttering on this word was less than on the word "Smith" but more than for "is" or "a." However, in this first reading, all words showed some stuttering.

Adaptation Trials						Communicative Stress
Fifth					A	Speaking alone
Fourth					B	Speaking to close friend
Third					C	Speaking to therapist
Second					D	Speaking to stranger
First					E	Speaking to audience
	Smith	is	a	stutterer		

Figure 10. **Schematic drawing showing interaction between phonemic fears and situational fears. The length of the vertical represents the severity of stuttering on that particular word in that situation.**

When the stutterer says the same sentence again on the second trial, he will stutter harder on "Smith" than on "stutter," as indicated by the amount of the vertical above the second baseline. However, he will not stutter as severely as he did on the first trial on either of these words since now we may ignore the portion below the second baseline. Note also that the words "is" and "a" have dropped out of the stuttering picture since they do not emerge above the second baseline. Some adaptation has occurred. On the third reading, looking at only the portion of the verticals above that baseline, we find the word "Smith" is the only one on which stuttering occurred, and the severity has lessened. The word "stutterer" is spoken fluently. On the fourth trial, all the words would be spoken fluently except for a short mild block on "Smith," and on the fifth trial no stuttering would emerge above the threshold.

Consider now the influence of situation fear. On the right side of the drawing the speaking situations are arbitrarily ranked from the least situation fear (the top horizontal baseline) to the greatest situation fear (the bottom baseline). If our hypothetical stutterer said the same sentence, "Smith is a stutterer" in each of these situations, we would note much the same effect that we found in the adaptation trials. When the situation fear is zero (Baseline A, when talking alone to himself) no stuttering verticals occur above that baseline, and he is completely fluent. When he says the same sentence to a friend, however, he has a short block on "Smith" as represented by the short segment above Baseline B. In speaking to the therapist, he still stutters only on Smith but has a longer or more severe block on it than he had with the friend. Now, moving downward to another baseline (C), he stutters on two words, on "Smith" and on "stutterer" when speaking to the stranger even though he said exactly the same words. However, it should be noted that he stuttered more severely on "Smith" than he did on "stutterer." The relationship between the two words was fairly constant, though both were similarly affected by the situational stress. Even in the most traumatic situation conceivable, in which the stutterer would show some abnormality on every single word, *Smith* would be stuttered most severely and the word *stutterer* would be next severe. *Is* would be short and mild, and the article *a* would be stuttered the least. We suspect that this order of severity reflects the differential conditioning of word fears, the cumulative memories of past unpleasantness, and positional and propositionality effects. The relative severity values of the particular words would vary of course with different stutterers.

Our schematic drawing is a generalized one. In actual testing it is difficult to maintain the constancy of any verbal utterance or to program the communicative stress appropriately. Nevertheless, we feel that there is a definite interaction between situational and word fears which is important both in understanding the nature of the disorder and in therapy. It is not enough merely to adapt the stutterer to situational stress and to extinguish situational fears; we must also reduce those which have become conditioned to the phonemic, positional, and other features of the words.

CORRELATION OF FEAR WITH FREQUENCY AND SEVERITY OF STUTTERING

The correlation between expectancy and the actual occurrence of stuttering has been demonstrated many times. When the product of situational and word fears is large and much fear is experienced, stuttering occurs more frequently and more severely than when the fear is low. Stutterers seem to be able, in a given situation, to predict how much stuttering they will have and how severe it will be. The correlation may not be high but it is certainly positive, perhaps because the fears they sense determine the outcome of the speech attempt. Any therapy worthy of the name should try to reduce this correlation. It therefore seems unwise to ask the stutterer merely to "bounce" or "prolong" until he can say the word. If his fear is strong, he will have to repeat the same syllable many more times or to prolong the first sound much more than if his fear is weak. These differential experiences will not be lost on the stutterer, and further fear conditioning will take place. We must try to reduce the correlation between fear and severity, not to maintain or enhance it.

OTHER PRECIPITATING CONDITIONS

Many other factors seem to play a role in the precipitation of stuttering. Some stutterers report being able to speak better when thoroughly fatigued; others speak worse. Some stutterers speak better when they are ill than when they are well. Some stutterers speak better when they speak swiftly; others when they speak slowly. Usually the amount of stuttering is reduced under masking noise, but there are many instances where noise, especially at the lower intensities, creates more severe and frequent stuttering. Many stutterers speak more fluently when thoroughly relaxed or under the influence of alcohol; others speak better when highly tensed and mobilizing all their attentional resources and much worse when intoxicated. Even the weather has been shown to produce differences in the amount of stuttering. One of the first things any worker with stutterers finds out is that individual variability dominates this problem.

The only plausible explanation for such variability is different learning experiences. In its advanced stages, stuttering and the expectation of it have become conditioned to many different constellations of stimuli. The group trends toward more stuttering with multiple, authoritative, or rejecting listeners merely reflect the stutterer's general history of hurt; the effects of the time pressure and propositionality in creating more stuttering merely testify to conditions under which past stuttering became more frustrating. In short, the general consistencies can be explained in terms of the nature of the disorder as an interference to communication and the way society responds to it. The individual differences reflect the distinctive personal histories of the stutterers, the particular stimulus configurations with which his stuttering behaviors have been associated. The important point is that the symptomatology of advanced stuttering, despite its inconsistencies and variability, is no product of blind chance. Stuttering may be awful but also it is lawful, not chaotic, no matter how bizarre it looks or sounds. It has simply been differentially conditioned.

OTHER COVERT REACTIONS

So far we have dealt only with the stutterer's feelings before the moment of stuttering. This section deals with those that follow it. Different stutterers report different reactions to the experience of fluency breaks and abnormality. Chief among these are the feelings that may be placed somewhere on the continuum of embarrassment-shame-guilt. As the stutterer scans his listener for signs of rejection or distress, he projects his own feelings of stigma onto that listener. His sensors are hyperactive and often pick up and misinterpret the listener's responses. We worked with a hard-bitten gold miner from Alaska once who, when stuttering, watched his listener with an intensity which can hardly be imagined. At the slightest evidence of a smile, no matter how casual or sympathetic or humorous, he punched that listener in the nose. We got to know the city jail very well during his treatment. This man had plenty of hostility but very little embarrassment. Most stutterers, however, are just as super-sensitive to penalty but respond instead with feelings of shame and humiliation. All these reactions vary in intensity with the duration or the abnormality of the stuttering. The wilder and more spasmodic the struggle, the more the embarrassment. Some of the guilt feelings arise, they tell us, because the stutterers have sullied or tortured their listener with their grotesque display; others because they have "imposed upon the listener and taken up valuable time." Doubtless, there are often deeper reasons than these. Whatever their cause, the most common covert reactions that follow the moment of stuttering are embarrassment, shame, and guilt.

There are also brief feelings of relief. They are usually short in duration but they are there. A specific moment of stuttering has run its course and is finished. The obstacle has been overcome. There is a fragment of tension reduction, alas very transitory, a flicker of temporary peace. This may precede the shame or the generation of new fears. That particular feeling of frustration and abnormality has been overpassed and for a brief instant there is momentary relief. We do not feel however that this is a major part of the stutterer's experience.

We have already mentioned another common covert reaction to the experience of stuttering—hostility. Hostility results partly from the aggressive feelings that accompany frustration and partly from the stutterer's natural resentment of the rejections and penalties shown by the listener. We hate our punishers. We get angry when we are blocked in carrying out a course of action. Many of our cases have revealed pronounced hostility once they felt it safe to do so. A few of them express their aggression overtly, but most seethe within. Vulnerable as they are to social penalty, they dare not add fuel to the flame of their distress by attacking their listeners; that would only bring on further penalty. Often the aggression is turned inward. Self-derogation, self-hatred often prevails and when it does the stuttering behavior is affected. We have seen stutterers bite themselves and hit their bodies in the throes of their struggle; we have seen them gag with symbolic revulsion. Even suicidal thoughts seem to appear more frequently than in the normal speaker. Profound dejection and depression are often the results of this self-attack.

It may seem that we have exaggerated the stutterer's feelings, that we have used only dark colors to draw the picture. Perhaps the stutterers we have known were the more severe ones. There may be many who consider the disorder only a minor nuisance. If so, they do not come to the speech clinic. Severe stuttering tends to make a person morbid. Once they trust you, most stutterers tell the same tale of fear, frustration, and shame. Here is one final account from one of our cases:

> In my thinking, and when I am alone, I can speak normally; but as soon as I am under threat or challenge, my world, my "facade" of normalcy collapses and leaves me to face the world of reality as a weak and too cowardly being behind a cellophane shell . . . it doesn't take much to trigger me off into my traditional reaction pattern.
>
> What's the matter with me. . . . I can't do anything right (at least to me). I've spent most of my life running away from everything, whether perceivable or not. I have little faith or trust in other people, much less in myself, and I don't feel that I am getting anywhere in the direction of planning and executing true goals and purposes of my life—rather, I survive from day to day, hour by hour, to the tyrannized by the real and imaginary dictates and reactions of others . . . instead of being the man that I want to be. I realize, to some extent, that I am sensitive, weak, and rather cowardly while still having big ambitions . . . , and yet I refuse in a thousand ways to lift myself from my life-sucking bog of self-imposed burden of resistance and resentment, yet my appetite for self-punishment seems to perpetuate itself in an unsatiable way.
>
> I have never—as far back as I can recall—been able, due to external pres-

sures and my own inner conflicts, to really be myself . . . either I've been a "man of a thousand faces" or else an instrument of someone else, whether they have realized it or not. Now, when I want to find myself, I don't even know where or how to look or proceed.

RESEARCH ON COVERT FEATURES OF STUTTERING

ANXIETY AND FEAR

The research on the emotional responses of stutterers has been mainly concerned with the relationship between fear and stuttering, although some of it focusses on general anxiety, shame, guilt, and hostility. Profound emotional reactions during stuttering were demonstrated long ago by Robbins (1920) who placed a tambour over the hole in the head of a trephined stutterer and recorded a marked increase in the brain volume during stuttering. This evidence of vascular change also occurred when the subject was startled by a sudden gunshot and other such stimuli. A close correlation was shown between this increase and blood pressure and pulse rate during the period just prior to as well as during the moment of stuttering. Fletcher (1914) anticipated Robbins' study by showing a plethysmographic decrease in the finger blood volume during speaking by stutterers and correctly ascribed this to the fear and attendant emotion. He also found marked increases in pulse rate. Travis, Tuttle, and Cowan (1936) demonstrated that rapid changes in blood pressure occurred during stuttering. Changes in heart rate have been shown by other investigators to accompany stuttering, but, as Ritzman (1934) and Palmer and Gillette (1938) discovered, these do not characteristically appear when stutterers are silent.

Breathing disturbances commonly accompany stuttering and contribute to the distress. Many researchers have called attention to these disruptions. Nadoleczny (1927) pneumographically recorded the breathing of stutterers before and during stuttering and found breath-holding characteristic of the expectancy period. These fixations of the respiratory musculatures were also noted by Travis (1927), Murray (1932), Fossler (1930), Travis (1936), and Van Riper (1936). These authors and others have shown that prolongations of the inspiration and expiration phases of the breathing during both stuttering and its anticipation also occur. Trumper (1928) and Twitmeyer (1930) found shallow breathing in stutterers.

In the early thirties, considerable research focused on incoordinations of respiration. Normally contractions of the thoracic and abdominal musculature are parallel during speech. Fletcher (1914), Henrickson (1936), and Morley (1937), however, found them to be out of phase or in complete antagonism in stuttering. Some horizontal asynchrony in the muscles of the respiration during stuttered speech was found by Travis (1936) and Mosier (1944), but Mosier also found that the same behaviors occurred in normal speakers under communicative stress. Intermittent inhalatory gasps can be heard in most recordings of stuttered speech, and Hill (1944), in his excellent survey of the literature, stresses their importance in supporting his view of stuttering as a contraction pattern of shock, startle, or surprise. We have not found them to occur consistently, however, and much stuttering can occur without them. Furthermore, breathing irregularities take place not only during the moment of stuttering but during its expectancy too. Stutterers complain of being unable to "get the air out"; they speak of "butterflies in their stomachs," a subjective experience that may reflect tremors of the diaphragm. In 1928 Trumper observed such tremors fluoroscopically, and Schilling (1960), using roentgenkymography, found that 16 of 35 stutterers showed clonic fluttering of the diaphragm even during silent breathing.

The subjective experience of breathing irregularities coupled with pronounced vascular changes can be very disturbing to the stutterer. Most of them are doubtless the results of emotionality and struggle. They do not seem to be marked in the very young stutterer. Bloodstein (1961) has shown that they increase with age, and Starbuck and Steer (1953) found that the respiratory irregularities of stutterers decrease with adaptation in repeated readings of the same material. Van Riper (1936) discovered that many of the abnormal respiratory patterns shown during overt stuttering were actually rehearsed during the silent period just before the speech attempt, and he attributed them to stereotyped learned behaviors. Moore (1938) was able to produce in normal speakers many of the same types of breathing anomalies shown in his stutterers by associating a severe electric shock with the utterance of certain words. Hill (1954), using a red light which had been previously conditioned to shock, also found such disintegrations.

Further evidence of the emotions experienced by stutterers comes from research using the galvanic skin response (GSR), electroencephalography (EEG), and electromyography (EMG). Umeda (1960) found significant differences in GSR changes from silent to oral reading in his stutterers but not in his normal speaking controls. Lingwall (1967) found that his adult stutterers had a higher frequency of GSR's just before the signal to speak isolated words than did his normal speakers but was unable to find any significant GSR differences during the actual speech attempts. Kline (1959) found that GSR and reaction times to stimulus words correlated significantly with frequency of stuttering. Taylor (1966) compared stutterers with themselves before and after moments of stuttering, using GSR and pulse rate, but found no significant differences. An interesting study indicating that the anxiety shown by stutterers is associated primarily with speaking was performed by Valyo (1964). He had his subjects alternate speech and silence for one minute periods. In silence, GSR recordings showed no differences between stutterers and normal speakers, but during speech the stutterers' GSR's doubled while the controls showed no change.

Brutten (1963) used the Palmar Sweat Index (PSI), a measure of anxiety, to investigate the covert behavior of stutterers, found a marked decrease in PSI during repeated readings of the same material (adaptation) and that this decrease was parallel to the decrease in expectancies of disfluency and to the number of disfluencies. He suggested that this was due either to anxiety reduction or to reactive inhibition. The normal speaking controls showed a similar decrease in nonfluencies but not the progressive decrease in palmar sweating. However, Gray and Brutten (1965), in a study of spontaneous recovery after adaptation found no direct relationship between changes in anxiety level as demonstrated by the PSI and changes in the frequency of stuttering. Hollander (1957) had stutterers reread a passage silently until adaptation occurred, then read it aloud. His argument was that if overt stuttering were related to expectancy, and if stutterers adapt in expectancy (and they did), then there should be a decrement in the subsequent overt stuttering. However, this did not occur. Karmen (1964) also used PSI in adaptation reading for 33 stutterers and their controls. There were no differences found either in initial PSI records, in adaptation rates, or in spontaneous recovery. If PSI is an index of general anxiety, not speech anxiety, stutterers seem to have no more of it than normal speakers.

Baron (1949) used an interesting, if oblique, approach to the problem of general anxiety, and found that when stutterers had to speak a given word one-half second after an eyelid conditioning trial, they conditioned much faster than the normal speaking controls. He attributed this facilitation to the speech anxiety felt by the stutterers. Karpf and Wischner (1960), in a similar experiment but using conditioned finger withdrawal, showed that stutterers conditioned faster than normals when speaking was done concurrently. Maxwell (1965) showed that the PSI was greater in an audience situation than when stutterers read to a single listener and that the PSI paralleled rather closely the amount of stuttering exhibited.

Emotion is often reflected in increased muscular tension, and there are many accounts of such tension in stuttering. The widespread use of relaxation methods in stuttering therapy suggests the importance of the stutterer's tension (or the therapists' belief in it). Jacobson (1938) showed long ago that anxiety is reflected in muscle tension, but the research is still sparse concerning tension and stuttering. Shackson (1936) using EMG found evidence of a latent tetany and muscle tremors of 50-60 per second in muscle-thickening records during stuttering. Brown and Shulman (1940) investigated the basal tension of stutterers in silence and found them no more tense than normal speakers under that condition, thus indicating that it could be speech anxiety rather than anxiety *per se* that was reflected in their usual tense struggling during speech. Although they were more concerned with the timing of the paired muscles than with the amount of tension, the EMG studies of both Travis (1934) and Williams (1955) showed evidence of increased tension during stuttering. Sheehan and Voas (1954) compared the masseter tension patterns during stuttering with those during normal speech and found that the tension built up to a peak just prior to the release.

Shrum (1967) failed to corroborate the peaking of tension at this point but did show that the tension was greater and lasted longer during stuttering than during fluency.

Evidence of strong emotion is often shown in dilatation of the pupils of the eye. Gardner (1937), using pupilometry found dilatation during all moments of stuttering in all of his subjects, but his normal speaking controls showed either no change at all or a narrowing. Luchsinger and Arnold (1965) report a later corroboration of these results. Marked incoordination of eye movements during stuttering in oral reading were noted by Denhardt in 1890 and were photographed by Murray (1932) and by Moser (1938). That the moment of stuttering or the fear of it can produce disruptions in motor patterns other than speech has been mentioned by several writers but Herren's (1931) research makes the point vividly. His subjects were required to repeatedly and rhythmically press bulbs which led to a kymograph. Normal speakers and stutterers (during their fluent periods) performed the activity well but the stutterers during stuttering showed marked interruptions and general disintegration. This breakdown appeared also when the feet were used.

In an EEG investigation, Knott and his colleagues (1959) discovered that their stutterers formed two dissimilar groups, one of which, on the Ulett measures, showed EEG responses characteristic of high anxiety, while the other did not. The same dichotomy (in severe stutterers) of highly anxious and mildly anxious subjects, as measured by PSI was also found by Karmen (1964).

SITUATION FEARS

Although stutterers are known to fear specific situations, these fears do not seem to arise from a realistic appraisal of potential listener reactions. Ainsworth (1939) showed that the breathing of normal speakers when listening to stuttering was affected empathically and in a different fashion than when listening to normal speech. Rosenberg and Curtiss (1954) reported that stuttering acted as a behavioral depressant for the listener, that the latter lost eye contact and became immobile when surprised by stuttering. McDonald and Frick (1954) had students listen to a three-minute tape of severe stuttering and report their reactions. Eight main categories were discovered: surprise, impatience, embarrassment, pity, amusement, curiosity, sympathy, and revulsion. Then they had a stutterer speak to store clerks who were subsequently interviewed, finding that amusement, revulsion, and impatience were reported very rarely but that pity or sympathy and curiosity, surprise, and embarrassment were common reactions.

The stutterer's fears are not always unrealistic, however. Perrin (1954) performed a sociometric analysis of the acceptance of speech defective children by their peers in grades one through six and found that even as early as the first grade 16 per cent of the speech defective children were considered isolates as compared to 4 per cent of the normal speaking children. Giolas and Williams (1958) had second graders listen to stories told with normal speech and with various types of stuttering behaviors. They preferred the persons who told the stories normally over those who stuttered while telling them.

Van Riper and Hull (1955) in a study performed in 1934, found an immediate increase in the frequency of stuttering after adaptation when the situation was changed by reading into a microphone or reading to an audience. Steer and Johnson (1936) replicated the study and reported as follows:

> . . . the least stuttering occurred in situations in which there was either a familiar audience (of one person) or no audience at all. The most stuttering occurred in situations in which the audience was unfamiliar, or indefinite (phonograph recording), or relatively large (two to at least eight persons) [p. 36].

Hahn (1940) required his subjects to read a prose selection in different social situations and found that they had more trouble speaking to a seen rather than to an unseen audience, but there were many individual differences. Porter (1939) had stutterers read while alone, with two, four, and eight listeners, and also to listeners evaluated as being hard or easy to talk to. She also found that individual stutterers differed one from another but that in general they stuttered less alone and more with one, two, and four or more listeners. No differences between four and eight listeners were significant. Those listeners evaluated as "hard to speak to" evoked more stuttering. She also mentions that the stutterers expected to stutter more than they really did. Eisenson and Wells (1942) had their stutterers read in unison with the experimenter into "live" and "dead" microphones and found a decreased frequency in the latter situation. Shulman (1945) showed that adaptation to the speaking situation was retarded when the size of the audience was increased. Lerman and Shames (1965) used the Discomfort-Relief Quotients, a presumed measure of anxiety, to evaluate stutterer's responses before entering situations of various difficulty but could find no relationships. Siegel and Haugen (1964) measured the adaptation rates of stuttering in situations of increasing and decreasing complexity. They found that adaptation slowed as the audience increased but that no clear cut reversal occurred when the size of the audience decreased. Young (1965) found that if 12 adolescent stutterers were not given prior information about the size of the audience to which they were speaking, no effect of audience variation occurred.

It has often been said that stutterers do not stutter when speaking alone to themselves or when singing. Although this is true more often than not, there is substantial evidence that some stutterers stutter in both conditions.

Witt (1925) found 8 per cent of the stutterers he examined who stuttered in singing, but Wiechmann and Richter (1966) surveyed 1582 stutterers and found only 2 per cent who did so. We once had a group of our stutterers, who had previously reported never having stuttered while singing, sing everything they said for a week. By the end of that time all were stuttering, not only in communicative singing, but also in singing songs, although there was less stuttering in the latter situation than in the former.

Travis (1928) found only a few individuals who stuttered when speaking to themselves. Other investigators have reported isolated instances of the same kind, but the most comprehensive investigation was done by Radol'-skii (1965), who studied 125 stutterers of various ages and found that most preschool stutterers had as much stuttering difficulty talking to themselves as to others, and that only 11 of the older ones showed absolutely no stuttering when alone and speaking with normal tempo. The author of the present text, in his youth stuttered severely when speaking to himself aloud and alone in the forest, and also recently, to his surprise, when reading a foreign language aloud to himself alone in his study. It was stuttering, not ambivalence or normal nonfluency. It is likely but not certain that in this solo stuttering, an imaginary critical audience exists. In this connection, Maddox (1938) found that when stutterers read while observing themselves in a mirror, they had more difficulty than when reading just to the experimenter. The degree of self-confrontation that exists when speaking alone may determine the degree of stuttering in this condition.

Some listeners are more punitive or potentially punitive than others. Berwick (1955) found that when stutterers read to photographs of listeners they had previously judged as punitive, an immediate increase in stuttering resulted after a series of adaptation readings to the experimenter. Less stuttering occurred than when reading to photographs of nonpunitive listeners. It is probable that some stutterers may be highly punitive listeners to their own stuttering. Sheehan, Hadley, and Gould (1967) had stutterers repeatedly read matched passages to their peers and to authority figures. The authority listeners produced more stuttering and a slower adaptation than the peers.

Renfrew's (1952) investigation of situation fears indicated great variaability from stutterer to stutterer with few features in common, but she also found considerable consistency for each individual stutterer. Similar results were reported by Bloodstein (1959). Oxtoby (1946) showed that there was very little transfer of adaptation from one situation to another. Shumak (1955) attempted to validate the Iowa Speech Situation Rating Sheet which lists 40 different speaking situations in which stutterers have difficulty speaking but was unable to do so. We urgently need some such measure of situation difficulty.

It is fairly well established that situations in which the need to accomplish communication is of great importance will be more feared and will evoke more stuttering than those in which communication is not so urgent.

Thus reading in unison with another speaker presents less difficulty for the stutterer, as the research of Barber (1939), Eisenson and Wells (1942), and Pattie and Knight (1944) have shown. In the Eisenson and Wells study, for example, when the subjects shifted from choral reading in unison to solo reading, the number of stutterings increased 60 per cent. The research on propositionality, to be reviewed later, also indicates that more stuttering occurs on strongly meaningful than on less meaningful speech.

Since communication always involves the dimension of time, it seems evident that those speaking situations in which time pressure is strong will be more feared than those in which it is not. Sheehan (1958) says:

> It is suggested that time pressure is a basic variable in stuttering, that it is through time pressure that the effect of interpersonal relations in stuttering is mediated. It is also through time pressure that anxiety and guilt and conflicts of all kinds come to play a part. When a stutterer feels in a subordinate or inferior role, or when speaking to an authority figure, he is likely to feel that he isn't really worthy of taking the other person's time (p. 143).

Stunden (1965) has demonstrated that stutterers were more vulnerable to time pressure than their controls.

WORD FEARS

In a respiratory study of stutterers' attempts on single words, Van Riper (1936) found evidences of rehearsal behavior during the period between word exposure and signal to speak. He also found a high inspiration-expiration ratio, a measure which is related to fear. He found further that although there is generally a high correspondence between the expectancy and the occurrence of stuttering, either can occur without the other. Johnson and Sinn (1937) had their stutterers do some adaptation reading, but after the first reading, they omitted all the words on which stuttering was expected. This procedure eliminated 98 per cent of the stutterings. Expectation occurred most generally on words previously stuttered. Milisen (1938), using both contextual and single words, found that in the sequential material (contextual) only 75 per cent of the stutterings were anticipated, as compared with 85 per cent for the single words. Of the words on which the stutterers signalled their prediction of stuttering, 61 per cent were stuttered in the contextual material as compared with 51 per cent for the single words. He concluded that stutterers were not able to anticipate all moments of stuttering.

Knott, Johnson, and Webster (1937) had their stutterers signal differently for certainty of stuttering, doubtful possibility, and certainty of fluency. They found a definite relationship between the degree of expectancy and stuttering. Eighty-eight per cent of anticipated (certain plus doubtful) words were stuttered and only 0.4 per cent of words for which fluency was expected showed stuttering. Sophisticated stutterers predicted less accurately than naive ones.

Johnson and Ainsworth (1938) had stutterers read silently, signalling expectancy or nonexpectancy on each word of a reading passage, and then do the same task again after two weeks. They found that the loci of expectancy on the second reading were generally the same and could not be accounted for by chance. Johnson and Solomon (1937) had stutterers mark copies of a reading passage to indicate words on which stuttering might occur. They found that stuttering occurred on 53 per cent of the words on which it had been anticipated and on only 10 per cent of those on which it had not. In an effort to account for the discrepancies between expectancy and occurrence of stuttering, Johnson and Solomon in the same study had 13 stutterers underline expected stutterings on different reading passages which were read immediately, then again after 15 minutes, after 15 more minutes, and after a one day interval. The percentage of anticipated and unanticipated stutterings remained much the same for all readings. Their conclusion that expectancy may operate at a low degree of consciousness seems forced from these data, but the article has been widely quoted. So also has the investigation by Johnson and Sinn (1937), who had their subjects reread a passage, speaking only the words on which no anticipation was present. They found that most of the unexpected stutterings occurred on words which had been stuttered in the previous reading. Milisen (1938) found that only three per cent of his stutterers were able to predict *all* of their stutterings and that the median stutterer could only predict 61 per cent, even when they were strongly shocked for failure to predict with accuracy.

Van Riper and Milisen (1939) showed that stutterers could predict with some accuracy the *duration* of their anticipated stutterings. Wischner (1952) showed that when stutterers *silently* read the same passage repeatedly and signalled expectancies of stuttering, a progressive decrease in the frequency of expectations occurred which appeared parallel to the adaptation effect usually shown by stutterers while speaking. Peins (1961) failed to corroborate the adaptation of expectancy, which had been reported by several other investigators. Martin and Haroldson (1967) had stutterers read a passage five times, rating each word on a five step expectancy scale. They found that words assigned a high expectancy value tended to be stuttered more consistently than those assigned a low expectancy. They state, however, that their data did not entirely support the frequently expressed view that in most instances stutterers can predict the occurrence of their blockings. In more than half of the instances where a word was assigned the highest expectancy value, no stuttering occurred. Lingwall (1967) reported that his GSR recordings, which are viewed by many as an indication of momentary fear or anxiety, showed no apparent relationship to given words or the ensuing stuttering on those words.

This review makes clear that the correlation between word fear or stuttering expectancy and the actual occurrence of stuttering is far from being perfect. Other factors besides word fear must play a part in its precipitation, although word fear may still have some significant effects. Any theory of stuttering which holds that anticipatory struggle comprises its essence must contend with these findings. The proponents of this view (Johnson, 1955; Bloodstein, 1960) have placed strong emphasis on marginal consciousness of approaching stuttering and upon a subliminal awareness of difficulty, to explain the exceptions. The evidence for this view is not too convincing.

CONSISTENCY OF WORD FEARS

Oblique support for the view that stuttering is always associated with expectancy comes from the studies of consistency. The loci of stuttering are not randomly distributed, nor are the loci of expectancies. Bloodstein (1959) has suggested that this consistency occurs because the memory of past unpleasantness is associated with certain features of the sound or word. The fact of consistency is well established: for the individual stutterer, more stuttering does occur on certain words than on other words (Johnson and Knott, 1937; Johnson and Sinn, 1937; Johnson and Millsapps, 1937; Shulman, 1945). Furthermore, the expectation of stuttering also shows the same consistency, as Johnson and Ainsworth (1938) demonstrated. Martin and Haroldson (1967) found that words with high expectancy ratings were stuttered more consistently than those with low expectancy. Words stuttered less consistently in a reading passage had lower expectancy ratings. The study by Endicott (1957) on recognition time is illuminating. He found, using a tachistoscopic presentation, that words on which stuttering had occurred took longer to perceive than those that had been spoken normally. The research by Goss (1948) revealed that the expectancy of stuttering operated on a time gradient, so that the probability of stuttering increased as the time interval between exposure of a stimulus word and the signal to speak was lengthened. Van Riper (1937) found that stutterers stuttered more on words they had just heard stuttered by another speaker than on those they had heard spoken fluently. Bloodstein (1960), finding the consistency effect even in young beginning stutterers who showed no other evidence of fear or avoidance, attributed it to vague word fears on the margin of consciousness. Substantial research by Goldman-Eisler (1958), and by McClay and Osgood (1959), and others has shown that normal speakers also show hesitation phenomena in a consistent fashion and at specific loci in the speech sequence and that they are due to factors other than fear. Neelley and Timmons (1967) found that both normal speaking children and young stutterers, aged five to eight, showed the consistency effect in rereading sentences although the stutterers were slightly more consistent. Silverman and Williams (1967) found that the loci of stuttering were on much the same words as the disfluencies of normal speakers, that the nonrandomness of disfluency is characteristic of all speakers, not just of stutterers. Schlesinger, Forte, Fried, and Melkman's (1965) research indicates that the consistency effect may be due in large part to information load as measured by transition probability, or to word familiarity as measured by word frequency, rather than to the fear of stuttering alone. Much of the older research on consistency is somewhat suspect since Tate and Cullinan (1962) have shown that simple percentage measures of consistency have little stability.

ADAPTATION AND WORD FEAR

The adaptation effect—the progressive reduction in the number of stutterings as a result of saying the same thing again—has been attributed, among other things, to a reduction in word fear. That adaptation does occur in most but not all stutterers in oral reading has been well established (Van Riper and Hull, 1955; Johnson and Knott, 1937; Sheehan, 1951; Wischner, 1952; Leutenneger, 1957, and others), and it also occurs to a lesser degree in spontaneous speech (Newman, 1934; Rousey, 1958). However, adaptation has also been shown for the occurrence and expectation of disfluencies of normal speakers (Brutten, 1963; Neelley and Timmons, 1967). This fact and the fact that adaptation can occur independently of such measures of emotion as the PSI in both normal speakers and stutterers (Gray, 1965; Maxwell and Brutten, 1964; and Brutten, 1963a) makes it difficult to accept the adaptation effect as being primarily determined by a decrement in word fear through deconfirmation. There are also stutterers who do not adapt (Van Riper and Hull, 1955; and Newman, 1963). Other explanations for the adaptation effect are available, as Wingate's excellent review (1963b), and his research (1966) have made clear.

CUES ASSOCIATED WITH WORD FEAR AND THE MOMENT OF STUTTERING

Most of the research deals primarily with the characteristics of the words on which stuttering actually occurs rather than those it is expected on. The presumption has been that if a person stutters on a given word, certain features of that word have served as cues to precipitate the antecedent fear. Our clinical experience has convinced us that this inference has some validity. Stutterers tell us that they scan approaching words for signals of trouble, that they expect to have more trouble on long words, unfamiliar words, very meaningful words, words on which they recall having severe stuttering. However, we know of no research which analyzes *expectancies* in terms of these multiple features.

PHONEMIC FEARS

As with word fears, the research has dealt not with expectancy, but with stuttering. If the correlation between stuttering and anticipation can be accepted, the studies on loci might be interpreted to mean that there is more phonemic fear on consonants than on vowels, on sounds in the initial rather than in the medial or final position of the word, and perhaps more on plosives than on continuants. Individual stutterers vary markedly from one another in the patterning of their loci, but they are fairly consistent within themselves from day to day. One study bearing directly on this problem was performed by Robbins (1936). He examined the phonemic perceptions of a small group of stutterers and found that initial consonants, plosives, and accented vowels were considered highly conspicuous. Bruner and Dowd (1958) have shown that for all speakers, the first part of a word carries more information than later parts. Connett (1955) was able to induce only slightly more stuttering on words beginning with /t/ by emphasizing its difficulty through suggestion.

FRUSTRATION, HOSTILITY, AND GUILT

Although there are many clinical descriptions of the stutterer's emotions other than fear and anxiety, the research is meager. Some of it deals with frustration. Burstscher (1952) surveyed the information available at that time and concluded that a low tolerance for frustration accounted for much of the secondary characteristics of stuttering. Murphy (1952) also found that stutterers were significantly less resistant to frustration than their controls in a listening task involving competing messages. He also found differences between stutterers and nonstutterers on the Rosenzweig Picture Frustration Test. Quarrington (1953), however, replicated Murphy's investigation and found no differences. Madison and Norman (1952) found significant differences between their subjects and controls on the Rosenzweig, the stutterers being more "intropunitive" and less "extropunitive" and having lower "obstacle dominance" scores. However, no significant differences, using the same test, were found by four other investigators: Hirsch (1950), Lowinger (1952), Seaman (1956), and Emerick (1966). Emerick makes the point that this test may be unsuitable for measuring the kind of frustration stutterers experience.

Closely related to frustration are aggression and hostility. Krugman (1946) found pronounced aggression in his Rorschachs on stutterers. Santostephano (1960) found that stutterers obtained significantly higher hostility scores than nonstutterers on the Rorschach Content Test. This investigator also created a laboratory stress situation designed to evoke hostility and found that the stutterers showed significantly more hostility than the controls. Feldstein and Jaffe (1962) used anger-producing interviews with normal speakers and found no significant increase in "ah" and "non-ah" speech disruptions when this emotion was produced. Perkins and Haugen (1965) permitted open aggressive responses for half of a group of stutterers and prevented them for the other half. They found that open aggression produced less stuttering and less anger. Adams and Dietze (1965) found significant difference in stutterers' and nonstutterers' reaction times to words connoting aggression, depression, and guilt, the stutterers responding more slowly. Sheehan, Cortese and Hadley (1962), using projective drawings, concluded tht guilt feelings occurred before, during, and subsequent to the moment of stuttering, and were most prevalent during the subsequent period.

RESEARCH ON THE LOCI OF STUTTERING

We have already made the point that phoneme and word fears do not occur randomly but are attached to certain cues, such as word position, word length, meaningfulness, phonemic characteristics, etc. In this section we review not the loci of the fears but the loci of the actual stutterings. As one might expect if learning is involved, the two sets of loci are fairly parallel. Many experimenters have explored this dimension of the problem in the hope that the location of the stutterings might help us understand their nature. Unfortunately, it seems that multiple factors interact to determine these loci, and it is difficult, in the individual stutterer, to assess the importance of the components, since the strength of any one factor depends on the person's past history of stuttering difficulty. For one stutterer, position (getting started) is most important; for another, the amount of information or uncertainty possessed by the word determines whether or not he will stutter on it; for a third, the phonemic characteristics of the word's first sound may be most crucial. The researches we report here obscure these differences since they are based on groups of stutterers.

WORD LENGTH AND FREQUENCY OF USAGE

Most of the research indicates that longer words are stuttered on more frequently than shorter ones whether measured by number of syllables or number of letters (Brown and Moren, 1942; Milisen, 1938; Hejna, 1955; Soderberg, 1966). Short words are also more frequently used and are more familiar than longer ones. Schlesinger, Melkman, and Levy (1966) found that when words of one, two, or three syllables were used, young stutterers had more difficulty as the word length increased, and less difficulty if the word had a high frequency of usage. Soderberg (1966) found both factors (length and frequency) to be important determiners but word length to be the more important factor. To account for this, explanations have been cast in terms of conspicuousness, coordinative loading, and the role of reenforcement.

LINGUISTIC CHARACTERISTICS

The linguistic characteristics of stuttered words have also been investigated. Propositional speech always seems to yield more stuttering than nonsense material, as Eisenson and Horowitz (1945) made clear. Bardrick and Sheehan (1956) had stutterers read one passage composed of numbers, another of ordinary meaningful prose, and a third of emotionally loaded words. The number of stutterings increased in that same order. In general, content (lexical) words such as nouns, verbs, adjectives, and adverbs are more frequently stuttered than function words such as conjunctions, prepositions, articles, possessive pronouns, etc. (Johnson and Brown, 1935; Brown, 1938; Hahn, 1942b; Hejna, 1955). However, as Quarrington, Conway, and Siegel (1962) have demonstrated, there is little agreement about the frequency of stuttering on the grammatical subclasses. Word length may account for the differences between lexical and function words, since lexical or content words are usually longer than function words. Taylor's (1966a) data supports this explanation. Lexical words also carry more information than function words and have greater statistical uncertainty in the speech sequence. Goldman-Eisler (1958) has shown that more hesitation pauses occur in normal speech before words of high information value and greater uncertainty than before words of low meaningful content and more certainty. Similar results were found by McClay and Osgood (1959) and Blankenship (1964). Soderberg (1967) found that prolongations occurred on lexical words while repetitions occurred with almost equal frequency on both lexical and function words. A study by Bloodstein and Gantwerk (1967) seems to corroborate Soderberg's results. They recorded the spontaneous speech of 13 young stutterers, ages two through six, and did not find the same sort of grammatical differences that had been previously demonstrated for adults. Much more stuttering occurred on conjunctions and personal pronouns than on nouns in these children. Presumably, though the authors did not mention it, stuttering at this early stage of development would be primarily repetitive and thus substantiate the Soderberg study. We need hesitation data on normal speaking children before these findings can be truly understood. Bloodstein and Gantwerk attribute their results to positional effects, since most of the stutterings occurred on the first words of sentences or clauses and commonly began with a pronoun or conjunction. It seems quite possible that once a stutterer begins to fear stuttering, he may then scan approaching utterances for words that are conspicuous by their length or meaningfulness and thus precipitate more stuttering on them.

POSITION OF THE WORD IN THE SENTENCE

Brown (1938) found more stuttering on the first word of a sentence, less on the second word, and even less on the third. This positional effect seems very well supported. Hejna (1955) found a gradual decrease in stutterings on consecutive words of a sentence in spontaneous speech but failed to find the most stuttering on the first word, explaining that in spontaneous speech, this word was often a starter word such as "Well" or "And," and not really a part of the sentence. Quarrington, Conway, and Siegel (1962) contrasted the amount of stuttering on first and final words of sentences, finding a significant difference in frequency with more stuttering on the initial words. Conway and Quarrington (1963) tried to control for other variables such as initial phonetic sound, grammatical class, and number of syllables by designing the sentences read by stutterers and also found that initial position had more stuttering than medial, and medial more than final position of words in the sentences. Quarrington (1965) found a correlation of .49 between position of the word within the sentence and decreasing frequency of stuttering. Taylor (1966b) showed that word position was a more important determiner of the loci of stuttering than either the length of the word or the phonetic characteristics of the syllables. Soderberg (1967) found more stuttering on the initial words of clauses than on subsequent words even though initial words were more typically function words and pronouns while final words were more often of the lexical class. Silverman and Williams (1967) found little differences between the loci of disfluencies in stutterers as compared with those of normal speakers except that the stutterers had more difficulties in the initial position, in getting started. Bloodstein and Gantwerk (1967) also found that very young stutterers had more trouble on the first words of their utterances.

PHONEMIC CHARACTERISTICS

Whether or not stuttering will occur seems to depend also on the characteristics of the first sound of the word, or the first sound of the syllable having primary accent. Johnson and Brown (1935) had stutterers read a long passage and then ranked the various speech sounds according to frequency of stuttering. Brown (1938) repeated the experiment using long lists of words out of context. He found that words beginning with consonants produced more stuttering than those beginning with vowels, although there was much individual variability about which sounds were difficult. Hahn (1942a) found a marked difference between consonants and vowels; only 2.9 per cent of the stutterings occurred on words beginning with a vowel. Quarrington, Conway, and Siegal (1962), using a special set of sentences in order to control for other factors, compared the occurrence of stuttering on four consonants, said by Johnson and Brown to be the most difficult ones, with four other consonants said to be least difficult. They found no significant differences in the amount of stuttering on the different sounds. Soderberg (1962) used word lists and found no significant differences in the frequency or duration of stutterings either between consonants and vowels, or between voiced and unvoiced consonants. His design, however, has been criticized by Taylor (1966a) as tending to minimize any vowel-consonant differences. Taylor (1966a), in her well-controlled study, found that consonants were stuttered much more frequently than vowels, but the particular consonantal contexts in which stuttering occurred were not those found by Brown or Hahn, no doubt because of individual variability.

The position of the sound in the word is of major importance in determining whether or not stuttering will occur on it. All investigators have found that more stuttering occurs on initial sounds or syllables than on later sounds or syllables. When stuttering does occur later in the word, it is usually on the syllable having primary or secondary accent. Froeschels (1961), on the basis of "many thousand cases," insisted that stutterers do not stutter "at the end of a word." Emerick (1963), however, describes a case showing such "final stuttering," although he agrees that it is rare. Attempts to explain why one consonant seems to evoke more stuttering than another have usually been expressed in terms of differential learning experiences (Van Riper, 1963). Since Fairbanks (1937), Hahn (1942a), and Taylor (1966b) failed to find any significant or consistent characteristics of the consonants on which stuttering occurs most often, either in complexity of coordination or in manner of production, it seems evident that if such factors exist they cannot be of major importance. The difference between consonants and vowels, however, is another matter and one which needs investigation.

COMBINATIONS OF FACTORS AFFECTING LOCI

Brown (1938) suggested that the locus of stuttering is determined, not by any one factor, but by all of them in combination. He felt that a word-weight could be achieved by combining word length, word position, grammatical structure, and the phonetic characteristic of the first sound. He showed that severe stutterers showed more stuttering when fewer of these characteristics occurred than mild stutterers. Oxtoby (1946) and Trotter

(1956) corroborated Brown's belief that the higher the word-weight, the more frequent the stuttering.

COMMENTARY

In conversation Kingsley had a painful hesitation in his speech, but in preaching, and in speaking with a set purpose, he was wholly free from it. He used to say that he could speak for God but not for himself (Duncan, 1949, p. 140).

A basic feature of stuttering behavior is that the stutterer is under time pressure to a great extent. He comes to learn to dread pauses, and the room settles around him with awful stillness when he begins to speak. The stutterer's block always seems longer than it really is, both to the stutterer and to his listeners (Sheehan, 1958, p. 143).

When a cue associated with a relatively great amount of past stuttering is introduced into what was previously a relatively "non-difficult" situation there is a statistically significant increase in frequency of stuttering in the latter situation (Johnson, Larson, and Knott, 1937, p. 108).

Excerpt from a letter from a Pakistani stutterer: "Dear Dr. Riper, there is a point I would like to tell you about my stammering. You see I am a Parsi by faith and our Holy Book is written in very old 'Pahlevi Script.' Now naturally, when I read our holy book, I never can understand a word of the script and incidently I *rarely* stammer while reading it."

Artificial sympathy is worse than indifference or open hostility. It is at once recognized by a stammerer: a counterfeit coin, even in a heap of coins, does not remain unconcealed from the expert eye of a cashier (Purohit, 1947, p. 420).

Some look at me with annoyance written on their faces and think it is a relief to them when I am gone (Boome and Richardson, 1932, p. 69).

Ridicule by others begets in the stammerer a habit of secrecy, of feeling himself cut off from his kindred, of brooding over his own thoughts, of fancying himself under a mysterious curse (A Minute Philosopher, 1859).

When a stammerer talks to a nonstammerer the latter at first gives him his full attention, but when the former begins to stammer the attention of the latter gets relaxed. For he thinks that the time is being unnecessarily wasted by stammering, therefore, he attends to some other object and when the stammerer is able to speak the sentence, he, not being able to decipher the broken words and sentences, requests him to speak again. One can very well imagine the difficulty the poor fellow with great difficulty has said what he had to say and is required to undergo the same difficulty once again. Nay the repetition proves to be more troublesome. For he is by now made to realize his shortcoming and is nervous enough to stammer more frequently and vigourously this time. No words can describe the difficulties and miseries of a stammerer; it can only be better understood by one who himself is a patient of the malady (Mathur, 1960, p. 59).

The nature of my stuttering problem consists mostly of word fears. I have learned to handle the stressful situations by forcing myself to be exposed to them. For example, I took a speech course and actively participated in class, which have reduced the anxiety that I used to feel.

I have had no real feelings of penalty, guilt, or hostility because of my personality. I try to see the brighter side of life and try to smile even if things go wrong.

As I stated in the first sentence, my word fears present the biggest problem. My tongue seems to forget where it should go next as in the word "any." I can form the initial sound but that is as far as I can get (A stutterer).

Because of his memory of past experience, the stammerer picks out bugaboo words as he talks. He becomes fearful of difficult words and ominous speech situations, and he develops speech aversion (Bluemel, 1957, p. 9).

I have exactly the same fears of Japanese sounds that I have of English sounds. It would be appropriate to say that English feared sounds were derived from Japanese feared sounds. I remember a long time ago that when I learned German I also had the same fears of German sounds that I had of Japanese sounds.

These are the pronounced feelings which arise when I stutter severely; disgust, disgrace, embarrassed, frustrated, angry, hostile, depressed, discouraged, inconvenience, disabled, stupid (Another stutterer).

Alice knew it was the Rabbit coming to look for her, and she trembled until she shook the house, quite forgetting that she was now a thousand times as large as the Rabbit and had no reason to be afraid of it (Lewis Carroll).

BIBLIOGRAPHY

Adams, M. R., and D. A. Dietze, "A Comparison of the Reaction Times of Stutterers and Nonstutterers to Items on a Word Association Test," *Journal of Speech and Hearing Research,* VIII (1965), 195–202.

Ainsworth, S. E., "Studies in the Psychology of Stuttering: Empathic Breathing of Auditors While Listening to Stuttered Speech," *Journal of Speech Disorders,* IV (1939), 149–156.

Barber, V. A., "Studies in the Psychology of Stuttering: XV, Chorus Reading as a Distraction in Stuttering," *Journal of Speech Disorders,* IV (1939), 371–83.

Bardrick, R. A., and J. G. Sheehan, "Emotional Loadings as a Source of Conflict in Stuttering," *American Psychologist*, XI (1956), 391 (abstract).

Baron, M., "The Effect on Eyelid Conditioning of a Speech Variable in Stutterers and Nonstutterers." Doctoral dissertation, State University of Iowa, 1949.

Berlinsky, S. L., "A Comparison of Stutterers and Nonstutterers in Four Conditions of Experimentally Induced Anxiety," *Dissertation Abstracts*, XIV (1954), 719 (abstract).

Berwick, N. H., "Stuttering in Response to Photographs of Certain Selected Listeners." In W. Johnson (ed.), *Stuttering in Children and Adults*. Minneapolis: University of Minnesota Press, 1955.

Blankenship, J., "Stuttering in Normal Speech," *Journal of Speech and Hearing Research*, VII (1964), 65–86.

Bloodstein, O., *A Handbook on Stuttering for Professional Workers*. Chicago: National Society for Crippled Children and Adults, 1959.

————. "Development of Stuttering," *Journal of Speech and Hearing Disorders*, XXV (1960), 219–37, 366–76; XXVI (1961), 67–82.

Bloodstein, O., and B. F. Gantwerk, "Grammatical Function in Relation to Stuttering in Young children," *Journal of Speech and Hearing Research*, X (1967) 786–89.

Bluemel, C. S., *The Riddle of Stuttering*. Danville, Ill.: Interstate, 1957.

Boome, E. J., and M. A. Richardson, *The Nature and Treatment of Stuttering*. New York: Dutton, 1932.

Brown, S. F., "Stuttering with Relation to Word Accent and Word Position," *Journal of Abnormal and Social Psychology*, XXXIII (1938), 112–20.

Brown, S. F., and A. Moren, "The Frequency of Stuttering in Relation to Word Length During Oral Reading," *Journal of Speech Disorders*, VII (1942), 153–59.

Brown, S. F., and E. E. Shulman, "Intramuscular Pressure in Stutterers and Nonstutterers," *Speech Monographs*, VII (1940), 63–74.

Bruner, J. S., and D. Dowd, "A Note on the Informativeness of Parts of Speech," *Language and Speech*, I (1958), 98–101.

Brutten, E. J., "Palmar Sweat Investigation of Disfluency and Expectancy Adaptation," *Journal of Speech and Hearing Research*, VI (1963a), 40–48.

————. "Fluency and Disfluency," *Asha*, III (1963b), 781 (abstract).

Brutten, E. J., and B. B. Gray, "Effects of Word Cue Removal on Adaptation and Adjacency: A Clinical Paradigm," *Journal of Speech and Hearing Disorders*, XXVI (1961), 385–89.

Burtscher, H. T., Jr., "The Operation of Frustration in the Transition to and the Development of Secondary Stuttering," *Speech Monographs*, XIX (1952), 191 (abstract).

Connett, M. H., "Experimentally Induced Changes in the Relative Frequency of Stuttering on a Specified Speech Sound." In W. Johnson (ed.), *Stuttering in Children and Adults*. Minneapolis: University of Minnesota Press, 1955.

Conway, J. K., and B. Quarrington, "Positional Effects in the Stuttering of Contextually Organized Verbal Material," *Journal of Abnormal and Social Psychology*, XLVII (1963), 299–303.

Cook, M., "Speech Disturbance and Length of Utterance," *Psychonomic Science*, X (1968), 125–26.

Denhardt, R., *Das Stottern: Eine Psychose*. Leipzig, 1890.

Duncan, M. H., "Home Adjustment of Stutterers Versus Non-stutterers," *Journal of Speech and Hearing Disorders,* XIV (1949), 255–59.

Eisenson, J., and E. Horowitz, "The Influence of Propositionality on Stuttering," *Journal of Speech Disorders,* X (1945), 193–97.

Eisenson, J., and C. Wells, "A Study of the Influences of Communicative Responsibility in a Choral Speech Situation For Stutterers," *Journal of Speech Disorders,* VII (1942), 259–62.

Emerick, L., "An Evaluation of Three Psychological Variables in Tonic and Clonic Stutterers and in Nonstutterers," *Dissertation Abstracts,* XXVIII (1-A), (1967), 317 (abstract).

Emerick, L., "A Clinical Observation on the 'Final' Stuttering," *Journal of Speech and Hearing Disorders,* XXVIII (1963), 194–95.

————. "Social Distance Scale for Stutterers," *Journal of Speech and Hearing Disorders,* XXV (1960), 408–9.

————. Personal communication, 1968.

Endicott, J., "An Exploratory Study of the Relationship Between Recognition Time of Stuttered and Nonstuttered Words," Master's thesis, Ohio University, 1957.

Fairbanks, G., "Some Correlates of Sound Difficulty in Stuttering," *Quarterly Journal of Speech,* XXIII (1937), 67–69.

Faling, J., personal communication, 1968.

Feldstein, S., and J. Jaffe. "The Relationship of Speech Disruption to the Experience of Anger," *Journal of Consulting Psychology,* XXVI (1962), 505–9.

Fletcher, J. M., "An Experimental Study of Stuttering," *American Journal of Psychology,* XXV (1914), 201–55.

Fossler, H. R., "Disturbances in Breathing During Stuttering," *Psychological Monographs,* XL (1930), 1–32.

Froeschels, E., "New Viewpoints on Stuttering," *Folia Phoniatrica,* XIII (1961), 187–201.

Gardner, W. H., "The Study of the Pupillary Reflex with Special Reference to Stuttering," *Psychological Monographs,* XLIX (1937), 1–31.

Giolas, T. G., and D. E. Williams, "Children's Reactions to Nonfluencies in Adult Speech," *Journal of Speech and Hearing Research,* I (1958), 86–93.

Goldman-Eisler, F., "Discussion and Further Comments." In E. R. Lenneberg, *New Directions in the Study of Language.* Cambridge, Mass.: M.I.T. Press, 1966.

————. "The Predictability of Words in Context and the Length of Pauses in Speech," *Language and Speech,* I (1958), 226–31.

Goss, A. E., "Stuttering Behavior and Anxiety as a Function of Experimental Training," *Journal of Speech Disorders,* XXI (1956), 343–51.

Gray, B. B., "The Relationship Between Anxiety Level, Fatigue, and Stuttering Adaptation," *Asha,* VI (1964), 416 (abstract).

Gray, B. B., and E. J. Brutten, "The Relationship Between Anxiety, Fatigue, and Spontaneous Recovery in Stuttering," *Behavior Research and Therapy,* II (1965), 251–59.

Hahn, E., "A Study of the Relationship Between Stuttering Occurrence and Phonetic Factors in Oral Reading," *Journal of Speech Disorders,* VII (1942a), 143–51.

————. "A Study of the Relationship Between Stuttering Occurrence and Grammatical Factors in Oral Reading," *Journal of Speech Disorders,* VII (1942b), 329–55.

―――. "A Study of the Relationship Between the Social Complexity of the Oral Reading Situation and the Severity of Stuttering," *Journal of Speech Disorders,* V, (1940), 5–14.

Hejna, R. F., "A Study of the Loci of Stuttering in Spontaneous Speech," *Dissertation Abstracts,* XV (1955) 1674–75 (abstract).

Henrikson, E. H., "Simultaneously Recorded Breathing and Vocal Disturbances of Stutterers," *Archives of Speech,* I (1936), 133–49.

Herren, R. Y., "The Effect of Stuttering on Voluntary Movement," *Journal of Experimental Psychology,* XIV (1931), 289–98.

Hill, H., "An Experimental Study of Disorganization of Speech and Manual Responses in Normal Subjects," *Journal of Speech and Hearing Disorders,* XIX (1954), 295–305.

―――. "An Interbehavioral Analysis of Several Aspects of Stuttering," *Journal of General Psychology,* XXXII (1945), 289–316.

―――. "An Experimental Study of Disorganization of Speech and Manual Responses in Normal Subjects," *Journal of Speech and Hearing Disorders,* XIX (1954), 295–305.

―――. "Stuttering: II. A Review and Integration of Physiological Data," *Journal of Speech Disorders,* IX (1944), 289–324.

Hirsch, B., "A Study of the Responses of Stutterers and Nonstutterers to Two Kinds of Personality Tests." Master's thesis, Fordham University, 1950.

Hollander, H., "An Investigation of the Effects of Silent Adaptation to Expectancy of Stuttering on Stuttering Behavior." Master's thesis, University of Pittsburgh, 1957.

Jacobson, E., *Progressive Relaxation.* Chicago: University of Chicago Press, 1938.

Johnson, W. (ed.), *Stuttering in Children and Adults: Thirty Years of Research at the University of Iowa.* Minneapolis: University of Minnesota Press, 1955.

―――. *The Onset of Stuttering.* Minneapolis: University of Minnesota Press, 1961.

Johnson, W., and S. Ainsworth, "Studies in the Psychology of Stuttering: X, Constancy of Loci of Expectancy of Stuttering," *Journal of Speech Disorders,* III (1938), 101–4.

Johnson, W., and S. F. Brown, "Stuttering in Relation to Various Speech Sounds," *Quarterly Journal of Speech,* XXI (1935), 481–96.

Johnson, W., and J. R. Knott, "Certain Objective Cues Related to the Precipitation of the Moment of Stuttering," *Journal of Speech Disorders,* II (1937) 17–19.

Johnson, W., R. P. Larson, and J. R. Knott, "Studies in the Psychology of Stuttering: III, Certain Objective Cues Related to the Precipitation of the Moment of Stuttering," *Journal of Speech Disorders,* II (1937) 105–9.

Johnson, W., and L. S. Millsapps, "Studies in the Psychology of Stuttering: VI, The Role of Cues Representative of Past Moments During Oral Reading," *Journal of Speech Disorders,* II (1937), 101–4.

Johnson, W., and A. Sinn, "Studies in the Psychology of Stuttering: V, Frequency of Stuttering with Expectation of Stuttering Controlled," *Journal of Speech Disorders,* II (1937), 98–100.

Johnson, W., and A. Solomon, "Studies in the Psychology of Stuttering: IV, A

Quantitative Study of Expectation of Stuttering as a Process Involving a Low Degree of Consciousness," *Journal of Speech Disorders,* II (1937), 95–97.

Karmen, J. L., "A Comparison Between Generalized Anxiety Adjustment and Adaptation of Stuttering Behavior," Doctoral dissertation, University of Arizona, 1964.

Karpf, B. V., and G. J. Wischner, "An Investigation of the Effect of Speech Anxiety (Drive) Upon the Conditioning of a Finger Withdrawal Response," *Asha,* II (1960), 367 (abstract).

Kazin, A., *A Walker in the Street.* New York: Harcourt, 1951.

Kline, D. F., "An Experimental Study of the Frequency of Stuttering in Relation to Certain Goal-Activity Drives in Basic Human Behavior," *Speech Monographs,* XXVI (1959), 137 (abstract).

Knott, J. R., R. E. Correll, and J. N. Shepherd, "Frequency Analysis of Electroencephalograms of Stutterers and Nonstutterers," *Journal of Speech and Hearing Research,* II (1959), 74–80.

Knott, J. R., W. Johnson, and M. Webster, "Studies in the Psychology of Stuttering: I, A Quantitative Evaluation of Expectation of Stuttering in Relation to the Occurrence of Stuttering," *Journal of Speech Disorders,* II (1937), 20–22.

Krugman, M., "Psychosomatic Study of Fifty Stuttering Children," *Journal of Orthopsychiatry,* XVI (1946), 127–33.

Lanyon, R. I., "Speech: Relation of Nonfluency to Information Value," *Science,* CLXIV (1969), 451–52.

Lerman, J. W., and G. H. Shames, "The Effect of Situational Difficulty on Stuttering," *Journal of Speech and Hearing Research,* VIII (1965), 271–80.

Leutenegger, R. R., "Adaptation and Recovery in the Oral Reading of Stutterers," *Journal of Speech Disorders,* XXII (1957), 276–87.

Lingwall, J. B., "Galvanic Skin Responses of Stutterers and Nonstutterers to Isolated Word Stimuli," convention address, A.S.H.A., 1967.

Lowinger, L., "The Psychodynamics of Stuttering: An Evaluation of the Factors of Aggression and Guilt Feelings in a Group of Institutionalized Children," *Dissertation Abstracts,* XII (1952), 725 (abstract).

Luchsinger, R., and G. E. Arnold, *Voice—Speech—Language.* Belmont, Cal.: Wadsworth, 1965.

Maddox, J. S., "Studies in the Psychology of Stuttering: VIII, The Role of Visual Cues in the Precipitation of Moments of Stuttering," *Journal of Speech Disorders,* III (1938), 90–94.

Madison, L., and R. A. Norman, "Comparison of the Performance of Stutterers and Nonstutterers on the Rosenzweig Picture Frustration Test," *Journal of Clinical Psychology,* VIII (1952), 179–83.

Martin, R. R., and S. K. Haroldson, "The Relationship Between Anticipation and Consistency of Stuttered Words," *Journal of Speech and Hearing Research,* X (1967), 323–27.

Mathur, M. L., *Causes and Cure of Stammering.* Jodhpur, India: Navyng, 1960.

Maxwell, D. L., "A Palmar Sweat Investigation of Stuttering Adaptation Under Two Levels of Audience Complexity." Master's thesis, Southern Illinois University, 1965.

Maxwell, D. L., and E. J. Brutten, "A Palmar-Sweat Investigation of Stuttering Adaptation and Spontaneous Recovery Under Two Levels of Audience Complexity," *Asha,* VI (1964), 416–17 (abstract).

McClay, H., and E. I. Osgood, "Hesitation Phenomena in Spontaneous English Speech," *Word,* XV (1959), 19–44.

McDonald, E., and J. Frick, "Store Clerks' Reactions to Stuttering," *Journal of Speech and Hearing Disorders,* XXIX (1954), 306–11.

Milisen, R., "Frequency of Stuttering with Anticipation of Stuttering Controlled," *Journal of Speech Disorders,* III (1938), 207–14.

Minute Philosopher, "The Irrationale of Speech," *Fraser's Magazine,* July, 1859, pp. 1–14.

Moore, W. E., "A Conditioned Reflex Study of Stuttering," *Journal of Speech Disorders,* III, (1938), 163–83.

Morley, A., "An Analysis of Associative and Predisposing Factors in the Symptomatology of Stuttering," *Psychological Monographs,* XLIX (1937), 50–107.

Moser, H. M., "A Qualitative Analysis of Eye-Movements During Stuttering," *Journal of Speech Disorders,* III (1938), 131–39.

Mosier, K. V., "A Study of the Horizontal Disintegration of Breathing During Normal and Abnormal Speech for Normal Speakers and Stutterers." Master's thesis, University of Indiana, 1944.

Murphy, A. T., "An Electroencephalographic Study of Frustration in Stutterers." Doctoral dissertation, University of Southern California, 1952.

Murray, E., "Disintegration of Breathing and Eye Movements in Stutterers During Silent Reading and Reasoning," *Psychological Monographs,* XLIII (1932), 218–275.

Nadoleczny, M., ["Stuttering as a Manifestation of a Spastic Coordination Neurosis"], *Archives of Psychiatry,* LXXXII (1927), 235–46.

Neelley, J. N., and R. J. Timmons, "Adaptation and Consistency in the Disfluent Speech Behavior of Young Stutterers and Nonstutterers," *Journal of Speech and Hearing Research,* X (1967), 250–56.

Newman, P. W., "Adaptation Performances of Individual Stutterers: Implications for Research," *Journal of Speech and Hearing Research,* VI (1963), 393–94.

———. "A Study of Adaptation and Recovery of the Stuttering Response in Self Formulated Speech," *Journal of Speech and Hearing Disorders,* XIX (1954), 312–21.

Oxtoby, E. T., "A Quantitative Study of Certain Phenomena Related to Expectancy of Stuttering." Doctoral dissertation, State University of Iowa, 1946.

Palmer, M., and A. M. Gillette, "Sex Differences in the Cardiac Rhythms of Stutterers," *Journal of Speech Disorders,* III (1938), 3–12.

Pattie, F. A., and B. B. Knight, "Why Does the Speech of Stutterers Improve in Chorus Reading," *Journal of Abnormal and Social Psychology,* XXXIX (1944), 362–67.

Peins, M., "Consistency Effect in Stuttering Expectancy," *Journal of Speech and Hearing Research,* IV (1961), 397–98.

Perkins, W. H., and C. Haugen, "The Relationship Between Frequency of Stuttering and Open Expression of Aggression," convention address, A.S.H.A., 1965.

Perrin, E. H., "Social Position of the Speech Defective Child," *Journal of Speech and Hearing Disorders,* XIX (1954), 250–52.

Porter, H.v.K. "Studies in the Psychology of Stuttering: XIV, Stuttering Phenomena in Relation to Size and Personnel of Audience," *Journal of Speech Disorders,* IV (1939), 323–33.

Purohit, S. N., "Why Stammerers Suffer," *Journal of Speech Disorders,* XII (1947), 419–20.

Quarrington, B., "Stuttering as a Function of the Information Value and Sentence Position of Words," *Journal of Abnormal Psychology,* LXX (1965), 221–24.

———. "The Performance of Stutterers on the Rosenzweig Picture Frustration Test," *Journal of Clinical Psychology,* IX (1953), 189–92.

Quarrington, B., J. Conway, and N. Siegel, "An Experimental Study of Some Properties of Stuttered Words," *Journal of Speech and Hearing Research,* V (1962), 387–94.

Razdol'skii, V. A., ["On the Speech of Stutterers When Alone"], *Zhurnal Nevropatologii i Psikhiatrii,* LXV (1965), 1717–20.

Renfrew, C. B., "A Questionnaire for Stutterers," *Speech* (London), XVI (1952); 21–24.

Ritzman, C. E., "A Comparative Cardiovascular and Metabolic Study of Stutterers and Nonstutterers," *Journal of Speech Disorders,* VIII (1943), 161–82.

Robbins, S. D., "Comparative Shock and Stammering," *American Journal of Physiology,* LII (1920), 168–81.

———. "Relative Attention Paid to Vowels and Consonants by Stammerers and Normal Speakers," *Proceedings of the American Association for the Study of Disorders of Speech,* VI (1936), 7–23.

Rosenberg, S., and J. Curtis, "The Effect of Stuttering on the Behavior of the Listener," *Journal of Abnormal Social Psychology,* XLIX (1954), 355–61.

Rousey, C. L., "Stuttering Severity During Prolonged Spontaneous Speech," *Journal of Speech and Hearing Research,* I (1958), 40–47.

Santostefano, S., "Anxiety and Hostility in Stuttering," *Journal of Speech and Hearing Research,* III (1960), 337–47.

Schilling, A., "Roentgen-Zwerchfell-Kymogramme bei Stottern," *Folia Phoniatrica,* XII (1960), 145–53.

Schlesinger, I. M., M. Forte, B. Fried, and R. Melkman, "Stuttering, Information Load, and Response Strength," *Journal of Speech and Hearing Disorders,* XXX (1965), 32–36.

Schlesinger, I. M., R. Melkman, and R. Levy, "Word Length and Frequency as Determinants of Stuttering," *Psychonomic Science,* VI (1966), 255–56.

Scripture, E. W., *Stuttering, Lisping, and Correction of the Speech of the Deaf.* New York: Macmillan, 1923.

Seaman, R., "A Study of the Responses of Stutterers to the Items of the Rosenzweig Picture Frustration Study." Master's thesis, Brooklyn College, 1956.

Shackson, R., "An Action Current Study of Muscle Contraction Latency with Special Reference to Latent Tetany in Stutterers," *Archives of Speech,* I (1936), 87–111.

Sheehan, J. G., "Conflict Theory of Stuttering." In J. Eisenson (ed.). *Stuttering: A Symposium.* New York: Harper, 1958.

———. "The Modification of Stuttering Through Nonreinforcement," *Journal of Abnormal and Social Psychology,* XLVI (1951), 51–63.

Sheehan, J. G., R. Cortese, and R. Hadley, "Guilt, Shame, and Tension in Graphic Projections of Stuttering," *Journal of Speech and Hearing Disorders,* XXXVII (1962), 129–39.

Sheehan, J. G., R. G. Hadley, and E. Gould, "Impact of Authority on Stuttering," *Journal of Abnormal Psychology,* LXII (1967), 290–93.

Sheehan, J. G., and R. B. Voas, "Tension Patterns During Stuttering in Relation to Conflict, Anxiety-Binding, and Reinforcement," *Speech Monographs,* XXI, (1954), 272–79.

Shrum, W. F., "A Study of the Speaking Behavior of Stutterers and Nonstutterers by Means of Multichannel Electromyography," convention address, A.S.H.A., 1967.

Shulman, E. A., "A Study of Certain Factors Influencing Variability of Stuttering." Doctoral dissertation, State University of Iowa, 1945.

Shumak, I. C., "A Speech Situation Rating Sheet for Stutterers." In Johnson, W. and Leutenneger, R. R. (eds.), *Stuttering in Children and Adults.* Minneapolis: University of Minnesota Press, 1955.

Siegel, G. M., and D. Haugen, "Audience Size and Variations in Stuttering Behavior," *Journal of Speech and Hearing Research,* VII (1964), 383–88.

Silverman, F. H., and D. E. Williams, "Loci of Disfluencies in the Speech of Non-stutterers During Oral Reading," *Journal of Speech and Hearing Research,* X (1967), 790–94.

Soderberg, G. A., "Linguistic Factors in Stuttering," *Journal of Speech and Hearing Research,* X (1967), 801–10.

———. "Phonetic Influences on Stuttering," *Journal of Speech and Hearing Research,* V (1962), 315–20.

———. "The Relations of Stuttering to Word Length and Word Frequency," *Journal of Speech and Hearing Research,* IX (1966), 584–89.

Starbuck, H., and M. D. Steer, "The Adaptation Effect in Stuttering Speech Behavior and Normal Speech," *Journal of Speech and Hearing Disorders,* XVIII (1953), 252–55.

Steer, M. D., and W. Johnson, "An Objective Study of the Relationship Between Psychological Factors and the Severity of Stuttering," *Journal of Abnormal and Social Psychology,* XXXI (1936), 36–46.

Stunden, A. A., "The Effects of Time Pressure as a Variable in the Verbal Behavior of Stutterers," *Dissertation Abstracts,* XXVI (1965), 1784–85 (abstract).

Tate, M. W., and W. L. Cullinan, "Measurement of Consistency of Stuttering," *Journal of Speech and Hearing Research,* V (1962), 272–83.

Taylor, J. A., "The Relationship of Anxiety to the Conditioned Eyelid Response," *Journal of Experimental Psychology,* XLI (1951), 81–92.

Taylor, I. K., "The Properties of Stuttered Words, *Journal of Verbal Learning and Behavior,* V (1966a), 112–18.

———. "What Words are Stuttered?" *Psychological Bulletin,* LXV (1966b), 233–42.

Travis, L. E., "Dissociation of the Homologous Muscle Function in Stuttering," *Archives of Neurology and Psychiatry,* XXX (1934), 127–33.

———. "The Influence of the Group Upon the Stutterer's Speech in Free Association," *Journal of Abnormal and Social Psychology,* XXIII (1928), 45–51.

———. "Disintegration of Breathing Movements During Stuttering," *Archives of Neurology and Psychiatry,* XVIII (1927), 673–90.

———. "The Unspeakable Feelings of People with Special Reference to Stuttering." In L. E. Travis (ed.), *Handbook of Speech Pathology.* New York: Appleton, 1957.

Travis, L. E., W. W. Tuttle, and D. W. Cowan, "A Study of Heart Rate During Stuttering," *Journal of Speech Disorders,* I (1936), 21–26.

Travis, V., "A Study of the Horizontal Disintegration of Breathing During Stuttering," *Archives of Speech,* I (1936), 157–70.

Trotter, W. D., "Relationship Between Severity of Stuttering and Word Conspicuousness," *Journal of Speech and Hearing Disorders,* XXI (1956), 198–201.

Trumper, M., "A Hematorespiratory Study of 101 Consecutive Cases of Stammering." Doctoral dissertation, University of Pennsylvania, 1928.

Tupper, M., "The Stammerer's Complaint." In J. Hunt, *Stammering and Stuttering.* 1861. Reprinted, New York: Hafner, 1967, p. 3.

Twitmeyer, E. B., "Stammering in Relation to Hemorespiratory Factors," *Quarterly Journal of Speech,* XVI (1930), 278–83.

Umeda, K., ["The Psychophysiological Study Upon Stutterers"] *Otology Fukuoka,* VI (1960), 377–91.

Valyo, R., "PGSR Responses of Stutterers and Nonstutterers During Periods of Silence and Verbalization," *Asha,* VI (1964), 422 (abstract).

Van Riper, C., *Speech Correction: Principles and Methods,* 4th Ed. Englewood Cliffs, N.J.: Prentice-Hall, 1963.

Van Riper, C., "The Influence of Empathic Response on Frequency of Stuttering." *Psychologic Monographs,* XLIX (1937), 244–46.

———. "Study of the Thoracic Breathing of Stutterers During Expectancy and Occurrence of Stuttering Spasms," *Journal of Speech Disorders,* I (1936), 61–72.

Van Riper, C., and C. J. Hull, "The Quantitative Measurement of the Effect of Certain Situations on Stuttering. In W. Johnson (ed.), *Stuttering in Children and Adults.* Minneapolis: University of Minnesota Press, 1955.

Van Riper, C., and R. L. Milisen, "A Study of the Predicted Duration of the Stutterers' Blocks as Related to their Actual Duration," *Journal of Speech Disorders,* IV (1939), 339–45.

Wiechmann, J., and E. Richter, "Die Haufigkeit des Stotterns beim Singen," *Folia Phoniatrica,* XVIII (1966), 435–46.

Williams, D. E., "Masseter Muscle Action Current Potentials in Stuttered and Nonstuttered Speech," *Journal of Speech and Hearing Disorders,* XX (1955), 242–61.

Wingate, M. E., "Stuttering Adaptation and Learning: I. The Relevance of Adaptation Studies to Stuttering as Learned Behavior," *Journal of Speech and Hearing Disorders,* XXXI (1966a), 148–56.

———. "Stuttering Adaptation and Learning: II. The Adequacy of Learning Principles in the Interpretation of Stuttering," *Journal of Speech and Hearing Disorders,* XXXI (1966b), 211–18.

———. "Evaluation and Stuttering," *Journal of Speech and Hearing Disorders,* XXVII (1962), 106–15; 244–57; 368–77.

———. "Stuttering Adaptation and Learning: I, The Relevance of Adaptation Studies to Stuttering as 'Learned' Behavior," *Journal of Speech and Hearing Disorders,* XXXI (1966), 148–56.

Wischner, G. J., "Anxiety Reduction as Reinforcement in Maladaptive Behavior: Evidence in Stutterer's Representations of the Moment of Difficulty," *Journal of Abnormal and Social Psychology,* XLVII (1952), 566–71.

Witt, M. H., "Statistische Erhebungen über den Einfluss des Singens und Flüsterns auf das Stottern," *Vox: Internationales Zentralblatt für Experimentalle Phonetik,* XI (1925), 41.

Young, M., "Audience Size, Perceived Situational Difficulty, and Stuttering Frequency," *Journal of Speech and Hearing Research,* VIII (1965), 401–7.

eight

THE SELF-CONCEPTS
OF STUTTERERS

We actively dislike the concept of self-concept. The abstraction is very difficult to make meaningful. Since the term *self-concept* has been used very loosely and in so many different ways it is hard to be sure we are really communicating when we use it. Psychological theories of the self have ranged from Moore's (1921) view of the self as the organized sum of all the individual's past experiences to Rogers' (1954) "the self the individual himself perceives, that is, his own attributes, feelings and behavior as observed subjectively and admitted to awareness (p. 85)." Tough old William James (1890) felt that the experience of the self was merely a complex of kinesthetic and organic sensations. Schilder (1950) stressed body image but did not omit the roles of emotion and evaluation in self-perception. With regard to the body image, he writes:

> The image of the human body means the picture of our own body which we form in our mind, that is to say, the way which the body appears to ourselves. These are sensations which are given to us. We see parts of the body surface. We have tactile, thermal, pain impressions. These are sensations which come from the muscles and their sheaths indicating the deformation of the muscle; sensations coming from the innervation of the muscles and sensations coming from the viscera. Beyond that there is the immediate experience that there is a unity of the body, a postural model of the body (p. 11).

Others have emphasized identity, continuity, evaluation, and social relationships as aspects of self-concept. Many writers protest the implication that the self-concept is unitary; they insist that we have as many selves as we have significant relationships. Others have said that we have "real-self" concepts and "ideal-self" concepts. Lowe (1961) reviewed the literature in an article called "Self-Concept: Fact or Artifact?" and came to no definite conclusions. Despite our distaste, however, we devote an entire chapter to the stutterer's self-concepts because there is no other hook on which to hang some very important information. Any therapist must deal with more than the stutterer's speech. Since stutterers have problems of identity, role, body image, and many other similar difficulties, we must try to understand them. We shall try to restrict our use of the term *self-concept* to self-awareness, self-identity, and self-evaluation, a restriction that probably won't restrict us much.

The literature on stuttering contains many statements to the effect that there is a unique "stuttering personality," although none of the various reviews of research have demonstrated that it exists. Nevertheless, although stutterers show a wide variety of personality patterns, perhaps as wide as that in the normal speaking population, there is no doubt that the person who says of himself, "I am a stutterer" formulates his self-concept in a way that implies compulsive deviancy. Such a self statement is almost as potent as a heroin user saying to himself for the first time: "I'm an addict." This self-identification as a member of a minority and deviant group has been demonstrated by Zelen, Sheehan, and Bugenthal (1954) and others. As stuttering develops, there comes a time when, as a result of his own communicative frustration and the social rejection he gets from others, the stutterer comes to label himself as such. He finds the label pinned on him over and over again. He is classified and grouped with other people who have trouble talking. With that label, he is given an identity as a deviant. It is a bad moment, one that will be repeated often. Wendell Johnson (1946) puts it vividly:

> It is likely that if you have never been regarded as a stutterer, you can come nowhere near appreciating the uncanny, crushing power of the social disapproval of whatever is regarded as stuttering. It is probably one of the most frightening, perplexing, and demoralizing influences to be found in our culture (p. 458).

Many groups and associations of stutterers, both here and abroad, have been organized to provide opportunities for social interaction and to minimize the deviancy. Few of them have survived very long, however, perhaps because of the stigma that is felt when an overt identification is made exceeds the relief gained. Many of the leaders of these groups, usually those with relatively more fluency but high degrees of situation fear, exploit their less fluent fellows by dominating the group meetings. In our experience they also tend to be highly punitive. Despite their loneliness, the severe stutterers soon find the situation intolerable, and unless new members appear the group breaks up. We know of two exceptions, one in Sweden, the Plus Club, and the National Council of Adult Stutterers based in Washington, D.C., which have existed for many years, and there may be others. In contrast to the prolific associations of other deviates, such as those for the blind, crippled, mentally retarded, or hard of hearing, where the deviancy is obvious and always present, stutterers' groups are based on a deviancy that is intermittent, easily disguised, and socially penalized, and the associations tend to be unstable. In this connection French (1966) writes:

> The fact is, and it is an important one, that stammerers cannot stand each other's company. For them there can be no equivalent of the invalid car rally [or] the homosexual bar. . . . Stammerers do not need each other— on the contrary, as I have mentioned before, they seek out and admire the fluent, as Moses was told by God to use Aaron and as Somerset Maugham needed his smooth, personable Gerald Huxton, his indispensable companion for twenty-five years (p. 74).

Indeed, the stutterer feels quite normal except when speaking—and even then provided he is not stuttering. The milder stutterer, as all clinicians soon discover, usually finds it very difficult even to look at another stutterer, especially one who stutters severely. Although he classifies himself as a stutterer, he has little pride or comfort in the fact. And his fluent intervals make group identification with other stutterers difficult.

THE BODY IMAGE

At the core of the self-concept is the body image. Here too there is conflict and ambivalence. When silent, the stutterer has no marked difference to reveal his deviancy. When speaking, his facial contortions, abnormal postures, and struggling suddenly present a most abnormal picture, not only to others but to himself. One stutterer, a beautiful girl, said,

> I'd rather be blind or deaf, or have a huge birthmark on my face, or be bald than stutter. Then I would always have the trouble and I could get used to it. I'll never be able to accept a face that only sometimes suddenly jumps around and makes horrible sounds. How can you learn to bear something that comes and goes so erratically?

Another said, "It's like as though my body changes its color. Sometimes it's all right, then suddenly it's black or purple. That's how it feels to stutter."

As Shearer (1961) asserted, conflicting body images may be present in the advanced stutterer. When silent, or when fluent, he looks pretty much like anyone else. Unlike the crippled, the image he presents to others at these times shows no deviancy. It is only when he stutters that he becomes, as one of our cases said, "a monster." It is only then that his deviancy appears.

Body image develops through the evaluations of others, through the adjectives they use and the comments they make about us. One stutterer said that when he was nine years old, a friend of his had said that he looked like a pig when he stuttered. Lip protrusion still occurred on the bilabials, but his body image was more important. "When I stutter I have a snout, not a mouth. I'm repulsive." A Q-Sort investigation, with items culled from a universe pertaining to the body image, would be, in our opinion, very revealing.

We have collected the self-drawings of many stuttering children. Some are quite normal, but there are others with no mouth at all, or with black scribbling where the mouth should be, one with feces-like sausages emerging from the lips, and some with earless heads. Most of the deviations occurred around the mouth, the rest of the body being drawn in the usual fashion. Fitzpatrick (1959) had adult stutterers draw themselves while speaking and also draw a picture of the ideal speaker. Marked differences were found, many of which concerned facial expression. The self-drawings showed clear distortion. The projective drawings in the Wischner (1952) and the Sheehan, Cortese, and Hadley studies (1962), although used in testing other hypotheses, have similar distortions around the mouth regions. According to Schilder (1950), whose work on body image is still the classic, the perception of our own body is focused on the areas around the openings into that body. The tension and spasmodic movements of the mouth experienced by advanced stutterers doubtless play some part in centering an awareness of abnormality in this region.

One must also explain the common finding that many stutterers are unable to describe exactly what their mouths are doing when they stutter. They find it hard to tell you about, or to duplicate, their abnormal mouth behaviors, even immediately after the moment of stuttering. Much training is necessary before they can do so. The perception seems to be couched in terms of affect, of generalized distress. Many stutterers and observers of stuttering have noted the marked dissociation which occurs at the moment of stuttering. A sort of black-out, an imperception, a blotting out of awareness seems to take place at the moment of the stuttering struggle and contortion. One stutterer said, "When I get stuck and my mouth starts jumping around, I slip out of my skin and fly up and sit on a limb until the word finally comes out. Then I return." In very severe stutterers, the dissociation is so extreme as to resemble a psychotic episode. It seems probable that this denial of the body image, even when transitory, must have a profound effect on the integration of the self-concept.

The body is not static, and it is the body image that provides continuity for the body in motion. The stutterer's body image, the essence of his identity, does not provide this continuity. Instead it flip-flops between normality and abnormality, and much of his basic insecurity stems from this inconsistency. Stutterers use various strategies to minimize the distress caused by these shifts in body image. Some of them try to strengthen the normal image by extreme and incessant carefulness in grooming. We have come to dub them "Dr. Jekyll stutterers" for they deny the "Mr. Hyde." Clinicians should see if this strategy is being used before asking a stutterer to watch himself in the mirror or to maintain eye contact with his listeners while stuttering. Such stutterers will resist and sabotage these assignments unless careful desensitization procedures are used first. They find it very difficult to confront their stuttering as a problem. They tend to deny it, to disguise it. They shut their eyes or look away when blocking. They intellectualize about their disorder in abstract terms. They show pronounced avoidance behavior. The clinician must understand that self-confrontation of the stuttering behavior for these persons poses a real threat to the very foundation of their identities. This is not to say that such stutterers should be spared the inevitable confrontation that therapy requires, but the clinician must understand the deep nature of the resistance. As Shearer (1961) writes:

> When confronted by recordings of their own stuttering, they are amazed and horrified. When required to face themselves in front of the mirror and stutter, they show marked reluctance and resistance. One case said that he "felt like Dr. Jekyll suddenly seeing Mr. Hyde" (p. 115).

Other stutterers solve their body image dilemma in the opposite way. They magnify their stuttering moments. They suffer visibly, almost revel in their verbal misery. Written accounts of their discomfort portray a morbidity so extreme as to seem pathological. Old wounds are probed over and over again to renew the ache. When they do pseudostuttering, they overdo it. They exaggerate most unrealistically the negative reactions of their listeners. Indeed, they often watch listeners closely for any hint of rejection. Whenever we find stutterers with good eye contact, we probe for evidence of this suspiciousness. Most of their stuttering behaviors consist of struggle reactions, facial contortions, and interruptor devices. These "Mr. Hyde stutterers" avoid situations more than they do words. They often prefer to be unkempt, even dirty. They resist reassurance by the therapist; their aspiration levels are low. They find it difficult to recognize that the fluent fraction of their speech output may have importance. They minimize their successes and maximize their failures. Their relapses are sudden, severe, and frequent. Again, the clinician must understand this behavior in terms of the body image problem. These stutterers don't want to be torn apart by intermittent fluency.

We are of course describing the extreme cases. Most stutterers are somewhere in between. Also, a given individual may oscillate back and forth along a continuum of self-identifications, and, during therapy, shift from his original position to its opposite. Any stutterer who shifts this way has a more favorable prognosis than one who does not. The therapist's task is to help the stutterer reconcile his two self-images and create an integrated one. Our own solution to this conflict, at the beginning of therapy, has been to promote the image of a fluent stutterer with a tolerable minimum of abnormality when it does occur and an appropriate appreciation of the fluency that always exists and can be facilitated. During therapy, this provides at least a temporary solution to the identity problem.

THE SOCIAL ASPECT OF THE STUTTERER'S SELF-CONCEPT

Our self-concepts contain much more than body image. They also include our notion of the way others see us. We construct our personal identities by internalizing the reactions and evaluations of the people who play important parts in our lives—parents, siblings, mates, friends, employers, and fellow workers. What we think we see in the eyes of others often determines what and whom we think we are. We live in a spider web of human relationships and must find our identities therein. Our own part of the web is tugged and distorted by the forces which affect any other part and, alas, we must remember most spider webs contain some spiders.

Much of the stutterer's abnormal speech behavior is based on the evaluations of others and the way he perceives them. If his parents react to his disfluencies with anxiety or rejection, then the stutterer will develop behaviors of avoidance and struggle, indicating that he has accepted their value judgments. If others find him unspeakable, he will soon find it difficult to speak. Conceptions of self emerge from social interaction. Even one's body image is affected by the responses made to it by others as Wright's (1960) review of physical disability has made clear. However, in a larger sense, we also view our identities in terms of our social status as defined by others and in terms of the roles we play in the social groups to which we belong.

THE SOCIAL STATUS OF THE STUTTERER

Since the organization of social groups depends on communication, stuttering impairs a person's ability to find or maintain a satisfying place in society as ours. Social status in our culture is determined largely by occupation, education, and evidence of success as measured by wealth and possessions, and by the number of people upon whom the person has claims.

Effective communication enhances the achievement of prestige in all of these, and stuttering, when severe, certainly interferes with it.

Many occupations require effective speech, and this fact screens out the stutterer or at least makes his participation very difficult. Any stutterer who wants to teach or be a salesman or a speech therapist must surmount formidable barriers. The vocational choices of stutterers have not been investigated thoroughly but, in general, the evidence indicates that stutterers usually choose vocations in which the lack of fluency will not jeopardize their success. This is not to say that stutterers prefer these occupations. Indeed, as Barbara (1954) maintains, they often see themselves as giants in chains. They dream of perfectionistic verbal achievements (the Demosthenes complex), and often they unrealistically prepare themeslves for vocations they are obviously not fitted for. It is true also that a few gifted stutterers with special opportunity and great motivation have managed to attain success in all occupations. One of the most successful salesmen we ever knew was a severe stutterer. "I have an advantage over other salesmen," he said, "The people I contact never forget me. I've learned to put them at ease and sometimes when they get too frustrated by my stuttering they give me a sale just to get rid of me." These exceptions only prove the rule. Many, if not most, stutterers are denied the social status that accompanies the more prestigious occupations and professions.

Social status, of course, is not always determined by wealth or occupation. The Chinese distinguish between two kinds of status: *mien* and *lien*. When they save *mien* (face), they preserve the reputation of the family; when they save *lien* (also face) they protect their personal integrity and reputation. Both types of status are affected by stuttering. We have worked with both Chinese and Japanese stutterers and found that our major difficulties concerned *mien*. A Chinese stutterer who could not bear to watch his stuttering on videotape or even to listen to it on an audiotape recording said, "Every time I stutter, nineteen generations of ancestors cry out from their graves." A black stutterer said,

> Whenever I stutter, you become whiter and I blacker. Whenever I stutter to a white man, I shame my whole race. If I could only get my race off my back, I could handle my mouth.

The daughter of a millionaire said that she had avoided practically all contact with her "social inferiors" though at considerable cost of effort and ingenuity.

> In my own set, when I stutter, no one flickers an eyelash. We all pretend that nothing has happened. Noblesse oblige, you know, and politesse, and the old tale of the Emperor's clothes. But when I have talked to clerks while shopping, or even to our chauffeur or yardmen, they stare, or stop what they are doing, or look pityingly and I can't bear it. So I find ways of never talking to anyone out of my class.

A successful business man said,

> If I know I can fire them or buy them, I don't mind my stuttering so much
> and I don't stutter so hard. I'm on top and they're down under. Don't give
> a damn what they think. It's my equals that bother me.

The last excerpt illustrates an important point in the status dynamics of
stuttering. As Sheehan, Hadley, and Gould (1967) have demonstrated, stutterers usually have more trouble speaking to authority figures or to their
superiors than to the people upon whom they have claims. They do not
expect as much rejection or penalty from the latter, and the rejection or
penalty they do receive is not as meaningful. Many stutterers know this
well. They do unwanted favors for others to put them in their debt; on the
job, in the family, or in the clinic, they do the dirty work, so that obliga-
tions are contracted. We have watched some of them weave complicated
webs of potlatch-like claims just so they could gain tolerance if not acceptance for their lack of fluency. Clinicians must always be aware of this tendency and beware of being entangled in the claim web.

SOCIAL IDENTITY
AND SOCIAL CONTROL

Self-evaluation depends only partly on social status as determined by family
position, occupation, wealth, or claims. It depends also on the attitudes and
evaluations of the people who are important to us and with whom we interact daily. Their expectations are powerful forces in shaping our self-concepts, positively or negatively. Not all the people with whom we interact are
equally important in this shaping process, but in each life there are always
a few special persons and groups whose acceptances, approvals, or rejections
are especially significant and potent in determining how we view ourselves.

One of the most important groups of course is the family. A large
amount of research, some of it conflicting in its conclusions, has been focused on parental reactions to stuttering. In general, it supports the common belief that parents tend to interpret stuttering as noxious behavior and
respond negatively to it. Kinstler (1961) has shown how important covert
rejection can be, and the autobiographies of most of our stutterers attest to
the traumatic effect of such parental reactions. Stutterers have been rejected, punished, mocked. They have been slapped and made to eat in the
kitchen when company came. Their stuttering has provoked family conflicts.
Their siblings have bedevilled them. Other stuttering children have been
pampered and overprotected, indeed almost encapsulated, by their parents
in the effort to spare them social penalty. This may cause other children in
the family to feel jealous resentment, which they may show in many different ways. In some families, stuttering is never mentioned or overtly re-

sponded to, although the covert negative reactions of the family members are quite obvious. When the stutterer is aware that he stutters, a family conspiracy of silence makes him feel that stuttering is somehow so evil it cannot even be mentioned. These reactions have ill effects on the still plastic self-concepts of those children. They make the child feel abnormal and socially unclean. They make him feel deviant.

Other significant persons and groups are found on the playground and at school. Although the research here is sparse, plenty of anecdotal accounts indicate that teasing, mockery, and rejection are common experiences for the child who stutters. Brook (1957), a British therapist, writes:

> . . . stammering is regarded as "socially taboo," "something nasty," or "something that just isn't acceptable." This attitude seems to be common to most countries and must have been handed down from ancient times. It is not merely to be explained away on the basis of sentiments passed on from parents to children. There seems to be something inherent in all of us (perhaps it springs from our racial unconscious) that causes us to view stammering, or the occasion of someone slipping on a banana skin, as something amusing (p. 105).

Stuttering has stimulus value. It is both visible and audible. Since it interferes with school recitations and the social play of children, it calls much unfavorable attention to itself, and few stutterers escape unscathed from the mockery and punishment of their peers. In the schoolroom or on the playground the child is on his own. There are no parents to protect him there; he feels the full force of the social controls against deviancy.

In adolescence, the stutterer's problems redouble. Try as he will to conform to the mores of his peer group in dress, hairdo, and rebellion, he finds it difficult to hold his own in the swift verbal interaction so important for this group. Adolescents are often the clinician's toughest cases. They cannot bear to confront their stuttering deviancy long enough to do anything about it. They resist being singled out. They want the security of peer group affiliation with an intensity which is almost overwhelming.

In adulthood, the important persons and groups are those of sexual partnership, marriage, and vocation. Here too, the stutterer feels the force of negative evaluation. Often he selects a sexual partner who evaluates his speech with unusual tolerance, one who is impelled, by insecurity or value judgment to seek a spouse who is not a threat.

> I happened by chance to be working with three boys and a girl two years ago, all of whom were about to be married. I was struck by the fact that all four of them maintained that they never stuttered at all with their prospective spouses. Do you suppose they chose spouses with whom they were fluent? Was it that the positive emotion of young love obliterated fear? Or were they evaluating their speech through rose-colored earmolds?

There is little research on the wives or husbands of stutterers, and it would be most interesting to discover their bases for marital choice. A few stutterers, especially those who have been enrolled in a speech clinic, marry other stutterers, but in general, the stutterer seeks a partner who can both accept him and protect him against communicative trauma and stress. We have seen some very good marriages which satisfied these criteria.

THE STIGMA OF STUTTERING

The end result of all these negative reactions from the important people and groups in the life of a stutterer is that he usually comes to conceive of himself not only as an inefficient speaker but as an undesirable and reprehensible one. Society classifies people according to its normative standards of behavior. In communication, a function essential to group cohesiveness, the stutterer violates the norms. His stuttering is an attribute that makes him different from others in an undesirable way. Such a discrediting attribute is what sociologists mean by stigma. It is a negative behavioral valence applied to deviancy by members of a society.

Stuttering, however, is only one of many attributes in a given person. The stutterer may be tall and good-looking or very athletic. He may be a good dancer, a fine writer, a brilliant scientist. All of us have differences, some of which are assets and others liabilities. Others accept us or reject us first on the basis of their own needs in a particular relationship situation, and second on the basis of the algebraic summation of our assets and liabilities. Although stuttering is considered a stigma of sorts, the stutterer may have other attributes that are highly valued by the people he knows, and these attributes permit group acceptance despite the stigma. He might be unable to join the college debate team because of the emphasis this group places on verbal fluency, but he might be readily accepted on the basketball team if he can shoot well enough or is eight feet tall. It should be noted, however, that since most groups maintain their cohesion through communication, the stigma of stuttering requires an inordinate amount of compensatory assets to cancel its effect. The pervasiveness of this stigma often causes the stutterer to accentuate this one feature of his personality so that it colors his whole self-concept. Whatever else he may be, and surely he is many things, he often comes to consider himself first and foremost as a stutterer. He is the Ancient Mariner and stuttering is his albatross.

Once a stutterer defines himself as a stutterer, as belonging to a special category of persons, the new role changes his perceptions in many ways. He is not just a boy, or a son, or an athlete, or a student, or any other of his cluster of roles. The adjective "stuttering" becomes attached to each designation. The stutterer-role permeates and influences all other roles because speech is important in social relationships. It modifies his expectancies of others and of himself. The research on aspiration level indicates that, with certain exceptions, stutterers aspire to levels lower than those of normal speakers, not only in speech but in other goal-setting activities. This is easy to understand when one realizes that the stutterer tries and fails to speak without stuttering hundreds of times each day. The cumulative influence of this repeated failure, and the many avoidances of speaking opportunities has a profound effect on his self-esteem. Helplessness, hopelessness, and worthlessness dominate his life.

When the stutterer assumes the role of stutterer the consequences can be devastating. Identity problems rear their ugly heads. Pretense, pseudo-identities, and counterfeit roles are attempted and fail with exposure. Self-alienation, denial, and disavowal take their turn with self-hatred, depression, or fantasies of self-glorification. "If only I didn't stutter . . ." said the giant feeling his chains. "If only I could speak," sang the hermit thrush. Obsessed with the need to protect themselves from hurt, some stutterers withdraw from social interaction to lick their wounds and build the walls that will later imprison them. Or they fasten like leeches to the few of their companions who do not punish them. There are a hundred habitual patterns of behavior which result from assuming the role of stutterer. We cannot mention them all but any competent clinician soon learns to diagnose and assess them carefully.

STIGMA VISIBILITY

Students of physical disability and deformity have a concept we should consider here. It is "visibility." A stigma is assessed according to its degree of visibility or obtrusiveness. Stutterers vary markedly, one from another, in terms of this visibility-audibility concept. One single, long blocking accompanied by bizarre facial contortions, jaw jerks, and limb movements, even though it is followed by five hundred fluently spoken words, constitutes a more "visible" stigma than 50 short prolongations or repetitions of a sound spoken without struggle. Stutterers learn this fact very soon and many of them escape from the consequences of their stuttering stigma by complicated rituals of avoidance and by "interiorizing" their stuttering. These interiorized stutterers have been described very vividly by Freund (1935) and Douglass and Quarrington (1952). We asked one such stutterer a question and had to wait minutes before he answered. Not an expression crossed his face. No attempt at speech was visible although a slight straining of the neck muscles indicated that he had heard me. Finally and suddenly he blurted the answer and said, "Oh, that was a long hard one." These interiorized stutterers seem to suffer even more than those whose behavior is overt. They operate communicatively in an incredible state of tension and vigilance. Their long, silent gaps distress not only their listeners but themselves. But they do manage to keep their stuttering stigma fairly invisible and inaudible by using tricks. They are very difficult cases for the clinician to help. It is interesting that Douglas and Quarrington found that the majority of their interiorized stutterers came from families striving for upward mobility.

SOCIAL EVALUATION AND
REACTIONS TO STUTTERING

Quite apart from the personal reactions of others to stuttering, which we have considered earlier, there are a number of stereotyped beliefs about the disorder, and most stutterers come to know them very well. One of these is that the stutterer is nervous, and needs calming. This belief probably comes from the nonfluency that most normal speakers exhibit under emotional stress. Perfect strangers will tell a stutterer to relax, to calm down, to take it easy. Another of these stereotypes is that stuttering is funny. Inevitably, the comic strips and television cartoons have exploited this, much to the suffering of stutterers who fail to see anything humorous about their disorder. Normally speaking children mock their stuttering playmates, call them "stutter-tongue" or sing the old song about K-K-K-Katy. There are many jokes about stuttering, a few of them even appropriate for polite company. There is another stereotype—that the stutterer is a bit insane or crazy. This one is usually reserved for those who show marked facial and bodily contortions. We have seen mothers snatch their children away from conversations with such stutterers. Another is that stuttering is a bad habit, like masturbation or thumb-sucking, which should be punished forthwith lest it continue. Another is that the stutterer is not very bright since he has not even learned to talk. Even babies learn to talk. Normally speaking persons who believe this speak very simply and carefully even to the adult stutterer and always a bit patronizingly. Many of our adult cases report that when they stutter upon asking directions to a bank or shop, the listeners will almost try to take them by the hand and take them there.

To dilute the demeaning impact which such listener reactions can have upon them, many stutterers develop intricate counterreactions. They restrict their social activity to groups that accept them, such as church organizations (or Boy Scouts), where they have the protection of an adult leader, or to clubs where they need take no active verbal part in the proceedings. When bidding for entrance into a new group, they contrive individual relationships with people who can later sponsor their membership without loss of group esteem. Stutterers often reconcile themselves to phantom membership, being present at the gatherings but never participating. Token belongingness is better than none, and they are careful not to run the risk of expulsion by opening their mouths. They become highly adept at scanning and evaluating the amount of group tolerance for their stuttering and do not exceed it.

A stutterer who feels like a marginal member of a social group may work hard at token identification. He may confine his utterance to the automatisms of small talk, or nonpropositional utterance. He often echoes what others have just said, begins to speak only under cover of the noises of their conversation, or uses many gestures and facial expressions to convey an impression of his interested participation. Or he may laugh a lot or even play the clown or fool to allay his hunger for social interaction. Some stutterers gain acceptance because they seem to be such good listeners. Other stutterers, in contrast, may pose as very taciturn individuals, speaking tersely, almost telegraphically, or starting to say something then pretending to think and hastily agreeing with the interlocutor who then finishes the sentence for them.

We have known stutterers who had become very adept in seeking entrance into new groups by mastering what might be called disclosure strategies. Even before they showed any actual stuttering they would, for example, casually or humorously comment upon the fact that they were stutterers. Or after the inadvertent disclosure of their impediment they would say something such as "Well, there I did it again. Thought I could keep from stuttering with you," or "Holy smoke, my tongue sure got tangled on that one, didn't it?" One of them, when asking a prospective employer for a job, would use this gambit: "Sir, could I have ten minutes of your valuable time to have a one minute conversation? I've got to say my name and introduce myself." Others have used a stuttering joke to break the ice and disarm a potential punisher. Others smile calmly after a moment of stuttering and repeat what they have previously said. They know an old truth, that the attitude of their listener is partly determined by the stutterer's own attitude. If the stutterer appears to accept his speaking disability without

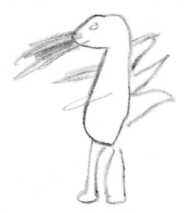

Figure 11. Self-drawing by a six-year-old boy. "During the time I'm saying it, I feel like a monster. Feel all hot when I stutter. Sometimes feel like I'm going to tip over when I say it that way."

emotional stress, the odds are that the listener will too. Stutterers become very skillful at computing odds, at estimating probabilities of listener responses.

ROLE BEHAVIOR IN STUTTERING

The self-concept may be visually schematized as a mulberry shaped lump. Its core is the body image, but clustering about that center are the various roles assumed by the person. Some of these roles are the more prominent bumps on our mulberry of the self. The outward contours change with time as new roles are acquired and old ones discarded. Our ever-changing social relationships demand that we change our patterns of behavior to fit them. We walk through a series of different social worlds in the course of a life time, each of which makes certain demands, and we adjust our behavior accordingly. We often have to bid for entrance into new groups; our acceptance depends on how well we satisfy the groups' criteria for membership. Stutterers have trouble doing this.

The stutterer does not live, like Kipling's wolf, "by his wild lone." He too, despite his difficulty in communication, must live in a social matrix. We have known a few hermit stutterers but only a few. Most stutterers do what all of us must do, experiment with new roles and shape our behavior in terms of group expectations. The stutterer, however, because of his communicative impediment is subject to narrower limits in his choice of roles than most of us are. Some of the limitations are imposed by others; we hope, for example that no stutterer serves as a traffic controller for any plane we might take. Some of the limits are self-imposed. We have known boys who refused to join the Boy Scouts because they knew they would stutter in saying the Scout oath or laws, youths who refused to be quarterbacks on football teams because they could not call signals fast enough, men who refused to get married for many reasons, all of which were based on their inability to communicate effectively. There are few social roles that do not require adequate speech. The stutterer soon learns and feels his limitations.

Nevertheless, most stutterers manage to acquire jobs and friends and mates and children, even though their choices (for all but the last of these) are more limited than for normal speakers. They have to work harder, tolerate more initial rejection, or accept a subordinate position in a new group. They must create compensatory assets in order to gain acceptance, and in general learn to live within their communicative limitations. A stutterer, once he has been able to master a new role and to know its satisfactions, often finds that role difficult to abandon, even when the social circumstances make it inappropriate. One stutterer, for example, reported his intense shame when he found himself clowning and laughing while telling a group of his friends that his brother had just been killed in an automobile accident. He had long used humor as a ploy to gain group acceptance. We know a stuttering scientist who spoiled one of our fly-fishing trips on the Gunnison River in Colorado by being unable to talk about anything except nuclear physics, even after he fell into a hole and wet his ears. It is our general impression that the more severe the stuttering, the fewer the roles undertaken. Perseveration in inappropriate social behavior may be largely due to the role rigidity created by stuttering.

At the same time, the stutterer also has a penchant for acting. Despite his difficulty in playing the new roles demanded by society, most stutterers speak more fluently when they escape from their real self-concepts by assuming phony roles. We have known stutterers to pass themselves off as policemen, ministers of the gospel, or visitors from foreign lands, and to be entirely fluent while playing these parts. Some very successful actors and actresses have been severe stutterers except on the stage or screen. Some stutterers are clergymen who are fluent only in the pulpit or in their ministerial robes. By playing false roles, these stutterers free themselves temporarily from their histories of stuttering, from their stuttering selves. By altering their language and denying their identities they escape from the control of the self-centered stimuli to which much of their stuttering behavior has been conditioned. However, the jeopardy of possible exposure often creates its own anxiety and this in turn more stuttering. Few stutterers are able to play such patently false roles long enough to incorporate them into their real self-concepts.

It is interesting to observe that when some stutterers in an unfamiliar situation, or as a result of therapy, are able to speak very fluently, they experience the same exposure-anxiety as when playing the false roles mentioned earlier. In them, the self-concept has become so colored by stuttering that prolonged and unexpected fluency is experienced as being almost traumatic. A role is a consistent pattern of behavior in a social context. Its use is governed primarily by group expectations. For years the adult stutterer has lived in groups which expected him to stutter and now suddenly he does not. Though relieved, he feels strange. Somehow, the integrity of the self feels threatened by that unexpected fluency. He does not feel like *him*. One stutterer said,

> Thank God! I'm glad that period of false fluency is over and I'm my old stuttering self again. The pressure was getting unbearable. Every new sentence, every new word I spoke, I thought would suddenly come out in the old horrible stuttering way and when they didn't, the pressure grew. I felt like a fake talking so easily and I knew it couldn't last. Odd as it may seem, now that I've relapsed, I feel calmer, more of a piece, even though I'm sorry it's gone.

Clinicians must deal with more than the speech of stutterers.

RESEARCH ON SELF-CONCEPT

The research dealing with the self-concepts of stutterers is scanty. An early investigation using questionnaires, interviews, and autobiographies by Johnson (1932) to study the stutterer's personality characteristics showed that wide varieties of personality patterns existed among his subjects. One of the first experiments on the problem, using the Q-Sort technique pioneered in England by Stephenson, was done by Fiedler and Wepman (1951) using ten stutterers (with only six nonstutterers as controls). They found no differences of statistical significance. A more thorough study using the Q-Sort was performed by Nelson (1955). It showed that the self-concepts of stutterers were more closely focused on stuttering than were those of a comparable group of student therapists. The stutterers tended to perceive themselves primarily in terms of their speech, i.e., as stutterers. Rahman (1956) also used this technique but compared real and ideal self-concepts of stutterers and their controls, finding some few differences (primarily those dealing with social interaction) in the real self-concepts but very few in ideal self-concepts. Essentially both groups were similar. Clark and Murray (1965) present three case studies showing the use of the Q-Sort and other self-concept measures in diagnosis and prognosis. In another publication Clark, (1965) illustrates the clinical use of the Illinois Index of Self Derogation, a stuttering Behavior Analysis Chart, and the Draw-a-Person test.

Another method of assessing the self-concepts of stutterers is the W-A-Y ("Who are you?") technique. Subjects are asked to answer this question repeatedly and differently each time. Zelen, Sheehan, and Bugenthal (1954) gave the test to 30 stutterers and 160 nonstutterers, finding some differences. One of the chief of these was in group membership. The stutterers conceived of themselves first as stutterers, (Sheehan, 1954) and then in terms of other roles. The role-perception of adolescent stutterers was investigated by Buscaglia (1963) using a modified form of the Sarbin-Hardyck Test. He found that the stutterers were less able to perceive their own life roles, and the life roles of others, than were the nonstutterers. He suggested that the differences reflected the social inadequacy of the stutterers. Other investigations of self-concept have used body image self-drawings (Clark, 1963; Fitzpatrick, 1959), the semantic differential (Hansen, 1964), and adjective checklists (Redwine, 1959) without yielding any firm conclusions about the self-concepts of stutterers as a group. Rieber (1963) presents a critical review of the general literature on stutterers' self-concepts.

COMMENTARY

When speaking, we must bypass the self. The stutterer cannot do this. He cannot forget his own body, his crooked mouth (Emonds, 1953–1954, p. 43).

. . . the longer the person has abnormal disfluencies, or the more gen-eralized his difficulties are in terms of words and situations, or the more these are brought to his attention in some way, then the more likely he is to develop a self-concept of being different—of being handicapped. His diffi-culties may be magnified by listener reaction or by self-imposed penalties, such as frustration. One of the more common ways to magnify the problem is to label the speaker a stutterer. It may also be magnified by subconscious psychological reasons for being dependent or for failing. Regardless of how it occurs, magnification of the disfluency increases the probability that the speaker will generalize from a self-concept of "I am a person who sometimes has difficulty speaking" to "I am a handicapped person" (Luper, 1968, p. 95).

In a very deep sense, the fundamental process around which the speaking, socializing, and total behavior of a person revolve is the *self process*. To a very considerable extent, a person's stuttering is determined by what he thinks of himself or of his "speech self," consciously or otherwise, (Murphy and Fitzsimons, 1960, p. 115).

I was a dancer with a divided face. One side, the right side, was serene; the hair nicely combed; the eye nice; the face unlined; the mouth just right. The other side, the left, was so different. The hair was in long, wild curls, the eye cocked and wild, face hard and lined, lipstick smeared and messy. I waited to see what would happen. I knew I would end up all one way or the other. I kept on dancing. Slowly the mouth became like the right side. Then the face changed to good side, then the hair changed until at the end the whole head and face were good except the left eye which remained a bit wild and watchful as if to say, "Ha, ha, you can't change me." (Travis, 1957, p. 956).

It is clear that the stutterer's role has a high degree of primacy in the sense that subjectively it pervades all his other roles. Although speech pathologists have emphasized the societal rejection of the stutterer, it is the internal rather than the external limits which seem to be more significant in explaining his [lack of] social participation (Lemert, 1951, p. 164).

Do you talk or think mainly about your stuttering as something that happens to you—or as something that you yourself do? Do you take for granted that you are a "stutterer," as though you were a native of Stutterania, perhaps a special kind of human being? (Johnson, 1961, p. 172).

It was Christmas eve. I remember that a cold wind was blowing and my teeth chattered as I rushed into the hardware store just before closing time. A group of clerks greeted me at the doorway. Gasping for breath, but smiling with eager anticipation, I proudly held out a shiny new silver dollar in the palm of my hand and tried to make known the object of my errand. "I want a kn-n-n-n" was as far as I got. The harder I tried the more severely I stut-tered. I felt the blood rush to my cheeks as I turned away from the clerks to look into the nearest counter, hoping that it contained pocketknives so that I could point to the gift I wanted. I saw only egg-beaters and strainers, so I tried again to say the word "knife" but in vain. Suddenly the men broke out in lusty laughter. I looked at them and tried to smile, but something seemed to choke me. I knew then that it would be useless to try to talk again, so I turned and ran out of the store, afraid not of the group of men, but of a new strange feeling of weakness and embarrassment which I had never experienced before. I lay awake for many hours, clutching the silver dollar, wondering why this had happened to me, and dreading to face the next day without the gift I so longed for. I was nine years old then and had been stuttering for more than two years, but until this incident occurred I had not become fully aware of the seriousness of my handicap. (Wedberg, 1937. From *The Stutterer Speaks* by Conrad Wedberg. Reprinted by permission of Expression Company, Publishers, Magnolia, Mass., pp. 24–25)

. . . there are few or no specialized roles available to stutterers, save perhaps that of a clown or entertainer. Fashioning their own roles is difficult because effective speech is a requirement for most social roles. Consequently they are reduced to filling conventional occupational roles usually below their educational or skills level, becoming, in a figurative sense, ridiculous or strangely silent hewers of wood and haulers of water (Lemert, 1967, p. 53).

The stutterer is usually a very nice fellow. You can always depend on him for a favor, like driving you someplace, letting you smoke his cigarettes, and never asking you for gas money. You'd really like to ask him to go out with the gang Friday night, but he just wouldn't fit in. He wouldn't enjoy himself (A stutterer).

BIBLIOGRAPHY

Barbara, D. A., *Stuttering: A Psychodynamic Approach to Its Understanding and Treatment*. New York: Julian, 1954.

Brook, F., *Stammering and Its Treatment*. London: Pitman, 1957.

Buscaglia, L. F., "An Experimental Study of the Sarbin-Hardyck Test as Indices of Role Perception for Adolescent Stutterers," *Speech Monographs*, XXX (1963), 243 (abstract).

Clark, R. M., "Techniques for Evaluating the Self-Concept of Stutterers," *De Therapia Vocis et Loquellae*, I (1965), 303–6.

———. "The Psychological Implications for Speech and Hearing Therapists of the Characteristics of Infantile Thinking and Body Image." In D. A. Barbara (ed.), *Psychological and Psychiatric Aspects of Speech and Hearing*. Springfield, Ill.: Thomas, 1960.

———. "The Self-Concept of Stutterers as Shown by Their Drawings," *Journal of the Australian College of Speech Therapy*, XIII (1963), 52–56.

Clark, R. M., and F. M. Murray, "Alterations in Self-Concept: A Barometer of Progress in Individuals Undergoing Therapy for Stuttering." In D. A. Barbara (ed.), *New Directions in Stuttering*. Springfield, Ill.: Thomas, 1965.

Douglass, E., and B. Quarrington, "The Differentiation of Interiorized and Exteriorized Stuttering," *Journal of Speech and Hearing Disorders,* XVII (1952), 377–85.

Emonds, P. L. F., "Het Stotteren," ["Stuttering"] *Gawein,* II (1953–1954), 1–17; 43–47.

Fiedler, F. E., and J. M. Wepman, "An Exploratory Investigation of the Self-Concept of Stutterers," *Journal of Speech and Hearing Disorders,* XVI (1951), 110–14.

Fitzpatrick, J. A., "An Investigation of the Body Image in Secondary Stutterers Revealed by Self-Drawings." Doctoral dissertation, Denver University, 1959.

French, P., "The Stammerer as Hero," *The Encounter,* XXVII (1966), 67–75.

Freund, H., "Über Inneres Stottern," *Zeitschrift Ohrenheilkunde,* LXIX, (1935), 146–48.

Hansen, R., "A Study of the Self-Concepts of Stutterers as Evaluated by a Semantic Differential Test." Master's thesis, Michigan State University, 1964.

Hanson, W., "The Self-Related Concept Discrepancies of Stutterers." Master's thesis, San Jose State College, 1961.

James, W., *Principles of Psychology,* Vol. I. New York: Holt, 1890.

Johnson, W., *People in Quandaries.* New York: Harper, 1946.

———. *Stuttering and What You Can Do About It.* Minneapolis: University of Minnesota Press, 1961.

———. "The Influence of Stuttering on the Personality," *University of Iowa Studies in Child Welfare,* V (1932), 1–140.

Kinstler, D. B., "Covert and Overt Maternal Rejection in Stuttering," *Journal of Speech and Hearing Disorders,* XXVI (1961), 145–55.

Lemert, E. M., *Human Deviance, Social Problems, and Social Control.* Englewood Cliffs, N. J.: Prentice-Hall, 1967.

———. *Social Pathology.* New York: McGraw-Hill, 1951.

Lowe, C. M., "The Self-Concept, Fact or Artifact?" *Psychological Bulletin,* LVIII (1961), 525–36.

Luper, H. L., "An Appraisal of Learning Theory Concepts in Understanding and Treating Stuttering." In H. H. Gregory (ed.), *Learning Theory and Stuttering Therapy.* Evanston: Northwestern University Press, 1968.

Moore, J. S., *The Foundations of Psychology.* Princeton: Princeton University Press, 1921.

Murphy, A. T., and R. M. Fitzsimons, *Stuttering and Personality Dynamics.* New York: Ronald, 1960.

Nelson, L., "An Investigation of the Changes in the Self-Concept of Stutterers." Master's thesis, Western Michigan University, 1955.

Rahman, P., "The Self-Concept and Ideal Self-Concept of Stutterers as Compared with Nonstutterers." Master's thesis, Brooklyn College, 1956.

Redwine, G. W., "An Experimental Study of the Relationship Between Self-Concepts of Fourth and Eighth Grade Stuttering and Nonstuttering Boys," *Speech Monographs,* XXVI (1959), 140–41 (abstract).

Rieber, R. W., "Stuttering and Self-Concept," *Journal of Psychology,* LV (1963), 307–11.

Rogers, C. B., and R. F. Diamond (eds.), *Psychotherapy and Personality Change.* Chicago: University of Chicago Press, 1954.

Schilder, P., *The Image and Appearance of the Human Body.* New York: International Universities Press, 1950.

Shearer, W. M., "A Theoretical Consideration of the Self-Concept and Body Image in Stuttering Therapy," *Asha,* III (1961), 115 (abstract).

Sheehan, J., "Self-Perception in Stuttering," *Journal of Clinical Psychology,* X (1954), 70–72.

Sheehan, J. G., P. Cortese, and R. Hadley, "Guilt, Shame, and Tension in Graphic Projections of Stuttering," *Journal of Speech and Hearing Disorders,* XXVII (1962) 129–39.

Sheehan, J., R. Hadley, and E. Gould, "Impact of Authority on Stuttering," *Journal of Abnormal Psychology,* LXXII (1967), 290–93.

Sheehan, J. G., S. L. Zelen, and J. F. T. Bugental, "Self-Perception in Stuttering," *Journal of Clinical Psychology,* X (1954), 70–72.

Starkweather, C. W., personal communication, 1970.

Travis, L. E., "The Unspeakable Feelings of People with Special Reference to Stuttering." In L. E. Travis (ed.), *Handbook of Speech Pathology.* New York: Appleton-Century, 1957.

Wedberg, C. F., *The Stutterer Speaks.* Magnolia, Mass: Expression Company, 1937.

Wischner, G. J., "An Experimental Approach to Expectancy and Anxiety in Stuttering Behavior," *Journal of Speech and Hearing Disorders,* XVII (1952), 139–54.

Wright, B. A., *Physical Disability: A Psychological Approach.* New York: Harper, 1960.

Zelen, S. L., Sheehan, J. G. and J. F. T. Bugental, "Self Perceptions in Stuttering." *Journal of Clinical Psychology,* X (1954), 70–72.

nine

THE SEVERITY OF
STUTTERING

Once when we were video recording an adult stutterer reading a
long passage for the first time, he only stuttered once and that
one time was on the first word. Later we measured the duration
of that moment of stuttering and it lasted only four tenths of a
second. Anyone who listened only to the sound track would have
been certain that the person was a normal speaker. And yet in
that four tenths of a second, his mouth gaped, his tongue pro-
truded tremorously, his eyeballs bulged, and his whole face was
contorted as he strained and struggled for utterance. Then he
suddenly stopped the struggle and said the word. If we had measured the severity of his stuttering only in terms of frequency or
duration, we would have concluded that he was a mild stutterer,
even though the young man said it was one of the worst blocks
he had ever experienced. We showed this segment of the videotape to a group of viewers and they unanimously agreed that it
was the speech of a very severe stutterer.

This example illustrates some of the difficulties in devising
adequate measures of severity. Another example may also be illuminating. A high school boy referred himself to our clinic saying that his stuttering was getting much worse. When we talked
to his parents and teachers, they were surprised. All of them said
he had improved greatly in previous weeks, that he now stuttered very rarely. One teacher did say that he was not reciting as
much as he used to but that when he did, she seldom heard him
stutter. What had occurred, of course, was that the youth had

begun to hide his stuttering, to develop silent struggling, and to avoid speaking whenever he felt that he might have trouble. Before, he had been fairly unconcerned about his stuttering; now he was deeply ashamed of it, a reaction that stemmed from an unfortunate experience. He had asked a pretty girl for a date, and she had responded flippantly, "I'm not so hard up that I have to date a stutterer like you." We cannot always rely on listener judgments in evaluating the severity of stuttering.

NEED FOR MEASURES
OF SEVERITY

We urgently need good measures of stuttering severity. We need them in research, for some of the conflicting results of different investigations of the same problem probably result from different severity mixes. One investigator, with an unusually large proportion of very severe stutterers among his subjects, for example, may find that their coordination is inferior, while another, with a large proportion of very mild stutterers in his group, will get conflicting results. The adaptation curves of very severe stutterers differ markedly from those of mild stutterers, and there are many other reasons why we have to control for severity in research samples.

Similarly, in clinical practice, we constantly evaluate the stutterer's performance. How bad a stutterer is he? Is he getting better or worse? Are our methods effective? During the initial examination, severity must be evaluated so that appropriate therapy plans can be devised, clinicians assigned, and schedules of appointments set up in terms of need. Some stuttering problems are so severe that they exceed our competence level, and so we seek the help of others. When we do so, our referral letter should include some statement of stuttering severity. Descriptive terms such as "very severe," "severe," "moderately severe," "mild," or "very mild" may not be sufficient and further descriptive material such as that found in the following quotation from Gregory (1968b) should be added.

> Cora was a moderately severe stutterer. She manifested some severely tonic blocks, especially on bilabial sounds, that lasted as long as seven seconds. Articulation was slurred, and she rambled as she spoke—both characteristics were thought to be secondary manifestations of stuttering. She blocked on most of the consonant sounds and often on medial and final syllables. There were contortions of the face, squinting of the eyes, and very poor eye contact. Her eyes would water as she spoke. During speech she said her head "was hot." In summary, Cora was very anxious and tense as she spoke (p. 41).

In this account (which admittedly need not represent the reality) Gregory states that Cora was a "moderately severe stutterer." Unfortunately we do not know the markings on his scale of severity, nor do we know its upper and lower extremes. From this description of her other behaviors, we would say that Cora should be called "severe" or "very severe," on a crude five-point scale such as that given above, but who are we to say that our estimates of severity or our terms representing severity are any better than those used by Gregory?

CLINICAL IMPRESSIONS OF SEVERITY

Although the phrases "very severe" and "very mild" might communicate the essence of a clinical impression, we are not so sure that this would be true for "moderate severity." Presumably, "moderate severity" describes the behavior of the average stutterer. But the average stutterer seen by a public school clinician would probably be less severe than one seen in a university clinic, and the latter less severe than one referred to a psychiatrist, so the population of each setting has to be taken into account too. Soderberg (1962) found that the majority of his 105 college stutterers were ranked as "mild" stutterers on the Iowa Scale of Severity and that the typical college stutterer actually has little overt speech difficulty in an oral reading situation. If, however, the samples had been taken from class recitation or job interviews, they would probably have shown more severity.

Our trouble in measuring severity lies first in this variability and second in the fact that we have no Bureau of Standards for stuttering. There is no standard stuttering kilo or centimeter. Each stutterer and each therapist has his own different internal yardstick, and what is worse, each one of them is more elastic than it is rigid. In measuring the severity of stuttering in a gay and very attractive girl, we may stretch our judgmental measuring stick a bit because of her other assets. Moreover, some clinicians' subjective scales of severity have only three divisions—severe, average, mild—while others have five, or seven, or nine. In this connection, we might morosely contemplate the study in which Cullinan, Prather, and Williams (1963) used seven different rating methods to evaluate the severity of tape-recorded samples of stuttered speech. Their judges evaluated each sample twice, using five-point, seven-point, and nine-point equal-appearing interval scales. A seven-point scale with well defined judgment markings and a direct-magnitude-estimation ratio scale were also used. They found that even with only one judge, no one method was reliable enough to serve as an adequate predictor of severity for an individual stutterer, and none of the seven methods seemed to be any better than the others. Results such as these cast much doubt on the accuracy of the working clinician's judgments of severity. Actually, of course, few clinicians would ever be content to describe the severity of a client's stuttering as a scale value or with an adjective. Instead, they add descriptions of the behavior. Thus Robinson (1968) describes his case as follows:

The overt stuttering he presented was of a relatively mild form consisting of two or three quick repetitions of word elements or, occasionally, brief fixations of articulatory postures accompanied by slight tremors. However, these signs of a stuttering problem were not evident frequently. He was admittedly clever at substitution and other verbal manipulations. Thus, he usually gave the impression of a person who stuttered only occasionally. He reported having many acquaintances and a few good friends who he was certain didn't know he was a stutterer. But he said his stuttering bothered him a great deal. It was very embarrassing, and he was always under a lot of tension and strain.

When he read aloud, the "sticky" blocks were more frequent and somewhat more pronounced and his embarrassment was obvious. Yet the overt stuttering certainly wasn't severe, and as we talked with him we felt that treatment would be relatively easy, particularly after we explained our treatment approach and emphasized the importance of having him test the validity of his concern about the stuttering by stuttering openly and freely (p. 70).

In this descriptive account, we note that Robinson mentions such factors as the frequency of the stuttering, its duration ("two or three repetitions" and "brief fixations"), its characteristic form, its visibility, and finally the subject's reactions of avoidance and embarrassment, all of which contributed to his impression of a "mild" degree of severity. In the following passage, note that Sheehan (1968) concentrates primarily on form and frequency in describing the case of Leonard who was:

. . . one of the severest stutterers I have ever encountered. Leonard's habitual pattern consisted of a violent tilting back of his head; rolling his eyes toward the ceiling; the muscles in his neck would stand out; he would become flushed; he would twist his face in a forced grimace; attempt various starters; some head jerks in an effort to release himself from the block; and also would accompany his stuttering with various bodily gestures. He had little fluency capacity and stuttered severely on almost every word. His name and words beginning with the same sound as his first and last names were especially difficult (p. 77).

In describing a "severe" stutterer, Gregory (1968a) mentions frequency, loci, form, and also the altered characteristics of the normal speech:

The client was a severe stutterer (oftentimes he blocked on every other word in conversational speech). He stuttered mostly on initial sounds, but there was also blocking on medial and final syllables of words. He displayed considerable tension of the lips, tongue, jaw, and larynx as he spoke. Starters such as "uh," "wa wa wa," and "well uh" were used frequently. A gasping type inhalation was involved in approximately one of every three blocks. Breaking through a speech block was sometimes accompanied by a slight leg movement. Fluent words, or occasional fluent phrases, were spoken in a slow, labored rate (p. 47).

RATING SCALES OF SEVERITY

In the effort to impose some pattern on the chaos of clinical judgments of severity, Lewis and Sherman (1951) developed the first rating scale based on principles which had been used in designing handwriting scales. This scale unfortunately required multiple judges and much time and effort to be useful even in group comparisons, and so it was never widely used clinically. Starbuck (1954) developed a filmed audiovisual scale in which samples of stutterers in the act of stuttering were arranged sequentially to represent differing degrees of severity. Starbuck showed that five factors varied significantly with each successive step on his scale. They were: total words spoken in a given time, number of blockings, facial grimaces, accompanying limb movement, and eye shift or eye-blink. In actual clinical use, this scale, like the Lewis and Sherman scale, proved difficult primarily because it is difficult to match one stutterer against another. They stutter too differently. When matched with the criterion sample, whether filmed or tape recorded, the differences in behavior are more marked than the similarities. Handwriting samples can be matched against a series of model specimens much more easily than can stuttering samples. At any rate, neither of these scales has had any extensive clinical use.

An instrument, however, which has been used very widely is the *Scale for Rating the Severity of Stuttering* published in Johnson, Darley, and Spriestersbach's *Diagnostic Methods in Speech Pathology* (1963). Although the authors strongly emphasize the limitations of this scale and term it a "rough measure only" many speech therapists use it, not only in diagnosis but also for measuring therapeutic progress. We can understand why they do so for in many ways it assembles in one instrument most of the real indications of stuttering severity. Seven scale values are given with descriptive legends for each. To illustrate, we quote those for Scale values 2 and 5:

> #2 *Mild*—stuttering on 1 to 2 per cent of words; tension barely perceptible; very few, if any, disfluencies last as long as a full second; patterns of disfluency simple; no conspicuous associated movements of body, arms, legs, or head.
> #5 *Moderate to severe*—stuttering on about 8 to 12 per cent of words; consistently noticeable tension; disfluencies average about 2 seconds in duration; a few distracting sounds and facial grimaces; a few distracting associated movements (p. 231).

This Iowa scale is, in our opinion, deficient because of the way the variables are grouped. Unfortunately, neither the amount of tension, nor the duration, number, or kind of associated struggle movements increase equally or proportionately with increased severity. How would we rank a stutterer, for example, who stutters on only two per cent of his words and thus would fit scale value 2 of mildness, but who also shows consistently noticeable tension every time he does stutter, which would classify him as moderately severe with a scale value of 5? As the research, which we shall summarize later, has shown, these variables are not highly correlated with one another, although the scale indicates that they should be. Again we face the problem of fit. Our stutterers just do not seem to fit into these categories on all the alleged features for any one step of the scale.

However, we have revised this Iowa scale so that it can be used as a profile. As such, it is very useful, especially for measuring changes during therapy. Therapy progress is seldom even. The stutterer may make gains in reducing the duration of his blocks at the same time that the frequency of his stuttering increases. Or he may begin to show longer stutterings but have eliminated much of the tension and struggle. By charting the client's status at different times during therapy on these profiles, the therapist is often able to shape the treatment appropriately. We provide such profiles in the accompanying figure 12.

A SEVERITY EQUATION

These profiles are far from satisfactory and we hunger for some sort of unitary measure. Perhaps none is possible, but we have made two preliminary attempts to achieve a first approximation. In one attempt, we placed thermistors on various parts of the body to get summated readings of heat output which might reflect the contributions of duration, frequency, tension, and overt or covert struggle as well as emotion, but the technology involved defeated us. In the other, using recorded samples of severe, moderate, and mild stutterers as judged by a listener panel, we computed the numerical values of the following items: frequency of individual moments of stuttering expressed as a percentage; their average duration; the duration of the most severe moment of stuttering; the average amount of tension and struggle as judged on a five-step scale; the extreme amount of tension and struggle exhibited on the most severe moment of stuttering as judged on that scale and the number of avoidance reactions shown. Although all of these values could be ascertained with some objectivity and reliability, their combination to yield a single measure of severity poses many problems. The items need differential weighting but the weights were unknown. Should the items be combined algebraically or multiplicatively, or even exponentially? With these questions in mind, we offer the following equation as a conceptual model illustrating the factors that combine in some way to make up stuttering severity. It is not a quantification, but hopefully it will stimulate the research upon which quantification rests.

$$S = aF + bD_1 + cD_2 + dT_1 + eT_2 + fA + gE$$

where

F = frequency of stuttered words as a percentage of spoken words.

D_1 = average duration of a stuttering moment.

D_2 = duration of the longest stuttering moment.
T_1 = average tension of a stuttering moment.
T_2 = amount of tension in the stuttering moment of greatest tension.
A = amount of avoidance.
E = amount of emotional involvement.

PROFILE OF STUTTERING SEVERITY

SCALE	FREQUENCY	TENSION-STRUGGLE	DURATION	POSTPONEMENT-AVOIDANCE
1.	Under 1%	None	Under $\frac{1}{2}$ sec.	None
2.	1 - 2%	Rare but present	Average $\frac{1}{2}$ sec.	Less than 5 %
3.	3 - 5%	Usual but mild	Average 1 sec.	5 - 10%
4.	6 - 8%	Severe	Average 2 sec.	11 - 20%
5.	9 - 12%	Very severe	Average 3 sec.	21 - 31 %
6.	13 - 25%	Overflow to eyes and limbs	Average 4 sec.	31 - 70%
7.	More than 25 %	Overflow to trunk	Longer than 5 sec.	More than 70%

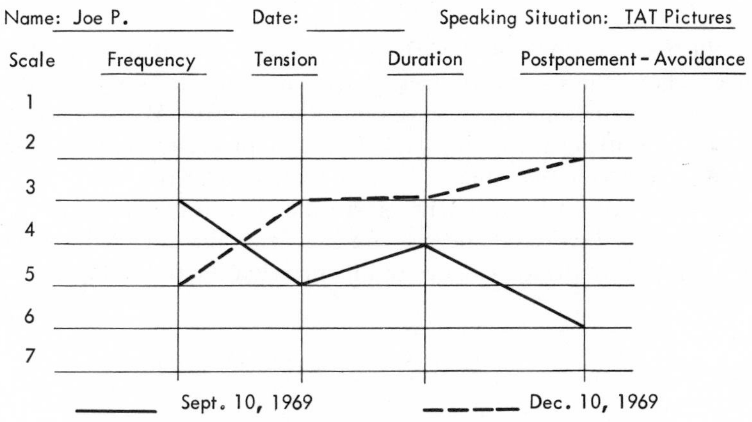

Figure 12. Profile of stuttering severity showing changes as a result of therapy.

Van Riper (1968) describes the diagnostic picture of a very severe stutterer. A portion of the account is given to demonstrate that an assessment of severity in terms of such an equation might be possible:

The symptomatic picture presented was as follows: Don stuttered on over 50 per cent of his words in oral reading and the percentage was much higher in propositional speech even in a relatively nonstressful situation. He showed very little adaptation on rereading or in repeating individual words, often an increase. There was no reduction in frequency under low frequency masking at 80 dB though there was some decrease in the duration of his blockings. The average duration of his moments of stuttering in oral reading was 4 seconds; the longest one was 28. In propositional speech the durations were longer. Occasionally he would just have to quit speaking.

Except for the use of "um but" or "oh" or "um" or "ah" which he used to get started, there were few avoidances, "I see no point in substituting an easier word like the other guys often do. I don't have any. If I try one, I get hung up on that too." As with most of the very severe stutterers, he had few specific phonemic or word fears, but his situation fears were very intense, often to the point of panic. Usually, Don plunged directly into the utterance, went into a prolonged tremor of the articulators, squeezed shut his eyes, jerked his jaw open very widely to interrupt the tremor, then did it again and again. Great tension accompanied this behavior and often it overflowed to the limbs and trunk. In his paroxysms, he would even stagger. Most of the grotesque behavior apparently seemed to serve as interruptor and escape devices. The tremors of the lips and jaws, which we were able to record electromyographically, ranged in frequency from 7 to 18 per second, with most of them oscillating at the first value. Often as a result of his longer blockings, he would become completely exhausted. Airflow was often interrupted at the laryngeal level as well as by the occluded tongue or lips. In some of his worst moments of stuttering, the tongue would protrude violently and show marked tremor (p. 101).

In the next sections of this chapter, we will try to describe how one might go about the diagnostic task of determining the weight of the components that contribute to the assessment of severity. We suspect that we will only be putting into words the kinds of processes that all therapists go through in arriving at their clinical impressions of the extent of a given stutterer's difficulty. We are fairly certain that we cannot cover all the diagnostic problems involved, and we are sure that no one will be entirely happy with the resulting evidence of our prescientific technology.

FREQUENCY OF STUTTERING

There is no doubt that one of the major contributors to a clinical impression of severity is the frequency of the moments of stuttering. The more often the stutterer stutters the more severe his problem seems to be. Although it is not the only factor, it is certainly one of the important ones. The stutterer reported by Bar (1967) who stuttered on 92.6 per cent of his words would be considered severe even if those stutterings were of short duration and contained little abnormality. All the research has shown positive correlations between frequency and rated severity, although they are not high enough to enable us to use frequency counts alone as the sole index of severity.

There are several difficulties in counting stutterings. In clinical practice, we can audiotape or videotape samples of the speech and then do our counting during several replays, a procedure which, as Aron (1967) and others have demonstrated, can yield highly reliable measures. As our summary of the research will show, combined audiovisual recordings yield higher frequency counts than either alone but audiotape recordings seem to be sufficient in most instances except when most of the stutterings are nonvocalized or are skillfully disguised.

VARIABILITY IN FREQUENCY

When estimating severity in the initial diagnosis or when ascertaining progress at different times during the course of therapy, it is important not to confine the speech samples to reading material. There are some very severe stutterers who can read with remarkable fluency. As we have seen, the amount of stuttering varies markedly in different speaking situations. The stutterer's performance in oral reading may not be representative of his real difficulty in communication. Sherman (1955) writes:

> Among a number of important considerations is the fact that stutterers typically vary from time to time in the severity of vocal characteristics of stuttering. They vary from day to day, from week to week, from month to month, regardless of whether they are undergoing therapy. . . . An improvement in the reading situation, for example, does not necessarily indicate that there is also a comparable improvement in the spontaneous speech situation (p. 15).

To cope with some of this situational variability, Johnson, Darley, and Spriestersbach (1963) recommended using the Job Task (talking for three minutes about the person's actual or preferred vocation) or the TAT-Task in which Card 10 from the Thematic Apperception Test is presented to the stutterer, and he is asked to talk for three minutes about what is happening in the picture. We have used these successfully as well as other methods. Our customary diagnostic routine is to use a reading passage, a paraphrase of material read silently, a narration of some personal experience, and some telephone calls to procure information. Occasionally we use Rotter's Incomplete Sentences Test (1950), in which the stutterer reads aloud the first part of each unfinished sentence and then completes it, a procedure that gives an immediate comparison of reading and spontaneous speech, and also introduces some emotional stress. As Moore (1954) showed, topics such as parents, family, and speech experiences tend to elicit more stuttering than other subjects, and in getting our sample of spontaneous speech we often bring these into the interview.

Cyclic variations in severity of stuttering have also been found by Quarrington (1956) and by Quarrington as reported by Sheehan (1969) in this passage:

> Quarrington has recently gathered data on 39 young stuttering children, mean age 4 years, 4 months, observed over a 1-year period. In 32 of these, stuttering persisted over the 1-year period, during which their mothers supplied daily ratings of the frequency of stuttering . . . the resulting data curves revealed the presence of significant periodicities (p. 453).

Pittenger (1940), however, found no cyclic patterns in a given reading situation. These variations should not, then, markedly affect severity ratings based on frequency counts, since the cycles reported by Quarrington range in length from two to six months. There is also a fascinating article by the Hungarians Hirschberg, Kovacs, Palotas and Szabo (1965) showing that certain "vago-tonic" stutterers stuttered more severely when a warm weather front passed over, while "sympathic-tonic" stutterers had more difficulty when a cold front came. Although we have not been able to assess the meteorology of stutterers, it is certain that more than a one-shot diagnosis of severity is needed. Stutterers are notoriously variable from situation to situation and from day to day, and repeated evaluations of severity are required no matter what methods are used to procure them.

SPEECH SAMPLING

It is also necessary to get a speech sample adequate in length for frequency counting. Obviously, too small a sample will not provide enough moments of stuttering to form any respectable basis for clinical judgment. Too large a sampling can be onerous. Our solution to the problem—probably not a very good one—is to use smaller samples for stutterers whose blockings are both frequent and full of struggle but larger ones for those with shorter and more repetitive behaviors. Generally speaking we seek a sampling of at least 400 words or ten moments of stuttering.

In order to survey the stutterer's difficulty, it is important to have reading materials that include words beginning with all of the different phonemes and also one contrived so that no one phoneme is loaded too heavily. Fairbanks' Rainbow Passage and that ancient composition entitled *Arthur the Young Rat* fulfill this criterion to some degree. The reason for using such material is that some stutterers have difficulty on only a few feared sounds, something to remember during initial interviews. An experienced therapist develops methods of eliciting spontaneous speech which also cover all the various phonemes, formulating his questions in such a way that the stutterer must use them all. Young and Prather (1962) found that 20-second samples of consecutive speech were sufficient for group analysis, but a much larger sample is necessary for diagnosing an individual case. Most clinical reading passages are 300-400 words long. If possible, the best technique is to talk long enough with the stutterer to evoke ten stuttering moments and then later, listen to a recording and count all the words he uttered to get a percentage. This procedure should be repeated in the telephone situation. Frequency counts are of course always expressed in percentages.

COUNTING FREQUENCIES

With some training, the therapist can learn to count and estimate percentages fairly well, even without the aid of a tape recording, when conversing with the stutterer or listening to him as he telephones. Usually it is necessary to watch as well as listen while counting stutterings. Many of the inaudible abnormal postures, tremors, or facial twitches which are characteristic components of severe blockings may be found in fleeting miniature when the visual record is scanned. They should not be ignored in a frequency count.*

Counting always presents the problem of what should be counted. Should we count normally spoken words that are preceded by obvious postponement, retrials, or accessory "ums" and "ers" or other avoidances? (Our answer (one of convenience) is yes. What do we do when confronted by oddly placed pauses such as "I'm going to the post . . . . . office?" We personally count such a gap as a moment of stuttering even when there are no overt signs of abnormality. Stuttering is not always overt. When doubt arises, we try only to be consistent. We count all doubtful items or none of them. When the stutterer blocks or repeats on almost every syllable of a monstrous word such as "diadochokinesis," we count six or seven stutterings rather than one—for surely the stutterer would too in assessing his own difficulty on that word. Many other clinicians (usually normal speakers) count only one.

ORGANIZING FREQUENCY DATA

After the counting is completed there are several sets of figures that have to be turned into percentages. A certain stutterer may stutter on 18 per cent of his words in oral reading, on 32 per cent in talking about the TAT pictures, and on 60 per cent when talking over the telephone. Which percentage should be used in the profile or equation? Although all three should

---

* One stutterer told this story when we called his attention to a tiny blocking which contained all the major features of his severe stuttering in miniature: "I guess you're right about that little block and I'm like the woman who upon marrying told her husband for the first time that she was already the mother of a baby. The man protested and became very angry. 'You should have told me that before we got married,' he shouted. Whereupon his wife answered, 'but it's only a little one.'"

be recorded in the case files, it is best to use the highest percentage as the component figure in assessing the disorder's general severity. This ensures against underestimation, for stutterers can be very skillful at disguising the true extent of their problem, at least during the initial interview. During the course of therapy, however, as we reassess the severity using the same test situations, we often plot all three measures on a progress chart, finding perhaps that the frequency in oral reading had shown an early decrease which was not paralleled by a similar decrease in spontaneous speech. Other workers often average all three figures or consistently use only the highest one.

In concluding this section, it should be noted again that the frequency with which a person stutters is only one of several factors that contribute to severity. It is an important one but there are others too. Aron (1967) comes to the same conclusion:

> It can be generalized from the results here that we should differentiate more clearly between the terms "frequency" and "severity" of stuttering. There is no doubt that the amount of frequency of stuttering will contribute to an impression of its severity, but it would also appear that frequency as such should not be regarded as an independent and accurate measure of severity (p. 32).

DURATION

Stuttering has been called a speech impediment because the flow of speech is intermittently interrupted. Whatever the behaviors are that interrupt speech, we must know how long they last, or how much time they take away from communication in order to estimate the size of that impediment. If two stutterers both repeat the first syllable and prolong the /m/ in the word "psychometric" the one who repeats the syllable four times and prolongs the /m/ four seconds will show more severity than one who repeats the first syllable only two times and prolongs the /m/ only two seconds. The duration of the individual moments of stuttering is one of the basic components of any adequate index of severity. Like tapeworms, longer stutterings are worse than shorter ones.

Although Lewis and Sherman (1951) stated that severity would be best measured by evaluating moments of stuttering generally rather than by counting frequencies, only a few workers have measured the duration of the individual moments of stuttering. Doubtless this is because it is difficult to time short segments of audiotape with a stopwatch or measure spectrographic recordings with a ruler. Instead, indirect measures of stuttering duration, such as reading rate, are used more widely on the assumption that the longer the stutterer takes to say his words, the longer it will take him to read a passage. Generally, this is true although there are some stutterers who show a burst of speed after a moment of stuttering to compensate for the gap. These individuals flee hastily from the scene of their verbal crime and thus spoil the use of overall reading rate as a measure of severity.

We have found little difficulty in timing the durations of individual moments of stuttering. Indeed, it is easier than counting frequencies once the therapist has trained himself to count silently in seconds with some accuracy. The author is able to measure accurately the durations of individual moments of stuttering in terms of hippopotamuses or hippopotami. He has learned to say the word "hippopotamus" covertly in exactly one second. The longest stuttering block he ever measured lasted for 32 hippopotamuses all in a row and then the poor devil quit talking. Thus Sheehan's (1946) results showed that the average duration of repetitive blocks in his subjects could be stated as one "hippopotamus-hippopot" (1.6 seconds) in our counting-system, and the average duration of the prolongations was "hippopotam" or .87 seconds. A two- or three-hippopotami blocking is usually felt and sensed as a moment of severe stuttering.

Among the advantages of timing the durations of the individual stutterings is that it gives an impression of both the average and extreme fluency impediments. We can assess the variability in terms of standard deviations about the means. We can understand how badly the stutterer stutters at his worst. Total reading times or reading measures do not provide this important information. Furthermore, the extremes of duration may be highly significant in evaluating the stutterer's progress. A stutterer who is no longer having his old long, hard blocks will feel that he has made progress even if the average frequency and duration have remained much the same. As we shall see, subjective estimates of severity made by the stutterer himself do not correlate very highly with those made by the clinician. There are various reasons for this discrepancy, but one of them is that stutterers often measure their severity by their worst difficulties, not by their average ones. In the equation of severity, the extreme and the average duration of stutterings should probably be given equal weight. In clinical profiles we use either the average or extreme durations or the summation of both. How valid these procedures are will be determined by future research.

In timing durations, live or videotaped speech samples are best, since the beginning of the speech attempt, though highly visible, may not be audible. One caution should be mentioned. Filled time always seems shorter than empty time. Unless we actually count durations in stopwatch seconds or African beasts, the silent blockings will always seem longer than those that are vocalized. Repetitive stutterings normally seem longer than fixations. Though we have no research on the subject, our own unpublished data show that 90 per cent of normal speaking college students evaluate four-second stutterings as very severe; two-second stutterings as severe; one-second stutterings as moderate in severity; and one-half-second stutterings as mild.

Clinicians should evaluate the stutterer's reports of having very long blocks with some reservations. They usually overestimate their duration.

Similarly, they also underestimate or completely fail to recognize the very short ones. This is reflected in the research of Ringel and Minifee (1966) who found that stutterers who were less able to make accurate judgments of time, either in silence or spontaneous speech, were the more severe.

TENSION AND STRUGGLE

As with measures of duration, we judge those moments of stuttering as more severe which are marked by tension or struggle. So does the stutterer. There is little research, but skilled clinicians can learn to make these judgments with some reliability as some of our own pilot studies with videotaped samples have shown. The presence of tremor, overflow movements, facial contortions, and even accompanying limb movements can be scanned, counted, and evaluated on improvised rating scales of severity. Again the clinician tries to estimate the amount of this tension and struggle shown on most of the moments of stuttering by a given stutterer, to compare this with that of other stutterers or with the picture remembered from earlier periods of therapy. Also, as with duration, we are interested in the most severe moments of tension and struggle, not just the average. Our research has shown a low but positive correlation between duration and tension judgments. That the correlation cannot be expected to be high is due to the fact that occasionally highly explosive and spasmodic blockings may be very short in duration. Electromyography can give objective measures of such tension for research purposes, but it is not very useful in routine clinical practice.

Severity can also be assessed in terms of visible abnormality though this is hard to quantify. Starbuck (1954) counted certain overt behaviors in devising his audiovisual scale of severity. In actual clinical practice this procedure is probably used very commonly in assessing severity. In his study of five days of continuous talking by stutterers, Rousey (1958) counted the number of visible symptoms (facial contortions, etc.) as one of his measures of severity and found the highest correlation (though it was only .62) between this item and the frequency of stuttering moments. The correlation was higher than that between frequency and either *rated* severity or the total output of words per eight hour day of talking. Clark and Murray (1962) suggest the use of a Behavior Analysis Chart in measuring therapeutic progress, i.e., severity.

COVERT RESPONSES

Here we have real difficulty trying to be objective. How can we possibly provide figures for profiles or an equation which can represent the levels of anxiety, frustration, or shame? Once again we have outdistanced our research. Measures such as the PSI (palmar sweat index) and the GSR (galvanic skin response) can give objective data, but they present many problems in interpretation and are not usually routinely available to the therapist. At present we are restricted largely to observation and inference. We can count how often the stutterer avoids words or postpones speech attempts. We can judge with some accuracy how reluctantly he enters a given speech situation. We can check his daily output of speech. We can see if he winces or blushes or averts his gaze or hangs his head when he stutters. We can listen to what he says about his problem as we carefully question him. An excellent exploratory procedure for eliciting covert reactions is to have the stutterer listen to a playback of his audio or video recording and then discuss the therapist's comments and checks on the enclosed form:

Therapist's Outline for Evaluating the Stutterers' Attitudes and Self-Reactions when Hearing His Recorded Speech or Seeing His Videotaped Speech.

1. Check your observations of the following items:
    A. Case's general activity became (heightened) (lessened) (remained the same) as when not listening to his recorded stuttering.
    B. Case (avoided) (did not avoid) eye contact with observer while listening to his recorded stuttering.
    C. Case showed a predominance of (seriousness) (nonchalance) (humor) (neutrality) (mixed emotions) while listening to his recorded speech.
    D. Case appeared to react (to certain details of his speech) (without any apparent reference to detailed aspects of his speech). State the details of his speech which were linked with his reactions.
    E. Case (remained silent while hearing his recorded speech) (interjected remarks—noting what they are) (showed typical gestures, facial expressions, etc.) (other ?).
    F. Case (flushed) (grinned) (fidgeted) (scowled) (other ?) while hearing himself stutter.
    G. Case (did) (did not) show empathic responses to certain details of his speech. Note what these responses are.
    H. Case (did) (did not) show reactions which indicated that he could anticipate or predict certain abnormalities to occur in the recorded speech. Note what these were.
    I. Case (did) (did not) voluntarily comment on his speech immediately following the hearing of his record. Note the comments, if any.
2. Ask the case the following questions and record his replies:
    A. Did you stutter (more) or (less) than you expected you would while making this recording?
    B. Did you regard your stuttering in this sample to be (more) or (less) severe than usual in this general type of situation?
    C. Did your stuttering in this recording seem (natural) or (different in some way) than expected? Explain.
    D. If you were to repeat this recording, do you think you would stutter (more), (less), (about the same), or (differently) than the first time? Explain.

E. Was listening to your recorded speech a (pleasant), (unpleasant), (amusing), (disturbing), (interesting), or (otherwise revealing) experience? Why?

By using this form, we can place most stutterers with reasonable accuracy on an internal scale of severity with respect to anxiety, frustration and shame. Numerical values may be placed on these covert reactions and entered into a profile or equation, although something within us always crieth fraud at the process. Better measures of these covert features of severity are badly needed.

Recently, several attempts have been made to give us the first mock-ups of such measures. While no one of them is adequate, all hold great promise, and we have profited from their use. The first of these, by Erickson (1969), consists of a Severity Scale and an Adjective Check List. A portion of the latter (the ACL) is included below. The items checked with an asterisk are those which significantly differentiated the more severe stutterers from those less severe on this severity scale.

Erickson Adjective Check List

Please check (√) the words in this list which best describe your characteristic feelings or behavior while you are talking with other persons in social conversation situations. Check as many or as few words as seem appropriate.

*__Sensitive	__Spontaneous	__Modest	__Eager
__Aggressive	__Thoughtful	__Fearful	__Secure
__Boisterous	__Irritable	*__Awkward	__Comfortable
__Domineering	*__Short-spoken	__Lively	__Calm
__Extroverted	__Argumentative	__Indifferent	__Expressive
__Forward	*__Insecure	__Responsive	*__Nervous
__Cheerful	*__Introverted	*__Uneasy	__Restless
*__Tense	__Passive	__Jovial	__Hostile
__Boastful	__Poised	__Aloof	__Talkative

Another pencil and paper instrument was devised by Lanyon (1967) using groups of mild and severe stutterers and normal-speaking controls to validate certain differentiating statements such as those in the table on page 235.

Another instrument is the *Perceptions of Stuttering Inventory* devised by Rothenberg (1963) and Woolf (1967). Its abbreviation is PSI which should not be confused with the Palmar Sweat Index. This PSI consists of a 60 item battery of behavioral statements concerning struggle, avoidance, and expectancy, and the stutterer is asked to check those that are characteristic or not characteristic of his own stuttering problem. On the basis of the scores, profiles of tendencies are constructed which can be used to assess degrees of severity in the different dimensions and also therapeutic progress.

THE STUTTERING SEVERITY (SS) SCALE, WITH
DIRECTIONS FOR SCORING INDICATED IN PARENTHESIS

Read each of the following statements. Decide whether each is true or false as applied to you. If a statement is true, or mostly true, as applied to you, cross out the letter T for that statement. If a statement is false, or not usually true, as applied to you, cross out the letter F.

Make an answer to every statement, even though some of them seem not to apply to you. [These are samples from the test.]

1. When I talk I often become short of breath. (T)
2. When I have a hard time talking, I tend to look away from my listener. (T)
3. I am sensitive about my speech problem. (T)
4. I worry about the fact that I stutter. (T)
5. If I want to, I can be very fluent. (F)
6. There is something wrong with my speech. (T)
7. When I can't say a word, there are little tricks I can use to help me. (T)
8. People notice that I talk differently. (T)
9. I avoid meeting some people because I'm afraid I might stutter. (T)
10. If I did not stutter, I would probably speak much more than I do. (T)

These instruments are useful to the practicing clinician in many ways, but we would hate to have to rely on them alone without any personal observation of the stutterer in action. We once had someone else get the scores on all three of these scales for five stutterers whom we knew, and then we tried to identify them blindly but missed on every one. Someday we will have good measures of stuttering severity. These are the best we have today.

SUBJECTIVE SEVERITY

In the conclusions to her study of the severity of stuttering, Aron (1967) makes this remarkable statement: "The clinical impression that stutterers are poor judges of their own speech performance was borne out by the results of this study." She asked stutterers to rate the severity of their own stuttering immediately after they had read a passage, and again 30 minutes later when listening to the recordings. She found that the stutterers' self-ratings did not correlate very highly with those of the judges nor with reading rate or frequency counts. What is more significant, when the stutterers were asked to compare their performance during testing with the general severity of their stuttering for the same day prior to the experiment, the correlations were insignificant (.04 – .32). From the experimenter's point of view, the stutterers were poor judges of their own severity, but it is also possible that, from the stutterers' point of view, the experimenter was the one making errors in judgment, no matter how objective her measures of frequency, word rate, or other data. Only the person with a bellyache knows how much it hurts. Aron recognized this point of view, stating that "the stutterer's feelings about his own performance should be viewed as a separate entity when comparing ratings and assessments of stuttering behavior." To cite just one of many similar observations in the literature, Naylor (1953) found no statistically significant relationship between his judges' evaluations of the severity of recorded samples of stuttering and the judgments of the stutterers who had recorded them. Indeed, they differed widely.

The clinician cannot afford to ignore the stutterer's subjective assessment of severity. For one thing it cannot be measured by the same yardstick at different times. In conditions where there is little time pressure for utterance, a moment of stuttering three or four seconds long would seem to the stutterer as being much less severe than a two-second blocking while trying to shout a warning to a child starting to cross a street in heavy traffic. Among familiar friends in casual conversation, ten moments of stuttering will seem less severe than three when answering a prospective employer's question, or than two while saying "I do" when getting married. Any clinician who thinks he can deny the validity of the stutterer's severity estimate is asking for resistance. Early in therapy, it is useful to ascertain the discrepancies between the stutterer's severity scale and our own. One way we do this is to sample enough of his moments of stuttering and ask him after each whether he would judge it to be more severe or less severe than his usual stuttering *in that particular speaking situation.* Later we ask him to demonstrate what he would consider a very severe, a severe, an average, or a mild "blocking," or we do the demonstrating. Through this exploration, we can get some crude idea of his internalized severity scale.

One should also recognize that during the course of therapy, the stutterer's severity yardsticks get shorter. One of our severe stutterers hardly recognized any three- or four-syllable repetition as a real moment of stuttering when he first came to us, for most of his difficulties consisted of very long (10-32 syllable) "runaways." Once he got in one of these reverberatory stutterings, he would yammer away almost endlessly before finally being able to continue. The little ones didn't count. However, four months later, he had improved so much that he would evaluate that same four-syllable repetition as being very severe. Clinicians often wonder why stutterers fail to recognize the very evident improvement they have made. They remain discouraged despite progress because their internal scales of severity have shrunk. It is for this reason that we always try to get audio- or videotapes at the beginning of therapy so that we can repeatedly show the stutterer his changes in severity.

Another observation should be of value to the beginning therapist. Stutterers do not base their subjective severity scales on oral reading but on live communication under pressure. Charting frequency counts or reading times at intervals during therapy will be considered by most stutterers a rather meaningless exercise. If they like you they will be polite, but their guts will cry nonsense. To them, oral reading in the laboratory or therapy room is only a remote and unreasonable facsimile of living speech.

REVIEW OF THE RESEARCH

RATINGS OF SEVERITY

In this review, we will necessarily have to cover some studies already reported. Lewis and Sherman (1951) were the first to devise a scale based on listener judgment of recorded samples of stuttering. It had face validity and sufficient reliability for research purposes when applied with groups of judges. Sherman (1955) used a nine step scale of equal-appearing intervals composed of three-minute samples, each one rated at 10 second intervals and concluded that a single judge could evaluate their severity with some reliability but that this reliability did not improve with training. Earlier, Sherman (1952) had discovered that five-minute samples could be rated with some reliability by a single judge. The reliability problem has been a difficult one, and it is even more troublesome when less objective scales are used. Also Sherman and McDermott (1958) found that different judges gave different ratings although a single judge could be consistent in his own ratings whether the sample included five, ten, fifteen, or twenty moments of stuttering.

Cullinan, Prather, and Williams (1963) compared ratings of severity on four-, five-, eight- and ten-point scales, using different instructions. They found that the reliability of the rating scale was not good enough to use in individual prediction, even when a judge used his own standard sample as a yardstick (direct magnitude estimation). A group of judges, however, using several judgments of the same sample, can achieve reliable mean scale values. All these studies used tape-recorded samples. Young (1961) showed that the relationship between Iowa Scale ratings and the frequency of stuttering (or the total time taken to read a standard passage) is not high enough to justify the use of the scale values instead of frequency counts or speaking time measures. Martin (1965) found that direct magnitude estimation scaling judgments could yield fairly stable judgments of severity if a large group of judges were used but not otherwise. Trotter and Kools (1955) had a group of judges listen to the *same* samples of recorded stuttering three times and then rate them in severity. Their mean scale values of severity decreased with each new listening session. They caution that this tendency may affect a clinician's estimation of progress. The stutterer may not really be improving. Aron (1967) did a very careful study of various measures of severity. She found that it was possible to make reliable ratings with a nine-point scale and recorded samples. The experimenter's three separate severity ratings of the same reading passages were highly correlated with each other (.93 to .98). Since her ratings agreed well with those of five other judges she felt they had validity.

In rating the severity of individual moments of stuttering on single words, Spielberger (1956) procured a test-retest correlation of .85. Sherman and McDermott (1958) showed that a single judge could rate the severity of stuttering on single words with fair reliability, but that other observers would not give similar scale values on the same single words. Trotter (1953) found that the rated severity of a word was related to its phonemic, grammatical, and positional features.

Much research and clinical observation indicate that judgments of severity based on oral reading alone are far from representative. Harris (1942), Dixon (1947), Cohen (1952), and many others have shown that marked discrepancies in severity occur between oral reading and spontaneous speech. Most recently, Aron (1967) found a "marked disparity" between her ratings of the oral reading and the spontaneous conversation of her stutterers.

Since most of the studies have used judgments of audio-recorded samples, some distortion may have been introduced by the inclusion of the visible behaviors so prominent in severe stutterers. Tuthill (1946) and Moller (1957) found no differences in rated severity by judges who both saw and heard the subjects and those who only heard the tape-recordings of the stutterers. Luper (1959), however, found that his judges rated movies of stuttering samples as more severe when run silently than when the same samples were shown with sound. Williams, Wark, and Minifie (1963) found that audio samples and combined audiovisual samples were judged similarly either on rating scale values or frequency counts. Martin (1965) showed that groups of speech clinicians, stutterers, and naive students all rated audiovisual samples of stuttering as higher in severity than they did when listening to the same samples by audio-recordings alone. It is possible that some of the discrepancy here may be due to different kinds of stuttering behaviors. Generally, although audio-recordings are probably satisfactory, the combined audiovisual samples are more useful in clinical practice.

FREQUENCY OF STUTTERING MOMENTS

Frequency counts have been used for years as a gross measure of severity, and they serve as the basic measure of progress in operant conditioning methods of therapy. Certainly, if no moments of stuttering occurred, the severity would be nil. The relationship between frequency and listener judgments of severity, however, is not as high as might be expected. The following table presents the correlations between frequency counts and ratings of severity from six studies:

Study	Correlation
Shulman (1945)	.57
Sherman and Trotter (1956)	.61
Rousey (1958)	.51
Young (1961)	.76 (part word disfluencies)
Young (1961) *	.83 (prolonged sounds)
Aron (1967)	.46 to .71

* In this connection, Prins and Lohr (1968) found that prolongations of sounds were the behaviors most highly correlated with other measures of severity.

Much variability in frequency counts occurs between reading and spontaneous speaking tasks. Sander (1961) discovered that, on the average, his stutterers stuttered on about 19 per cent of their words in spontaneous speaking but only on about 10 per cent in oral reading. The large standard deviations, however, demonstrated that a wide range of individual frequency counts was involved. Young (1961) found that his stutterers had a mean frequency count (also with wide variations) of 13 per cent for spontaneous speaking. Frequency norms expressed in deciles for oral reading and two Job Tasks are provided by Johnson, Darley, and Spriestersbach (1963). Frequency, however, is not the sole measure of severity as indicated by the findings of Berlin and Berlin (1964), who presented simulated samples of stuttering which were identical in frequency but differed in form. Listeners to these different kinds of stuttering judged them as differing in severity. Also, Cullinan (1963), found that frequency counts were not sufficiently stable from day to day to serve as adequate measures.

RATE OF UTTERANCE
AS A MEASURE OF DURATION

Since stuttering interrupts the forward flow of speech, it is not surprising to find that much research has focussed on the rate of speaking or oral reading as expressed usually in words per minute.* Pittelman (1942) and Roberts (1949) were among the first to try to verify this measure. Pittelman used passages that differed in emotionality. Stutterers read more slowly than inferior speakers or normal speakers on both types of materials, and all groups read the emotional passage more slowly than the nonemotional one. Roberts used adaptation reading of the same passage by both her stutterers and a control group and also measured total phonation times as well as reading times. She found, as did Pittelman, that stutterers read a passage slower than the normal speakers but more swiftly with each successive reading. What this indicates, of course, is that the frequency and/or duration of the stutterer's repetitions and voiced prolongations decreased as adaptation occurred. Meyer (1944) found that generally the reading rate

* Minifee and Cooker (1964) concluded that counting syllables rather than words was a better measure since on polysyllabic words, stutterers could stutter more than once.

could be used as a crude index of severity. Bloodstein (1944) discovered that stutterers read more slowly than normal speakers not only for the whole passage but also for those segments of the passage on which they were fluent. Johnson and Colley (1945) found that frequency and duration were not highly related. Dixon (1947) revealed that, in adaptation readings, the reading times decreased proportionately with the decrease in numbers of stutterings. Liebman (1956) and Quarrington (1959) showed that test-retests of reading times correlated only about .69, thus indicating that such measures of severity were of small clinical use. Cullinan (1963) found the same thing, reporting that the overall reading rate was not stable enough to represent an individual stutterer's behavior.

Some of the more recent investigations have shown a positive relationship between reading and speaking times and other measures of severity. These may be summarized as follows:

Study		*Correlation*
Young (1961)	Speaking rate and frequency	.59
Sander (1961)	Speaking rate and frequency	.81
Bloodstein (1944)	Reading rate and frequency	.88
Young (1961)	Reading rate and frequency	.68
Sander (1961)	Reading rate and frequency	.86
Aron (1967)	Reading rate and frequency	.64 to .70
Young 1961)	Reading rate and scale judgments	.68
Aron (1967)	Reading rate and scale judgments	.72 to .88

Boehmler (1966) approached the matter differently in a pilot study. He measured the duration of silences and pause times for stutterers and normal speakers. The more severe stutterers showed more silent pauses and in different places than the less severe ones or the normal speakers. Mahl and Schultze (1964) summarize a series of studies related to silent pauses and other hesitation phenomena as a measure of anxiety in the speech of psychoneurotics and other individuals with emotional problems. In general they feel that such behaviors can be used to measure severity of emotional disorders.

ADAPTATION AND CONSISTENCY
AS MEASURES OF SEVERITY

Johnson and Brown (1935) and Shulman (1945) report that the more severe stutterers had greater consistency in the loci of their stuttering. Leibman (1956), like Shulman, found a correlation of about .68 between consistency and severity, but he concluded that his consistency measures were too unreliable to yield accurate results. Tate, Cullinan, and Ahlstrand (1961) showed that of five different ways of measuring adaptation none was reliable or stable enough to use in measuring stuttering performance. Cullinan (1963) found that computing the weighted percentages of adaptation was the best method, but even this had a reliability of only .70. Lanyon (1965) found no significant relationship between this percentage measure of adaptation and the amount of improvement shown by stutterers at Iowa after a year of therapy. He also found that consistency (the tendency for stuttering to occur on the same words) was not related to improvement. Agnello (1966) found that if stuttering occurs on a certain kind of syllable consistently, it tends to be more severe. Leith (1954) points out various difficulties in identifying moments of stuttering in adaptation readings and questions the validity of adaptation measures.

Van Riper and Hull (1955) reported that the more severe stutterers had higher initial scores, higher plateaus, and more gradual rates of adaptation than those of milder stutterers. Luper (1950) however, found no relationship between adaptation rate and severity as judged by observers at the beginning and end of treatment. Brown (1945) suggested that we use word-weight measures of the loci of stuttering as indices of severity. Mild stutterers would require combined cues from position, length, grammatical class, and initial sound before stuttering on a given word; moderate stutterers would require only two or three of these, and severe stutterers only one to precipitate stuttering.

OTHER MEASURES OF SEVERITY

Froeschels and Rieber (1963) reported that stutterers who could not respond to visual and auditory signals to stop talking during a moment of stuttering were the more difficult cases. They showed greater "imperceptiveness." Ringel and Minifie (1966) found that those stutterers who were less able to make accurate judgments of time (protensity), either in silence or in spontaneous speech or oral reading, were more severe than those who could estimate time more accurately. Electromyography as a measure of the tension of individual moments of stuttering has been investigated by Shrum (1967). Brutten (1963) has suggested that a lack of decrement in palmar sweat measurements during adaptation readings may indicate greater severity. Attitude scales such as the Ammons-Johnson (1944) do not have enough reliability to use clinically except for exploration. The amount of time actually spent in talking each day has been suggested by Johnson, Darley, and Spriestersbach (1963) as a possible measure of severity, and Trotter and Brown (1958) showed that daily talking time increased as a result of therapy from an average of 26 minutes to 44 minutes per day. Naylor (1953) and others showed that the more severe stutterers spoke better under delayed auditory feedback than did the milder ones. Milisen (1938) found that severe stutterers were more able to predict the occurrence of stutterings than were the milder ones. The research of Leith (1954) suggests that the use of phonation time ratios and measures of pitch variability might be used to get some estimate of blockage and spontaneity.

Eventually we may have a battery of evaluative measures for severity which combine a few or many of these various factors. Young (1961) and Soderberg (1962) have suggested such a battery. Young even attempted to achieve a regression equation which would combine several factors but felt that it was not applicable to individual diagnosis.

COMMENTARY

All therapists whether of one school of stuttering or another must be interested in observations of the person who stutters, observations which when tabulated will provide a better overall picture of the speech behavior than is gained from the average case report. These observations, however, need not involve highly accurate measurements of overt symptoms or attitudes, because the conditions change so markedly from one period to another and from one situation to another. Nevertheless, each therapist needs information regarding the nature and frequency of the overt stuttering symptoms, as well as other types of speech interruptions. He needs information about the withdrawal behavior which occurs in relation to each type of interruption. It is important that he have some measure of the severity of the disorder in different situations, as well as of the attitudes toward the disorder (Milisen, 1957, pp. 298–299).

The stuttering was severe and frequent. It was characterized by prolonged struggle behavior, tremors, and numerous repeated attempts to initiate the beginning sounds or syllables of troublesome words. Word and situation avoidance occurred only infrequently. Louise reported going through several phases in which she worked to hide the stuttering with substitutions and careful phrasing and by avoiding feared situations when she could, but she said it never really worked out well. She said she got tired of trying to think up ways of talking to avoid stuttering and there were too many situations to avoid. She didn't want to become a recluse. In fact, she said that she really liked to talk, so she had become reconciled to the stuttering and just tried to avoid thinking about "the awful faces" she made when it occurred.

Louise said that she had some recollection of stuttering occasionally in the early grades in school, but that it was no problem until the junior high years. It apparently had become much worse then. She would not recite in classes, and her grades, which up to that time had been a source of great pride for her, became the cause of much frustration and embarrassment. This pattern continued through high school. She even failed one course because she refused to present an oral report (Robinson, 1968, p. 65).

. . . it is by no means to be overlooked or underemphasized that the sorts of listener judgments represented by ratings, however rough and even wildly unscientific they may be, are among the most substantial facts of life that stutterers face hour after hour, day in and day out. They are therefore extremely important—regardless of their precision or reliability as gauged by laboratory standards. It is, for all practical purposes, impossible to disregard them in working with stutterers clinically (Johnson, Darley, and Spriestersbach, 1963, pp. 261–262).

The problems encountered in measuring stuttering severity are similar to those surrounding the assessment of many areas of psychological or behavioral malfunctioning. Consider the disorder of schizophrenia. A diagnostician could, after one or more interviews, give his schizophrenic patient an implicit severity rating—for example, "moderately schizophrenic but not hospitalizable." In making such a rating, the diagnostician might have made an intuitive integration of all the information provided by the patient, or he might have simply counted instances of observable schizophrenic behavior and utilized a "frequency" score.

Such behavior by a diagnostician of schizophrenia would suffer from the same limitations which are inherent in the methods typically used to assess stuttering severity—whether by the clinical judgment of a single expert or by counting instances of stuttering behavior in a single speech sample. These disadvantages stem largely from *inadequate sampling* of the person's behavior. In the case of stuttering, such limitations have been largely obscured by the deceptive reliability and simplicity with which instances of stuttering behavior can be counted (Lanyon, 1967, p. 836).

Note that the PSI [Perceptions of Stuttering Inventory] judgments of severity are based on behavior, extending to *several* dimensions of stuttering, *as perceived* by the stutterer. Thus, the PSI has given the clinician another basis for judging severity and for making the recommendations for management which follow from such judgments. In the past, the clinician's estimate of stuttering severity may have been limited by what he could observe of overt struggle and may not have included *how the stutterer perceives his stuttering*. Furthermore, the two may not be consonant. The writer has examined adult stutterers whose speech behavior contradicted their report of how they stuttered; while their overt speech presented little or no evidence of disfluencies or struggle, they regarded their stuttering as severe or moderately severe and their PSI profiles were of corresponding severity (Woolf, 1967, p. 163).

Efforts to evaluate severity of stuttering as it appears to the stutterer have included measurement of (a) emotional and psychological reactions to stuttering, (b) the effects of penalty felt by the stutterer to be attached to his stuttering spasms, (c) the relations between severity of stuttering and personal adjustment, and (d) the effects on stuttering of anxiety, fear, dread, shame, and other attitudes (Naylor, 1953, p. 34).

The degree of severity of stuttering can probably be best assessed by determining the reaction of the individual toward it. If he is not "anxious" about his speech, the number of fluency breaks is relatively unimportant; if he is seriously concerned about minor deviations from normal fluency which may not even be obvious to the casual listener, he cannot be considered a "mild stutterer"—he has a serious problem (West, Ansberry, and Carr, 1957, p. 428).

BIBLIOGRAPHY

Agnello, J. G., "Some Acoustic and Pause Characteristics of Nonfluencies in the Speech of Stutterers," Technical Report National Institute of Mental Health, Grant No. 11067–01, 1966.

Ammons, R., and W. Johnson, "Studies in the Psychology of Stuttering: The Construction and Association of a Test of Attitude Toward Stuttering," *Journal of Speech Disorders*, IX (1944), 39–49.

Aron, M. L., "The Relationships Between Measurements of Stuttering Behavior," *Journal of the South African Logopedic Society*, XIV (1967), 15–34.

Bar, A., "Effects of Listening Instructions on Attention to Manner and Content of Stutterers' Speech," *Journal of Speech and Hearing Research*, X (1967), 87–92.

Barr, W., "A Quantitative Study of the Specific Phenomena Observed in Stuttering," *Journal of Speech Disorders*, V (1940), 277–80.

Berlin, S., and C. Berlin, "Acceptability of Stuttering Control Patterns," *Journal of Speech and Hearing Disorders*, XXIX (1964), 436–41.

Bloodstein, O., "The Relationship Between Oral Reading Rate and Severity of Stuttering," *Journal of Speech Disorders*, IX (1944), 161–73.

Boehmler, R., "A Normative Study of Durational Distributions of Speech and Silence Intervals During Oral Reading, convention address, A.S.H.A., 1966.

————. "A Quantitative Study of the Extensional Definition of Stuttering with Special Reference to the Audible Designata," *Speech Monographs*, XXI, (1954), 205 (abstract).

————. "Listener Responses to Nonfluencies," *Journal of Speech and Hearing Research*, I (1958), 132–41.

Brown, S. F., "The Loci of Stutterings in the Speech Sequence," *Journal of Speech Disorders*, X (1945), 181–92.

Brutten, E. J., "Palmar Sweat Investigation of Disfluency and Expectancy Adaptation," *Journal of Speech and Hearing Research*, VI (1963), 40–48.

Clark, R. M., and F. P. Murray, "The Use of the Self-Concept as an Adjunct to Diagnosis and Therapy." In D. A. Barbara (ed.), *The Psychotherapy of Stuttering*. Springfield, Ill.: Thomas, 1962.

Cohen, E., "A Comparison of Oral and Spontaneous Speech of Stutterers with Special Reference to the Adaptation and Consistency Effects." Doctoral dissertation, State University of Iowa, 1952.

Conway, J. K., and B. Quarrington, "Positional Effects in the Stuttering of Contextually Organized Verbal Material," *Journal of Abnormal and Social Psychology*, LXVII (1963), 299–303.

Cullinan, W. L., "Stability of Consistency Measures in Stuttering, *Journal of Speech and Hearing Research*, VI (1963), 134–38.

Cullinan, W. L., E. M. Prather, and D. E. Williams, "Comparison of Procedures for Scaling Severity of Stuttering," *Journal of Speech and Hearing Research*, VI (1963), 187–94.

Dixon, C., "The Amount and Rate of Adaptation of Stuttering in Different Oral Reading Situations." Master's thesis, State University of Iowa, 1947.

Emerick, L. L., "Extensional Definition and Attitude Toward Stuttering," *Journal of Speech and Hearing Research*, III (1960), 181–86.

Erickson, R. L., "Assessing Communication Attitudes Among Stutterers," *Journal of Speech and Hearing Research*, XII (1969), 711–24.

Froeschels, E., and R. W. Rieber, "The Problem of Auditory and Visual Impercivity in Stutterers," *Folia Phoniatrica*, XV (1963), 13–20.

Goldiamond, I., "Stuttering and Fluency as Manipulatable Operant Response Classes." In L. Krasner and L. P. Ullman (eds.), *Research in Behavior Modification*. New York: Holt, Rinehart and Winston, 1965.

Gregory, H., "A Clinical Failure: Fred." In H. Luper (ed.), *Stuttering: Successes and Failures in Therapy*. Memphis: Speech Foundation of America, 1968a.

———. "A Clinical Success: Cora," In H. Luper (ed.), *Stuttering: Successes and Failures in Therapy*. Memphis: Speech Foundation of America, 1968b.

Harris, W. E., "A Study of the Transfer of the Adaptation Effect in Stuttering," *Journal of Speech Disorders*, VII (1942), 209–21.

Hirschberg, J., E. Kovacs, S. Palotas, and S. Szabo, ["Meteoropathological Observations of Stuttering Persons,"] *De Therapia Vocis et Loquellae*, II (1965), 357–58.

Johnson, W. "Measurements of Oral Reading and Speaking Rate and Disfluency of Adult Male and Female Stutterers," *Journal of Speech and Hearing Disorders*, Monograph Supplement VII (1961). 1–20.

Johnson, E., and S. F. Brown, "Stuttering in Relation to Various Speech Sounds," *Quarterly Journal of Speech*, XXI (1935), 481–96.

Johnson, W., and W. Colley, "The Relationship Between Frequency and Duration of Moments of Stuttering," *Journal of Speech Disorders*, X (1945), 35–38.

Johnson, W., F. L. Darley, and D. C. Spriestersbach, *Diagnostic Methods in Speech Pathology*. New York: Harper and Row, 1963.

Lanyon, R. I., "The Measurement of Stuttering Severity," *Journal of Speech and Hearing Research*, X (1967), 836–43.

———. "The Relationship of Adaptation and Consistency to Improvement in Stuttering Therapy," *Journal of Speech and Hearing Research*, VIII (1965), 263–69.

Leibman, J., "The Test-Retest Reliability of Adaptation and Consistency Scores." Master's thesis, Brooklyn College, 1956.

Leith, W. R., "An Investigation of the Adaptation Phenomenon and Certain Concomitant Voice Alterations in Stutterers and Non-Stutterers," *Dissertation Abstracts*, XIV (1954), 2156–57.

Lewis, D., and D. Sherman, "Measuring Severity of Stuttering," *Journal of Speech and Hearing Disorders*, XVI (1951), 320–26.

Luper, H. L., "A Study of the Relationship Between Stuttering Adaptation and Improvement During Speech Therapy." Master's thesis, Ohio State University, 1950.

———. "Consistency of Stuttering in Relation to the Goal Gradient Hypothesis," *Journal of Speech Disorders*, XXI (1956), 336–42.

———. "Relative Severity of Stuttering Ratings from Visual and Auditory Presentations of the Same Speech Sample," *Southern Speech Journal*, XXV (1959), 107–14.

Mahl, G. F., and G. Schultze, "Psychological Research in the Extra Linguistic Area." In T. A. Sebeok (ed.), *Approaches to Semiotics*. The Hague: Mouton & Co., 1964.

Martin, R., "Direct Magnitude-Estimation Judgments of Stuttering Severity Using

Audible and Audible-Visible Speech Samples," *Speech Monographs,* XXXII (1965), 169–77.

Meyer, B. C., "Psychology of Stuttering: Relationship Between Oral Reading Rate and Severity of Stuttering," *Journal of Speech Disorders,* IX (1944), 161–73.

Milisen, R., "Frequency of Stuttering with Anticipation of Stuttering Controlled," *Journal of Speech Disorders,* III (1938), 207–14.

————. "Methods of Evaluation and Diagnosis of Speech Disorders." In L. E. Travis (ed.), *A Handbook of Speech Pathology.* New York: Appleton-Century-Crofts, 1957.

Minifee, F. D., and H. S. Cooker, "A Disfluency Index," *Journal of Speech and Hearing Disorders,* XXIX (1964), 189–93.

Moller, H., "A Preliminary Investigation of the Effects of Secondary Characteristics Upon Judged Severity." Master's thesis, Queens College, 1957.

Moore, W. E., "Relations of Stuttering in Spontaneous Speech to Speech Content and to Adaptation," *Journal of Speech and Hearing Disorders,* XIX (1954), 208–16.

Naylor, R. V., "A Comparative Study of Methods of Estimating the Severity of Stuttering," *Journal of Speech and Hearing Disorders,* XVIII (1953), 30–37.

Pittelman, R. K., "A Comparative Study of Oral Reading Rate of Superior, Normal, and Stuttering Speakers." Master's thesis, Purdue University, 1942.

Pittenger, K. L., "A Study of the Duration of Temporal Intervals Between Successive Moments of Stuttering," *Journal of Speech Disorders,* V (1940), 333–41.

Prins, T. D., and F. E. Lohr, "A Study of the Behavioral Components of Stuttered Speech," Final Report Project No. 6-2382. Grant No. OEG -3-6-062382-1882. U. S. Department of Health, Education and Welfare, 1968.

Quarrington, B., "Cyclic Variations in Stuttering Frequency and Severity and Some Related Forms of Variation," *Canadian Journal of Psychology,* X (1956), 178–83.

————. "Measures of Stuttering Adaptation," *Journal of Speech and Hearing Research,* II (1959), 105–12.

Ringel, R., and F. Minifie, "Protensity Estimates of Stutterers and Nonstutterers," *Journal of Speech and Hearing Research,* IX (1966), 289–96.

Roberts, P. P., "Speech Sound Time and Oral Reading Time of College Stutterers and Nonstutterers." Master's thesis, Purdue University, 1949.

Robinson, F. B., "A Clinical Failure: Harry." In H. Luper (ed.), *Stuttering: Successes and Failures in Therapy.* Memphis: Speech Foundation of America, 1968.

Rothenberg, L. P., "An Exploratory Study of Adult Stutterers' Perceptions of Their Stuttering and Their Perceptions of the Processes and Outcomes of Stuttering Therapy," quoted in G. Woolf, "The Assessment of Stuttering as Struggle, Avoidance and Expectancy," *British Journal of Disorders of Communication,* II (1967), 158–71.

Rotter, J. B., and J. E. Rafferty, *Manual for the Rotter Incomplete Sentences Blank, College Form.* New York: Psychological Corporation, 1950.

Rousey, C. L., "Stuttering Severity During Prolonged Spontaneous Speech," *Journal of Speech and Hearing Research,* I (1958), 40–47.

Sander, E. L., "Reliability of the Iowa Speech Disfluency Test," *Journal of Speech and Hearing Disorders,* Monograph Supplement VII (1961), 21–30.

Sheehan, J. G., "A Clinical Success: Leonard." In H. Luper (ed.), *Stuttering:*

Successes and Failures in Therapy. Memphis: Speech Foundation of America, 1968.

————. "A Study of the Phenomena of Stuttering." Master's thesis, University of Michigan, 1946.

————. "Cyclic Variation in Stuttering," *Journal of Abnormal Psychology*, LXXIV (1969), 452–53.

————. "Modification of Stuttering Through Nonreinforcement," *Journal of Abnormal and Social Psychology*, XLVI (1951), 51–63.

————. "Rorschach Prognosis in Psychotherapy and Speech Therapy," *Journal of Speech and Hearing Disorders*, XIX (1954), 217–19.

Sheehan, J. G., and R. B. Voas, "Tension Patterns During Stuttering in Relation to Conflict, Anxiety Binding, and Reinforcement," *Speech Monographs*, XXI (1954), 272–79.

Sherman, D., "Clinical and Experimental Use of the Iowa Scale of Severity of Stuttering," *Journal of Speech and Hearing Disorders*, XVII (1952), 316–20.

————. "Reliability and Utility of Individual Ratings of Audible Characteristics of Stuttering," *Journal of Speech and Hearing Disorders*, IX (1955), 11–16.

Sherman, D., and R. McDermott, "Individual Ratings of Severity of Moments of Stuttering," *Journal of Speech and Hearing Research*, I (1958), 61–67.

Sherman, D., and W. D. Trotter, "Correlation Between Two Measures of the Severity of Stuttering," *Journal of Speech and Hearing Disorders*, XXI (1956), 426–29.

Shrum, W. F., "A Study of the Speaking Behavior of Stutterers and Nonstutterers by Means of Electromyography," convention address, A. S. H. A., 1967.

Shulman, E. A., "A Study of Certain Factors Influencing Variability of Stuttering." Doctoral dissertation, State University of Iowa, 1945.

Shumak, C., "A Speech Situation Rating Sheet for Stutterers." In W. Johnson (ed.), *Stuttering in Children and Adults*, Minneapolis: University of Minnesota Press, 1955.

Snidecor, J. C., "Tension and Facial Appearance in Stuttering." In W. Johnson (ed.), *Stuttering in Children and Adults*. Minneapolis: University of Minnesota Press, 1955.

Soderberg, G., "What is 'Average' Stuttering?" *Journal of Speech and Hearing Disorders*, XXVII (1962), 85–86.

Spielberger, C. D., "The Effects of Stuttering Behavior and Response Set on Recognition Thresholds," *Journal of Personality*, XXV (1956), 33–45.

Starbuck, H. B., "Determination of Severity of Stuttering and Construction of an Audio-Visual Scale." Doctoral dissertation, Purdue University, 1954.

Tate, M. W., and W. L. Cullinan, "Measurement of Consistency of Stuttering," *Journal of Speech and Hearing Research*, V (1962), 272–83.

Tate, M. W., W. L. Cullinan, and A. Ahlstrand, "Measurement of Adaptation in Stuttering," *Journal of Speech and Hearing Research*, IV (1961), 321–29.

Trotter, W. D., "A Study of the Severity of the Individual Moments of Stuttering Under the Conditions of Successive Readings of the Same Material." Doctoral dissertation, State University of Iowa, 1953.

Trotter, W., and L. Brown, "Speaking Time Behavior Before and After Speech Therapy," *Journal of Speech and Hearing Research*, I (1958), 48–51.

Trotter, W. D., and J. A. Kools, "Listener Adaptation to the Severity of Stuttering," *Journal of Speech and Hearing Disorders*, XX (1955), 385–87.

Tuthill, C. E., "A Quantitative Study of Extensional Meaning with Special Reference to Stuttering," *Speech Monographs*, XIII (1946), 81–98.

Van Riper, C., "A Clinical Success: Don." In H. Luper (ed.), *Stuttering: Successes and Failures in Therapy*. Memphis: Speech Foundation of America, 1968.

Van Riper, C., and C. J. Hull, "The Quantitative Measurement of the Effect of Certain Situations on Stuttering." In W. Johnson (ed.), *Stuttering in Children and Adults*. Minneapolis: University of Minnesota Press, 1955.

Van Riper, C., and R. Milisen, "A Study of the Predicted Duration of the Stutterer's Blocks as Related to Their Actual Duration," *Journal of Speech Disorders*, IV (1939), 339–45.

West, R., M. Ansberry, and A. Carr, *The Rehabilitation of Speech*. New York: Harper, 1957.

Williams, D. E., M. Wark, and F. D. Minifie, "Ratings of Stuttering by Audio, Visual, and Audiovisual Cues," *Journal of Speech and Hearing Research*, VI (1963), 91–100.

Woolf, G., "The Assessment of Stuttering as Struggle, Avoidance, and Expectancy," *British Journal of Disorders in Communication*, II (1967), 158–71.

Young, M. A., "Predicting Ratings of Severity of Stuttering," *Journal of Speech and Hearing Disorders*, Monograph Supplement VII (1961), 31–54.

Young, M. A., and E. M. Prather, "Measuring Severity of Stuttering Using Short Segments of Speech," *Journal of Speech and Hearing Research*, V (1962), 256–62.

ten

TYPES OF
STUTTERERS

The need to make sense out of the differences in etiology and symptomatology that characterize stuttering has led to many different categorizations of subgroups or types of stutterers. The hypothesis that the population of stutterers is not homogeneous, that it includes subgroups that can be differentiated, is an extremely attractive one. It would account for many of the direct contradictions found in the research. It might explain why some stutterers profit from a certain kind of therapy while others do not. Such a hypothesis might offer a reasonable explanation for the incredible variety of stuttering—perhaps the disorder is like a lake into which many different waters finally flow. It seems possible, even plausible, that breaks in the flow of speech might be caused by different things. If differing subpopulations of stutterers could be discovered, each having its own well defined cluster of features which contrast it with the other subpopulations, then many of our theoretical and clinical problems might be resolved.

Over 80 years ago Ssikorski (1889) made a statement which is still echoed today:

> The varieties of stuttering are so many and complex that the person interested in this neurosis must ask himself whether it is a single disorder or a number of disorders which have been grouped together because they have been insufficiently analyzed. The overt behaviors differ so much that it seems almost impossible to compare and classify the symptoms (p. 44).

Nevertheless, we must tackle typology with some caution. Kretschmer's (1925) effort to classify human beings into distinct physical types (asthenic, pyknic, etc.) created more problems than it solved, and Sheldon's later typology studies (1954), which correlated endomorphic, ectomorphic, and mesomorphic characteristics with personality traits has been shown by Tyler (1956) and others to be very vulnerable. There is some evidence to support the belief that some individuals tend toward more heightened sympathetic and others toward more parasympathetic arousal in terms of automatic balance and that these "constitutional" differences may be stable (Wenger and Wellington, 1943), but the differences exist on a continuum, and it is difficult to use them meaningfully to yield well defined types. Typology has found much more support in the European than in the American literature on stuttering, and it is possible that our skepticism has prevented us from recognizing that subgroups of stutterers may actually exist.

Among many others, St. Onge and Calvert (1964) have strongly challenged the assumption that all stutterers are peas from the same pod. In their critical article they wax both vehement and eloquent:

> For example, it appears well within the realm of possibility that a population of dysrhythmic speakers could be found who possess no organic or psychological signs whatever, aside from markedly dysrhythmic speech. We usually do not know how many stutterers have or do not have serious organic or psychogenic signs, because investigators seldom trouble to perform the necessary diagnostic refinements. If some stutterers exist without other signs, perhaps the presence of an idiopathic group could be established. Alternatively, is there a group of stutterers whose pathology is primarily psychic, but in whom the dysrhythmia of speech looms large, and other and possibly more significant psychological signs are subordinated? Is there a psychogenic stutterer without organic signs? Also, is there a predominantly organic stutterer who on careful neurological examination would show many positive signs? The painful fact is that after over 2,000 studies we cannot answer these relatively simple questions with a substantial statement of how stutterers distribute themselves on either the psychological or organic side (p. 164).

TYPES OF STUTTERING:
THE LITERATURE

But first let us review the literature. Most of it consists of arbitrary classifications based on clinical impressions. Stutterers have been grouped in terms of similar etiologies, similar stuttering behavior patterns, and similar therapeutic problems.

ETIOLOGICAL TYPES

One of the first efforts to distinguish different types of stutterers by their causes was that by Hieronymous Mercurialis (1530-1606). In his book on childhood diseases he describes two distinct stuttering types: *balbuties naturalis*, an organic disorder due to brain hyperexcitability, and *balbuties accidentalis* caused by fright and other emotions and made worse by them. This dichotomy is still represented today. Very soon, however, the number of subclassifications grew as observers of stuttering found more and more apparent etiologies of stuttering. In his youth, this author translated an ancient and obscure German booklet, now lost, but which intrigued him greatly because it contained 99 different etiological and symptomatic varieties of stuttering, each with a Greek or Latin name. Why couldn't that author have found the hundreth variety if only for purposes of closure? Perhaps it was indeed later discovered by Emerick (1968) who, with tongue in cheek, described a case of "spasmophemia porcus" in which the child began to stutter after his father's pigs got loose in the back seat of an automobile when he was taking them to market. Hunt (1861) lists 21 different etiological types of stuttering including "pneumognathoglossocheilomanis," a term that might cause anyone to hesitate. Klencke (1860), a contemporary of Hunt, was more conservative. He listed only five types: nervous, respiratory, constitutional, emotional, and habitual.

The incredible proliferation of types of stuttering finally led to a sensible counterreaction, so that Schulthess (1830) used only three classes: ideopathic (unknown etiology), symptomatic, and sympathetic, and Wyneken (1868) used ideopathic, deuteropathic (result of disease), and symptomatic (result of brain lesions). Throughout the literature we find this same magical triad of typology. (Why must we always classify things in threes?) In the twentieth century, Brill (1923), who defined stuttering as a psychoneurotic symptom, described three types: depressive, psychoneurotic, and psychopathic. Many authors with widely different ideas of the origin and nature of stuttering have found three categories.

MODERN ETIOLOGICAL TYPES

Our forerunners would not be particularly surprised to find typological classifications still popular today. They would feel quite comfortable in the six-fold typology given by Luchsinger and Arnold (1965): 1. The organically and inherited type with a strong cluttering component; 2. symptomatic stuttering in which the disorder reflects the disturbance caused by organic brain lesion; 3. developmental stuttering due to psychological shock or imitation during the speech learning period; 4. physiological stuttering arising from normal nonfluency; 5. traumatic stuttering resulting from great stress such as that produced by combat experience; and 6. hysterical stuttering. Luchsinger and Arnold present this classification without any research evidence, and it is presumably based on clinical impressions and case history material.

Another similar classification is given by Zaliouk and Zaliouk (1965). They examined 58 Israelic stutterers aged 6 to 15 years using a variety of tests and anamnesic inquiries. Though their data are not presented in a form which permits any real evaluation, they concluded that their stutterers fell into six groups, each having a unique and typical profile: tachylalic, spastic dysphonic, delayed language type, poor coordination type, dyslexic-dysgraphic type, and psychogenic type. We provide in the following quotations sample descriptions of two of their types:

> *Tachylalic stutterers:* The speech pattern of this group was characterized by its excessive rate (5-7 words per second), while other motor patterns were equally very rapid, such as writing, walking, eating, etc. Most tachylalic children had other members of the family with either a similar type of stuttering or at least rapid speech and motor patterns. The speech was typical, mostly the clonic (cluttering) form of stuttering, or blurred speech with arhythmia and generally shallow breathing. Most of these children had extrovert personalities, and were hardly conscious of their speech defect, at least it did not interfere with their social and speaking activities. There were 11 (eleven) such cases. . . . *Laterality-Motor Stuttering:* The common symptoms of this group were: lack of motor dominance, ambilaterality, reversed laterality, and poor motor coordination. The stuttering pattern was associated in many cases with other speech defects such as: dyslalias, blurred speech, rhinolalia. There were 7 (seven) such cases (p. 437).

In the Netherlands, Grewel (1960) has devised a most elaborate and detailed set of stuttering subgroups. He says, "Stuttering is not a unitary disorder. There are different varieties of stuttering and different manifestations termed stuttering. These have different causes, different symptoms, and different courses of development." Grewel describes a large number of subvarieties of broken speech which are often included in the stuttering category and cites cases representative of many of them. Among these are to be found the developmental form of stuttering (normal child disfluencies); the tachylalic; the cluttering type; a pseudocluttering variety in which auditory perception is impaired; a paraphrasic and paliphemic type in which the person finds difficulty in the encoding of speech; a neurotic variety in which fears of any kind precipitate stuttering behaviors; a type (school stuttering) marked by blockings confined to reading and spelling in the school situation; a pubertal form in which sexual conflicts are reflected in the speech; hysterical stuttering with predominantly oral symptoms; and others. Grewel also distinguishes between these conditions and the broken speech resembling stuttering shown in epilepsy and aphasia or dysarthria. He insists that careful diagnosis should lead to different forms of treatment for the different kinds of problems encountered. Thus for "literal" or "letter" stuttering which he describes as a "remarkable form of neurotic stuttering characterized by loci confined to the first letter of 'bad' or 'filthy' words or the person's own name and by a strong evidence of guilt and shame," Grewel maintains that for this group any speaking exercises would be useless and that psychotherapy would be the treatment of choice.

With some relief we move to Russia to find Amirov (1960) using only two types: excitatory and inhibitory, both based on Pavlovian conditioning theory. In Austria, Trojan and Wiehs (1963) use four classes: a neuropathic; a poorly coordinated type; a sensory variety with impaired auditory and kinesthetic perception such as is found in cluttering; and a psychopathological type. Four clinical types described by Freund (1966) are frequently found in the current literature. He writes, "We believe that by far the most common clinical variety of stuttering is that which shows all the characteristics of an expectancy neurosis." However, Freund also describes "another variety of stuttering—the hysterical type. It presents a different clinical picture both in diagnosis and therapy from that of the expectancy-neurosis type. Often it shows opposing features." (Some of these features are late and sudden onset, stereotypy, exhibitionism, lack of affect, etc.) Freund's other two types are based on cluttering and brain damage.

We conclude this section on etiological stuttering types by returning to St. Onge (1963), who tentatively offers a triad of major alternatives to the view that stuttering is a unitary disorder, a position he finds unsupportable. Again the magical number three crops up, but it is perhaps of some interest that the three kinds of stutterers he describes seem to have their common items drawn from all the other collections. St. Onge's three types are as follows: "(a) the stutterer with no organic or psychogenic signs but who is simply phobic about speech; (b) the psychogenic stutterer for whom stuttering is a useful symptom of a larger disorder; and (c) the organic stutterer who is nonfluent because of organicity, or through organicity is unable to tolerate the normal fears associated with speaking." If we weren't all jaundiced by too many memories of the old mountain of nonsense written about stuttering, the fairly good consensus on these three types would be impressive, but we must remember that these typological statements were based on clinical impressions as remembered in arm chairs. They sound reasonable enough, but what real evidence do we have that these types exist or, for that matter, whether any subgroups of stutterers exist?

RESEARCH ON TYPES OF STUTTERING

In most of the research on types of stuttering, the subjects are analyzed to determine the presence or absence of certain phenomena. Usually these investigations consider only a single feature or at most two. For example, Fritzell, Peterson, and Sellden (1965) described two subgroups of children one of which showed paroxysmal EEG activity and the other of which did not. Similarly, Weiss (1967) found a subgroup of stutterers showing evidence of latent tetany and another group that did not. And Zerneri (1965) tested 102 stutterers under DAF and classified as organic all those who showed no disrupting effect of the delay. And Baldan (1965) distinguished subgroups of stutterers in terms of their reactions to motor-facial tests or induced nystagmus. Are these really subgroups? Such findings only show that differences exist among stutterers. One difference is hardly a sufficient criterion by which to distinguish a "type." These observations of differences do, of course, provide the material out of which distinctive clusters of features may yet be distilled to provide a basis for types or for a general syndrome.

In a few experiments the investigators deliberately selected subgroups of stutterers differing on certain designated features and then tested to see if these groups also differed on other related features. Graham and Brumlik (1961), for example, compared the stuttering behaviors of a small subgroup of stutterers known to have epileptiform spike discharges in their EEGs with two other groups, one of which had other abnormal EEGs and the other normal brainwave tracings. Those with the spikes had very mild and infrequent stutterings; those with the other kinds of abnormal EEGs had the most severe stutterings. Some showed no abnormality. The number of subjects was too small to permit any definitive conclusions, and we include the study here only to illustrate a possible methodology for future efforts to determine types. Gregory (1964) pioneered another possible method for defining subgroups. In his investigation of possible neural deficits in the auditory feedback system, he examined the performance of those subjects who scored lower than the lowest scoring normal speakers on his three basic filtered-speech tests to see if these same individuals also did poorly on tests of diadochokinesis, the Heath Railwalking Test, the MMPI, etc. He failed to find any positive evidence for the existence of definite subgroups, but his method is interesting. Brankel (1961) suggests that it would also be important to test stutterers on several functions *simultaneously* (breathing, EEGs etc.) if we hope to get the data we need to determine types.

BASIC RESEARCH

The only truly comprehensive investigation of the typology of stutterers is a doctoral dissertation performed by Asa Berlin (1954). Although regrettably it was never published, it is probably the most definitive study that has been done, and it could well serve as a model for the future research which is so needed. At most we can only briefly present a glimpse of this work. Berlin selected three *mutually exclusive* groups of stutterers: those with pronounced family histories, those with definite evidence of brain damage, and those with psychogenic problems as defined by high scores on the MMPI. He then administered a questionnaire covering a large number of items about onset, speech symptoms, illnesses, and home environment, and he also gave the subjects certain tests of laterality and diadochokinesis. Berlin failed to find any hard evidence for the presence of different types, although a slight trend in the data indicated that a familial, perhaps organic, subgroup might be discerned. Berlin's study should be repeated with many other kinds of characteristics (adaptation types, EEG types, responses to masking and DAF, responses to certain drugs, speech characteristics, response to contingent punishment, arousal patterns and the like), and the sample of subjects should not be confined to adult stutterers. A better categorization of the groups and less reliance on questionnaire data would also be necessary. We hope this research will be done. The only other respectable source of data bearing on typology is the study of Andrews and Harris (1964). By submitting their vast amount of data to factorial analysis, they were able to procure four possible factors that seemed to play an important part in the persistence of stuttering: a hereditary familial factor, a history of delayed speech, poor emotional home environment, and a "general lack of capacity to think, talk, and behave" appropriately (whatever that means). Andrews and Harris feel that there are definite subgroups in the population of stutterers and hope that future research will locate and define them. So do we.

TYPES IN TERMS OF SYMPTOMS

Stuttering has been called a syndrome, meaning a set of symptoms that characterize a malady. This medical model may or may not be appropriate to stuttering. Certainly if stuttering is no more than a collection of learned behaviors, as some contend, the term syndrome must be stretched considerably. Nevertheless, there seem to be certain clusters of stuttering behaviors that lend themselves to categorization. Probably the most notable of these are found in two dichotomies, the first is divided into clonic and tonic stutterers, and the second into *interiorized* (masked unvocalized, or hidden) and *exteriorized* (vocalized) stutterers. Other symptomatological classes have also been described.

TONIC AND CLONIC STUTTERING

The terms *tonus* and *clonus* come from physiology, clonus referring to oscillatory and tonus to sustained contraction of muscle. Using these two terms to represent the wide variety of repetitive and fixatory behaviors of stutterers adds little precision to the description, but they have had wide usage, especially in Europe. One of the major difficulties lies in the overlap. Few pure clonic or pure tonic stutterers are to be found. According to Bloodstein (1960), even in young children, where repetitive stuttering behaviors apparently predominate, the presence of prolongations and "tonic blockings" are commonly discerned. In older stutterers, both clonic and tonic behaviors are usually seen in the same individual. Clonic repetitions predominate on stop consonants while tonic fixations occur more on continuants; in some stutterers, however, the reverse is true. Moreover, a moment of stuttering on a single word may include both tonic and clonic components. Finally, even the most tonic of all tonic fixations will show rhythmic alternations of tension in the accompanying tremors, if the latter are examined electromyographically. Is this clonus? Fletcher (1928), discussing tonic and clonic forms of stuttering says, "The fundamental difficulty in each of these cases is precisely the same . . . [any differences in symptoms are] purely incidental and superficial having nothing whatsoever to do with the basic character of this disorder."

Most modern investigators have accepted the impreciseness of the categories. Thus Froeschels (1943) (who did much to make the terms popular and who views tonus as the result of the child's struggle once he comes to believe that speech is difficult has added the terms *tonoclonus* and *clonotonus* to take care of the varying predominance of the two features. Most of those who have conducted research with clonic and tonic stutterers have had to use the adverbial phrases "predominantly clonic" and "predominantly tonic" in defining their different groups of subjects since they were unable to isolate any pure types.

At any rate, there are four major studies which sought to relate the type of stuttering (tonic or clonic) to personality differences. They are by Matha (1938) in France, and Krugman (1946), Diamond (1953), and Emerick (1966) in the United States. The first three of these investigators failed to use matched controls and had other deficiencies in experimental design and in the interpretation of data, but they all found in general that the tonic stutterers tended to be more withdrawing and sensitive while the clonic ones were more extraverted and outgoing. Emerick's study was designed and controlled better, and he found no differences between his groups in responses to frustration or in goal setting. The sparseness of research, along with the imprecision of criteria, scarcely allows us to feel that clonic and tonic types of stutterers are useful categories. Certainly we should suspect the conclusions of Otsuki (1953) who found tonic stuttering to reflect masculinity and clonic stuttering femininity.

TYPES IN TERMS
OF COVERT FEATURES

Several experiments have been designed to discover different types of stutterers with respect to anxiety, hostility, and other emotional aspects of the problem. Krantz (1954) explored 120 adult stutterers with a variety of tests to determine whether subgroups could be found with respect to manifest anxiety, hostility, and rigidity. She was unable to find any and concluded also that stutterers were far from constituting a homogeneous population. Gray and Karmen (1967) used the Palmar Sweat Index as a measure of anxiety during adaptation readings. They felt they had perhaps discovered subgroups of stutterers which differed in frequency of stuttering as related to nonverbal anxiety levels. Something of the same sort was found by Knott, Correll, and Shepherd (1959), who discovered two groups of stutterers whose EEGs differed from each other even more than either one differed from those of normal speakers. These authors attributed the variance to distinct differences in emotionality as reflected in the brainwaves. In England, Renfrew (1952) used Bloodstein's (1949) questionnaire to see if there were different types of stutterers in terms of the situations that evoked the most and least fluency. No discrete types of stutterers were found, and she concluded that, "The situations which cause difficulty to each stammerer seem to be entirely individual and linked with his own special problems." This sad survey of the little we know about different patterns of covert features of stuttering certainly does not make us particularly optimistic that any real types of stutterers can be discerned by examining their emotional responses.

Another approach to a typology based on symptoms is found in Robinson's (1964, pp. 100-101) four common patterns of clinical problems shown by advanced stutterers. While he does not hold that these patterns represent all kinds of clinical problems, he feels that they are common ones, and he offers a somewhat different kind of therapy for each. No research has yet determined whether his four types are truly exclusive, but many clinicians feel they have some face validity. His schema is as follows:

FOUR COMMON PATTERNS OF CLINICAL PROBLEMS

		Common and Prominent	*Relatively Rare*
Pattern I	Overt:	Devices to avoid, hide, disguise, deny, circumlocute. Ritualistic behavior; speech on residual air.	Long uninterrupted prolongations or repetitions or tremors. Facial contortions, "convulsive" movements.
	Covert:	Embarrassment, shame, specific word fears, some guilt.	Frustration, anger, hostility.
Pattern II	Overt:	Struggling, facial contortions, tremors, "convulsive" mannerisms, compulsive stuttering and talking.	Avoidance, postponement, disguise, giving up.

		Common and Prominent	Relatively Rare
	Covert:	Frustration, anger, aggression, some guilt.	Embarrassment, word or situation fears, anxiety.
Pattern III	Overt:	Hesitancy, retrials, halfhearted attempts, abulia.	Struggle, severe contortions or tremors, disguise rituals.
	Covert:	Anxiety, frustration.	Hostility, guilt.
Pattern IV	Overt:	Weak speech attempts, extended prolongations or silent blocks, abulia.	Aggressive speech attempts, struggle, tremors, facial contortions.
	Covert:	Impotence, helplessness, frustration, low ego strength, guilt, anxiety, suggestibility.	Outwardly expressed hostility.

INTERIORIZED AND EXTERIORIZED STUTTERERS

Another attempt to distinguish types of stutterers in terms of characteristic behavior patterns is based on visibility and audibility. The most familiar of these attempts was that by Douglass and Quarrington (1952) in which, through observation, they differentiated two types of stutterers, the interiorized and exteriorized, in terms of the relative prominence of overt or covert features. According to these authors, the interiorized stutterer is the one who is able to conceal the overt manifestations of the disorder though at the price of constant vigilance, avoidance, and anxiety. This type is said to demonstrate a different course of development and different personality characteristics. The exteriorized stutterer is outgoing and extravertive, and his stuttering abnormality is readily apparent to the listener. No real research has since corroborated these findings of presumed types except for another study by Quarrington and Douglass (1960) and a negative finding by Doust (1956). Quarrington and Douglass compared vocalized and nonvocalized stutterers under one condition in which they were being heard and another in which they were not heard by listeners. They write, "The diagnosis of V (vocalized) or NV (nonvocalized) condition was made by an experienced speech pathologist after observing spontaneous and test-speech behavior of the subjects. Subjects who did not show a marked predominance of NV or V blocks were not included in this investigation." The NV (nonvocalized) stutterers showed a greater reduction of stuttering when they were not being listened to. Doust (1956) had a group of "nonvocalized-interiorized" and a group of "vocalized-exteriorized" stutterers undergo stress by using a breath-holding technique. He found no difference between the groups although they both differed from normals and neurotics. It is our general impression that interiorized-nonvocalized and exteriorized-vocalized forms of stuttering should be regarded not as different basic types but rather as different ways of responding to the same disorder, either because of different learning experiences or because of different personality patterns.

OTHER DIFFERENTIATING CHARACTERISTICS

Newman (1963) found a subgroup of stutterers who did not show the characteristic adaptation curve and suggested that these might comprise a different type of stutterer. Chevrie-Muller 1963), using glottography, found two groups—one which showed impaired laryngeal functioning and the other which did not. Murray (1966) similarly found two groups of stutterers, those who became fluent under masking and those who did not. Soderberg (1968) reviewed the research on delayed auditory feedback with stutterers and found possible evidence for types of stutterers in terms of their response to the delay. Other studies in this same vein have found marked differences among stutterers in motor coordination, in EEG abnormalities, in response to electronystography or photic stimulation, etc.

All that these studies seem to show is that there is a lack of homogeneity in the population of stutterers. However, if different stuttering subtypes exist, it should be possible to tell one from another on more than a single trait or factor. There should at least be clusters of characteristic factors with minimal overlap between clusters. At present most of the research demonstrates only that stutterers differ one from another on one or two factors. There are many hints that subgroups of stutterers may yet be discovered, but at the present time we can only conclude that the typologies of stuttering based on etiology or symptomatology which have been proposed so far have little scientific evidence to support them.

DEVELOPMENTAL TYPES

Labels have also been bestowed on patterns of behavior that reflect the course of the disorder's growth. We have already seen some of these, since few writers have been able to keep from using developmental differences in contriving their categories. Thus Froeschels (1952) distinguishes between physiological stuttering (normal childhood disfluency), imitative stuttering, and genuine stuttering. Bluemel (1932) adopted the terms "primary" and "secondary" to describe the marked differences between early and fully developed stuttering. Van Riper (1954) inserted a third variety "transitional stuttering" as a convenient term for stutterers in the developmental stage in which frustration and struggle behavior are shown but not fear and avoidance. Still later, Bloodstein (1960) provided a fourfold classification based on developmental characteristics. Dostalova and Dosuzkov (1965) return to the Latin and give us three types: *Balbuties praecox, Balbuties vulgaris,* and *Balbuties tarda.* That's enough. Any more would be vulgaris.

COMMENTARY

Virtually all of our research studies lump together any and all individuals who reveal rhythmic disorders of speech, using curious aggregations of morons, psychotics, prepsychotics, neurotics, epileptics, etc. These problems are often casually combined with others having dysrhythmic speech who lack any additional signs. Most serious research studies on stuttering offer no clues whatever that the tester had any difficulties in selecting who should be included or excluded or on what grounds the elections were made, except of course that they stuttered (St. Onge, 1963, p. 196).

If types of stutterers do exist, the first job must be the selection of items which may play a primary role in the determination of a specific type of stuttering (Berlin, 1954, p. 23).

Studies concerned with the syndromic aspects of stuttering should rigorously exclude stutterers of mixed symptomatology to achieve, for research purposes, a pure population (St. Onge, 1963, p. 197).

On delving further into the etiology and pathogenesis of stuttering, one finds that it is not a nosological entity; different types of stuttering are evoked by different pathogenic factors. Most often stuttering is a functional ailment, like neurosis, in this case a logoneurosis. Far less often it is a syndrome in the clinical picture of organic cerebral lesions such as encephalitis, extrapyramidal disorders and the like (Daskalov, 1962, p. 1049).

Two types of muscular spasms are to be observed, a tonic contraction of the muscles which results in a complete block of speech, and which is sometimes called stammering, and the clonic or repetitive spasm which gives rise to the typical stutter. There seems to be no valid reason to attempt to separate these two conditions since close observation will show them to be intimately intermingled in almost all cases (Orton, 1937, p. 123).

It has been discovered that tonic and clonic stammering are physiologically and pathologically distinct phenomena. This will open new horizons in the study of these two disorders. From the psychological point of view, subjects suffering from these two types of stammering present very different personality characteristics (De Parrel, 1965, p. 113).

If we term the iterations (syllabic repetitions) "clonus" and the pressure symptoms "tonus," then the combination of the two may be called "clonotonus" and "tonoclonus" respectively, depending on which sign is the most prominent. It seems evident that the tonic component is due to an attempt on the part of the child to overcome the iterations (Froeschels, 1943, p. 149).

The behavior of the two types, interiorized and exteriorized stutterers, is to be differentiated in numerous ways. They both fear entering speaking situations but mainly for different reasons. The interiorized stutterer's main concern is to avoid stuttering and he will sacrifice expression or any other subgoal for achievement of his main goal if necessary. To the exteriorized stutterer, however, oral expression is the main goal and avoidance of stuttering a subgoal. Another difference is that with any exteriorized stutterer who has been studied, one can predict with surprising accuracy what stuttering patterns he is likely to display under given speaking conditions. A similar prediction is not possible, however, with the interiorized stutterer. He does not characteristically react in a stereotyped voluntary manner, but uses his devices with much diversity and dexterity as seems appropriate to the circumstances and it is impossible to make accurate predictions as to his likely behavior in any given circumstances (Douglass and Quarrington, 1952, pp. 381–382)."

The interiorized secondary stutterer, of which we speak, is characterized by acute and constant awareness of his speech difficulty and of stuttering threats contained in speaking situations. Constant preparedness, constant vigilance to guard against revelation of his stutter, complete avoidance of possible situations anticipated as threatening are all attitudes evidenced. Every eventuality must be anticipated so that he can either avoid the danger entirely or meet it fully prepared. To be caught unprepared would be a tragedy. He plans, of course, to speak but little, to fulfill the minimum demands of his society in the way of oral expression. Should the general situation be perceived as a threatening one, he may keep quiet and wait for safe "moments" in which to slip in a word or a short statement. He soon becomes quite clever at protecting himself against the risk of stuttering; a ready nod of assent is frequently used in order to be agreeable and thereby not provoke argument which might lead him into verbal battle. If and when stuttering moments seem imminent he has readily available a reservoir of devices calculated to disguise stuttering (Douglass and Quarrington, 1952, p. 379).

My observations have shown that the clinical picture of stammering neurosis in some patients is dominated by paroxysmal phenomena in the muscles of the articulatory or vocal apparatus, combined with an increased tone of the body musculature as a whole; in other patients by a disorder of vocal breathing; and in a third group by neurotic features, with a fear of speaking and with other phobias arising in response to the speech defect.

This clinical classification of stammerers, by introducing some degree of precision into our concepts of the nature of stammering, will help in the development of correct methods of treatment and contribute towards determining the choice of treatment and the prognosis of stammering in each concrete case (Kochergina, 1965, p. 374).

There are at present 58 classifications of depression, based upon a mixture of etiology and symptomatology (Dunlop, 1964, p. 108).

BIBLIOGRAPHY

Amirov, R. Z., ["Trigeminal, Tricomponent Method of Studying Higher Nervous Activity in Man"], *Zhurnal Vysshei Nervonoï Deiatel'nosti*, X (1960), 468–72.

Andrews, G., and M. Harris, *The Syndrome of Stuttering*. London: Heinemann, 1964.

Baldan, G., ["Study of the Vestibular Function in a Group of Stutterers: Electronystagmographic Researches"], *De Therapia Vocis et Loquellae*, I (1965), 349–51.

Berlin, A. J., "An Exploratory Attempt to Isolate Types of Stuttering." Doctoral dissertation, Northwestern University, 1954.

Bloodstein, O., "Conditions under which Stuttering is Reduced or Absent," *Journal of Speech and Hearing Disorders*, XIV (1949), 295–303.

————. "Development of Stuttering," *Journal of Speech and Hearing Disorders*, XXV (1960), 219–37.

Bluemel, C. S., "Primary and Secondary Stammering," *Quarterly Journal of Speech*, XVIII (1932), 187–200.

Brankel, O., ["Pneumotachographic Studies in Stutterers"], *Folia Phoniatrica*, XIII (1961), 136–43.

Brill, A. A., "Speech Disturbances in Nervous Mental Diseases," *Quarterly Journal of Speech*, IX (1923), 129–35.

Chevrie-Muller, C., ["A Study of Laryngeal Function in Stutterers by the Glotto-Graphic Method"], *Proceedings, VIIe Congrès de la Société Français de Médecine de la Voix et de la Parole*, Paris (1963).

Daskalov, D., "Basic Principles and Methods of Prevention and Treatment of Stuttering," *Nevropatologii e Psikhiatrii imeni S.S. Korsakova*, LXII (1962), 1047–52.

Denhardt, R., *Das Stottern: eine Psychose*. Leipzig: Ernst Keil's Nachfolger, 1890.

De Parrel, S., *Speech Disorders*. Oxford: Pergamon Press, 1965.

Diamond, M., "Personality Differences Between Tonic and Clonic Stutterers." Doctoral dissertation, Syracuse University, 1953.

Dostalova, N., and T. Dosuzkov, "Über die drei Hauptformen des Neurotische Stotterns," *De Therapia Vocis et Loquellae*, I (1965), 273–76.

Douglass, E., and B. Quarrington, "The Differentiation of Interiorized and Exteriorized Stuttering," *Journal of Speech and Hearing Disorders*, XVII (1952), 372–88.

Doust, J. W. L., "Stress and Psychopathology in Stutterers," *Canadian Journal of Psychology*, X (1956), 31–37.

Dunlop, E., "The Choice of Antidepressants in Various Types of Depression," *Psychosomatic Medicine*, V (1964), 107–110.

Emerick, L. L., "A Study of Psychological Traits in Tonic and Clonic Stutterers." Doctoral dissertation, Michigan State University, 1966.

Emerick, L. L., "A Clinical Success: Mark." In H. Luper (ed.), *Stuttering: Successes and Failures in Therapy,* Memphis: Speech Foundation of America, 1968.

Fletcher, J. M., *The Problem of Stuttering.* New York: Longmans Green, 1928.

Freund, H., "Inneres Stottern und Einstalbewegungen," *Zeitschrift für Neurologie und Psychiatrie,* VI (1932), 1243–45.

———. *Psychopathology and the Problems of Stuttering.* Springfield, Ill.: Thomas, 1966.

Fritzell, B., I. Peterson, and U. Sellden, "An EEG Study of Stuttering and Nonstuttering School Children," *De Therapia Vocis et Loquellae,* I (1965), 343–46.

Froeschels, E., "Pathology and Therapy of Stuttering," *Nervous Child,* II (1943), 148–61.

———. "The Significance of Symptomatology for the Understanding of the Essence of Stuttering," *Folia Phoniatrica,* IV (1952), 217–30.

Graham, J. K., and J. Brumlik, "Neurologic and Encephalographic Abnormalities in Stuttering and Matched Nonstuttering Adults," *Asha,* III (1961), 342 (abstract).

Gregory, H. H., "Stuttering and Auditory Central Nervous System Disorder," *Journal of Speech and Hearing Research,* VII (1964), 335–41.

Grewel, F., "Balbutiés (Stotteren)" *Logopaedie et Foniatrie,* XXXII (1960), 109–15; 125–28; 145–52; 165–68.

Gray, B. B., and J. L. Karmen, "The Relationship Between Nonverbal Anxiety and Stuttering Adaptation," *Journal of Communication Disorders,* I (1967), 141–51.

Hunt, J., *Stammering and Stuttering, Their Nature and Treatment.* (Original Edition, 1861). Reprinted. New York: Hafner, 1967.

Klencke, H., *Die Heilung des Stotterns.* Leipzig, 1860.

Knott, J. R., R. E. Correll, and J. N. Shepherd, "Frequency Analysis of Electroencephalograms of Stutterers and Nonstutterers," *Journal of Speech and Hearing Research,* II (1959), 74–80.

Kochergina, V. S., ["Drug Treatment of Stammering in Adults"], *Zhurnal Nevropathologii i. Psikhiatrii imeni S. S. Korsakova,* LXV (1965), 753–56.

Krantz, J., "A Study of the Interrelationships Among Manifest Anxiety, Manifest Hostility, Rigidity, Duration of Severity, and Severity of Stuttering Within a Group of Stutterers." Master's thesis, Pennsylvania State University, 1954.

Kretschmer, E., *Physique and Character.* New York: Harcourt, 1925.

Krugman, M., "Psychosomatic Study of Fifty Stuttering Children," *American Journal of Orthopsychiatry,* XVI (1946), 127–33.

Landolt, H., and R. Luchsinger, ["Language Disorder, Stuttering and Chronic Organic Psychosyndrome; Electroencephalographic Results and Studies of Pathology of Speech."] *Deutsche Medizinische Wochenshrift,* LXXIX (1954), 1012–15.

Luchsinger, R., and G. E. Arnold, *Voice–Speech–Language.* Belmont, Cal.: Wadsworth, 1965.

Matha, L., "Demonstration de Technique Rééducation des Troubles Psychoneuro-moteurs du Type Bégaiement Tonique," *Revue Française de Phoniatrie,* XXIII (1938), 99–126.

Murray, F. P., "The Effects of Variably Presented Noise Upon the Speech of Stutterers." Doctoral dissertation. Denver University, 1966.

Newman, P. W., "Adaptation Performances of Individual Stutterers: Implications for Research," *Journal of Speech and Hearing Research,* VI (1963), 393–94.

Orton, S. T., *Reading, Writing, and Speech Problems of Children.* New York: Norton and Co., 1937.

Otsuki, K., ["A Habit of Stuttering"], 1953, abstract no. 101 in G. Kamiyama, *A Handbook for the Study of Stuttering.* Tokyo: Kongo Shuppan, 1967.

Quarrington, B., and E. Douglass, "Audibility Avoidance in Nonvocalized Stutterers," *Journal of Speech and Hearing Disorders,* XXV (1960), 358–65.

Renfrew, C. B., "A Questionnaire for Stutterers," *Speech* (London), XVI (1952), 21–24.

Robinson, F. B., *Introduction to Stuttering.* Englewood Cliffs, N. J.: Prentice-Hall, 1964.

Schulthess, R., *Das Stammeln und Stottern.* Zurich: Hana Borg, 1830.

Sheldon, W. H., *Atlas of Men: A Guide for Somatotyping the Adult Male at all Ages.* New York: Harper, 1954.

Soderberg, G. A., "Delayed Auditory Feedback and Stuttering," *Journal of Speech and Hearing Disorders,* XXXIII (1968), 260–67.

Ssikorski, J. A., *Über das Stottern.* Berlin: Hirschwald, 1889.

St. Onge, K., "The Stuttering Syndrome," *Journal of Speech and Hearing Research,* VI (1963), 195–97.

St. Onge, K., and J. J. Calvert, "Stuttering Research," *Quarterly Journal of Speech,* L (1964), 159–65.

Trojan, L., and H. Weihs, "Studien zur Stottertherapie," *Folia Phoniatrica,* XV (1963), 42–67.

Tyler, L. E., *The Psychology of Human Differences,* 2nd Ed. New York: Appleton-Century, 1956.

Van Riper, C., *Speech Correction: Principles and Methods,* Third Ed., Englewood Cliffs, N.J.: Prentice-Hall, 1954.

———. *Speech Correction: Principles and Methods,* 4th Ed. Englewood Cliffs, N.J.: Prentice-Hall, 1963.

Weiss, B., [Neuromuscular Excitability in Stutterers"], *Folia Phoniatrica,* XIX (1967), 117–24.

Wenger, M. A., and M. Wellington, "The Measurement of Autonomic Balance in Children: Method and Normative Data," *Psychosomatic Medicine,* V (1943), 241–53.

Wolf, A. A., and E. G. Wolf, "Feedback Processes in the Theory of Certain Speech Disorders," *Speech Pathology and Therapy,* II (1959), 48–55.

Wyneken, C., "Über das Stottern und dessen Heilung," *Zeitschrift für Rationelle Medicin,* XXXI (1968), 1–29.

Zaliouk, D., and A. Zaliouk, "Stuttering: A Differential Approach in Diagnosis and Therapy," *De Therapia Vocis et Loquellae,* I (1965), 437–41.

Zerneri, L., "Tentative d'Applicazione Delle Voci Retardata (DAF) Della Terapia Della Bulbuzie," *Bollettino Della Societa Italiana Di Fonetica, Fonentria e Audiologia,* XIX (1965), 125–30.

eleven

STUTTERING
AS A NEUROSIS

A huge amount of the literature on stuttering is devoted to the neurotic aspects of the disorder. However, since many of the authors who consider stuttering a neurosis have divergent opinions about what kind of neurosis it is presumed to be, it is necessary first to clarify what is usually meant by the term. Neurotic behavior usually presents three major characteristics—unpleasant feelings, inability to understand or to accept the feelings, and symptoms or patterns of behavior that symbolize and maintain them. Many adult stutterers fulfill these three criteria of neurosis. Do not forget, however, that most beginning stutterers, and some adult ones, show very marked and deviate speech behaviors without apparently manifesting any of these characteristics. The questions immediately presented are: If stuttering is neurotic in nature, is it a primary neurosis or a secondary one? Is the neurosis the source of the stutterer's difficulties or is it the consequence? Are all stutterers neurotic?

First let us explore the nature of neurotic behavior more closely. For many years, experimental neuroses have been produced in animals. Early in this century Pavlov trained dogs to make discriminations between such stimuli as circles and ellipses. When the differences between these stimuli were gradually reduced to the point where the discrimination was difficult or impossible, the dogs developed maladaptive and persistent behaviors which made them unfit for further conditioning. Since then, many other workers have created similar experimental neuroses.

They have been produced in sheep by Liddell (1964) and in cats by Masserman (1943). They have also been deliberately produced in children by Watson and Rayner (1920) and by Krasnogorski (1925). The purpose in all these experiments is to set up a conflict between drives or cues so that an overt *adaptive* response could not be accomplished. When no appropriate responses can be made in such a conflict situation, strong autonomic responses occur as evidenced by cardiovascular changes, pupillary dilation, respiratory effects, and a variety of inappropriate motor behaviors. These autonomic responses and maladaptive motor patterns generalized rapidly to other stimuli and, once conditioned, were very difficult to extinguish.

Liddell describes a sheep made neurotic by conditioning:

> Here we see the diffused, agitated pattern of the classical experimental neurosis, continual head movement, bleating, left foreleg overreacting to the metronome. He had been taught to give no reaction to the metronome at 50 beats per minute, but here it shows that he cannot inhibit, and all differentiation between signals for shock and for no shock has been eliminated. The heart beat is irregular, with many premature beats. Moreover the heart of this animal is disturbed in the barn at night. The animal also loses its normal gregariousness and when alarmed by marauding dogs, will not run off with the flock but in another direction, and the neurotic sheep will often be mauled by the dogs (pp. 133–134).

Human neuroses generally have as their core an emotional upheaval of anxiety that seems unrelated to the stimuli which trigger it. All of us know fear and anxiety. When we are threatened by a dangerous situation, the autonomic response of anxiety is adaptive and useful. It is when apprehensiveness occurs in situations which should not normally produce it that we have neurotic anxiety. The symptoms of neuroses, so widely variable, are viewed by many writers as defenses against the distress of this unexplainable and inappropriate anxiety. In behavioral terms, they are nonadjustive habits which are continually reinforced by a temporary anxiety reduction. Mowrer (1950) has discussed neurosis in similar terms. Indeed, he speaks of the "neurotic paradox," wherein behavior which is obviously more punishing than satisfying seems to persist, and behavior which apparently ought to produce desirable consequences is abandoned. His main solution for the paradox is that neurotic behavior makes sense if we consider the timing of the rewards or punishments. If the rewards come later and are greater than the punishment, the maladaptive "neurotic" behavior will continue.

It is obvious that many of the behaviors of confirmed stuttering would fit these descriptions. It is not so clear that the original stuttering presents this picture or that it originates in such conflict situations in the majority of cases. We have studied very carefully the situations in which children began to stutter and have done so very soon after it appeared. A few of them demonstrated very clearly, so clearly that we cannot explain the origin in any other way, that the disorder had its roots in such situations and seemed to be the result of conflict-produced emotion. But this neurotic origin did *not* appear in most of the 44 children we were able to follow from onset to maturity (see Chapter V).

Neurotic anxieties and neurotic behaviors usually arise in conflict situations. Strong incompatible urges or responses compete, and when the conflict cannot be resolved, anxiety is generated. Dollard and Miller (1950) say that "an intense emotional conflict is the necessary basis for neurotic behavior." The suffering that comes from unresolved conflicts impels the person to react in various ways; those coinciding with a decrease in the suffering, however momentary, will tend to persist as neurotic symptoms.

It should also be pointed out that neuroses can also originate in trap situations, those in which the animal or person is repeatedly punished without being able to avoid or escape or react appropriately. For example, Liddell conditioned his sheep to flex its foreleg on the fifth or tenth or fifteenth beat of a metronome by administering the shock at these intervals. However, when he tried to condition them to an interval of 30 beats, the animal became "neurotic." The crucial factor in the production of neurosis may not always be unresolved conflict. It may also be centered in the inability of the animal to respond so as to minimize anticipated punishment. This has been shown by the experiments of Wolpe (1958) in which cats were confined in a cage and subjected to intermittent shocks that they could not escape. These cats demonstrated the same sort of persistent disturbed behaviors (crouching, random clawing, howling, and the autonomic responses of pupillary dilation, hair erection, etc.) which Masserman (1934) had previously termed neurotic and attributed to conflict. Thus, the feeling of helplessness due to communicative frustration may be as important as the ambivalence of conflict in the production of neurotic anxiety, and certainly the stutterer experiences great communicative frustration.

In his own words Coriat (1931) states a psychoanalytic view:

> The anxiety in stammerers when they attempt or prepare to speak is not due to anticipation or to anxiety over a specific situation, but is caused by the fear of the ego being overwhelmed by the all-powerful auto-eroticism. This is particularly shown by the fact that stammerers frequently have literal dreams of nursing. Stammering becomes, therefore, a form of gratification of the original oral libido which continues as a post-natal gratification in talking. The confirmed stammerer tenaciously retains his earliest source of pleasure, that is, nursing; he reacts to the original oral binding of the mouth through a repetition compulsion localized in the speech mechanism, that is, in the tongue, lip, and jaw movements of the original physiological nursing mechanism (p. 155).

There are various views of the nature of the neurosis in stuttering. Even the psychoanalytic interpretations differ. Though Freud was unable to relieve the stuttering in one of his early cases, Frau Emmy, and felt that psychoanalysis was not an appropriate method for treating the disorder; many of his followers have not agreed. Stuttering has usually been regarded by the psychoanalysts as symptomatic of conflicts which have been resolved by fixations at anal or oral levels. To Coriat (1931), stuttering was the compromise symptom which partially solved the conflict between the instinctual need to remain an infantile suckling and the ego-need for more appropriate behavior. The anxiety, he felt, was due to the ego's fear of being "overwhelmed by the all-powerful oral eroticism." Stuttering behavior, according to Coriat, is related to the sucking and biting reactions of the infant at the nipple. Since speech also involves the lips and tongue, the compulsive repetition of movements performed by these organs allows even the adult stutterer to get his perverted oral pleasure as he talks.

Fenichel (1945), in contrast with Coriat, finds the essential conflict on anal rather than oral fixations. Stuttering is a pregenital conversion (hysterical) neurosis in that the early problems dealing with the retention and expulsion of the feces have been displaced upwards into the sphincters of the mouth. For the stutterer, according to Fenichel, speaking affords an opportunity to smear and soil his listener aggressively and with relative impunity. The attendant anxiety felt by the stutterer is due to his unconscious realization of the symbolic nature of his symptoms.

Heilpern (1941) presents a vivid picture:

> The patient's strong anal fixation is not surprising when one learns about his parent's personality. She made a habit of conversing with him when he was on the toilet. For a long time, even after he had begun to attend school, she examined his stools daily. In a rage, she once threw two quarters into the toilet, and then promised repentantly a piece of cake as a reward to him who would recover the money. The boy, almost grown up, did it. Humorous gifts, popular in this family, are toy chamber pots with little sausages in them. The mother can produce flatus voluntarily and does so jokingly to congratulate the father on the morning of his birthday. When she is in a rage, she pours out the chamber pot or even defecates on the floor (p. 97).

Glauber (1958) also rejected Coriat's restricted belief that the stutterer experiences perverted pleasure from his (stuttering) "act of nursing at an illusory nipple," as the complete explanation of the disorder. Instead, the basic conflict is between the id and the superego, the battleground lying in the ego-function of speech, for speech not only employs the oral pleasure-seeking (sucking) and aggression (biting), but it also serves as the basic mechanism for being able to live in a world of others. According to Glauber, it is the anxiety generated by all these conflicting drives that causes the stutterer to speak so haltingly. The result of this conflict is that the ego remains weak and arrested in its development and so does its most important function—speech. Stuttering as a symptom of the neurotic conflict shows features of regression as well as fixation and, at times, it reflects the person's need to defend himself against both of these solutions as well as the anxiety they create.

Barbara (1954), who has written much on stuttering, is one representative of the neoanalytic school, and much of his theory appears based on the position of Karen Horney. The basic conflict lies in the child's inadequate interpersonal relationships. Parental mishandling or perfectionistic demands or the lack of consistent tender loving care produces competing needs to comply, to avoid, or to react aggressively. Because these are incompatible with each other, ambivalence results and anxiety is generated. Since speech is the main vehicle for acquiring and maintaining interpersonal relationships, it reflects this ambivalence and anxiety in the form of hesitancy or stuttering. Barbara says:

> I feel that the symptom and the greater part of the ritual of stuttering itself is a major attempt toward an unconscious magical gesture with the purpose of symbolically demonstrating to others how the person who stutters suffers and is victimized (1954, p. 204).

Barbara also shows how a secondary stuttering neurosis can become overlaid on the primary one. Stutterers develop distinctive personality patterns (e.g., the Demosthenes complex) to prevent the anxiety from overwhelming them. In his fantasies:

> . . . as the individual who stutters soars to godlike heights, he is of necessity driven away from his real self. He becomes blinded by the compulsive need to have to prove himself—to become his Demosthenes image of himself (Barbara, 1954, p. 110).

Several other well known American authors have used psychoanalytic principles in formulating their concepts of stuttering, although they have freed themselves somewhat from psychoanalytic terminology. Travis (1957), for example, as a result of his clinical experiences, considers the stutterer as one who is still caught in the conflict between the repressed urges to suck, eat, evacuate, and explore sexual pleasures and the parentally induced but reluctantly accepted inhibitions of these forbidden needs. Through stuttering the incompatabilities of love, hate, and fear can be resolved. It allows the stutterer to vent his forbidden impulses and to be punished for them without allowing them to be recognized for what they really are. Thereby the anxiety can be kept within bearable limits. The stutterer has difficulty in speaking because he has unspeakable feelings.

Murphy and Fitzsimons (1960) see stuttering as a "learned, nonintegrative, self-defensive reaction to anxiety or fear of threatening circumstances with which the person feels incapable of coping." The child becomes hesitant in speech as well as in other functions because he has been belittled, dominated, rejected, and suppressed by the important persons (parents, etc.) in his environment and so fails to integrate his self-concept. The anxiety and guilt stemming from his feelings of inadequacy in interpersonal relationships make him hesitant in these interactions with others. Since this takes place at a critical stage in the child's development, this interpersonal hesitancy becomes reflected in his speaking, for speech always involves the display of the self. These authors seem to have applied to stuttering some of the concepts of the interpersonal theory of neurosis formulated by Harry Stack Sullivan. We present a brief quotation summarizing their position:

> We have maintained that the seeds of stuttering behavior are imbedded in the soil of early socialization experiences, and that stuttering's tap roots are intertwined most intimately with parent-child relationships. When nonverbal or verbal communicative or developmental task breakdowns germinate in these processes, the resulting disruptions to self-differentiation and integration are experienced by the child as feelings of apprehension or dread. . . . Stuttering can be defined as "what a person is." It tells us that self-defensive processes are in action, that anxieties or fears of diffused or specific character are operating, that the person is attempting not only to protect himself but to prove and improve himself also (Murphy and Fitzsimons, 1960, pp. 171–72).

Sheehan (1954; 1958) attempts to reconcile the psychoanalytic and learning theory points of view. He states that stuttering is one of the "neurotic reactions of a neurotic age." "It is a fault in the social presentation of the self, a self-role conflict." Applying the conflict theory of Dollard and Miller, Sheehan sees the disorder as a double approach-avoidance conflict with the stuttering repetitions and prolongations representing the precarious equilibrium between these two drives to speak and to keep silent. According to Sheehan, the approach-avoidance conflicts can occur on several levels: (1) the word level, (2) the situation level, (3) the expression of antagonistic emotions, (4) the level of interpersonal relationships (e.g., status), and (5) the ego-protective level. Anxiety can be generated by conflict at any of these levels, and stuttering is maintained by anxiety reduction since once the stuttering (which has become the symptomatic focus of all these fears) has occurred, the fear subsides. Guilt also plays a part in the generation of these conflicts. Sheehan feels that guilt serves as one of the original sources of the fear and the need to avoid speaking:

> Primary guilt would refer to the constellation of feelings which was behind the original appearance of stuttering, which the symptom formation has the function of handling. Secondary guilt refers to the feelings the stutterer develops as a result of his inevitable knowledge that his blocks are distressing to others, more so at times than to himself (1958, p. 135).

Sheehan also stresses the expressive nature of the symptom in advanced stuttering. The stutterer unconsciously chooses the type of stuttering which will best express his basic attitudes toward himself and toward his listeners.

Freund (1966) describes four major varieties of stuttering, two of which are neurotic in nature. The most common form of stuttering, according to Freund, belongs in the category of expectancy neuroses such as writer's cramp, stage fright, intermittent aphonia, certain forms of impotence, and other similar problems. The stutterer "experiences strange difficulties in the performance of an automatic skill (speaking) which previously he had been able to carry out with the greatest of ease." These difficulties may arise from many different stress factors (interpersonal conflicts, difficulties in verbal formulation and recall, physical and emotional traumatic experiences, social ambivalence, fear of listener reactions, and many others), but Freund stresses that the expectancy neurosis typically found in stutterers develops *after* the experience of communicative failure, not before. Freund writes:

> All of these forms of expectancy neurotic disturbances including stuttering have as a common characteristic that they are based upon actual "primary" traumatic experiences of failure in the performance of a learned skill or a simple motor or sensory act, often, though not necessarily, in socially embarrassing situations. The anticipation of their dreaded recurrence leads them, via inhibition, etc., to the establishment of a vicious spiral. In opposition to the phonophobias, the dread here is not of a symbolic nature but is based upon actual experience (1966, pp. 37–38).*

The traumatic experiences of feeling blocked, of helplessness, of inability to cope, are sensed as a reflection of personal inadequacy, and the stutterer learns various defensive behaviors to protect his ego from being overwhelmed by the consequent anxiety. Freund points out clearly that the Freudian concepts of neurosis do not account for "the secondary 'neurotic' phase of actual stuttering—with the pathological defense system erected against the recurrence of communicative failure." Since the neurosis in "common stuttering" is born only after traumatic communicative failure has been experienced, it must be viewed as quite different from the "transference neuroses" of the psychoanalytic school. It is an expectancy neurosis.

We share with Freund the belief that the neurosis in confirmed stuttering most usually belongs in the category of expectancy neuroses. Unlike Freund, we do not feel that there is always a basic neurotic predisposition, and we cannot agree with this statement of his position:

> We feel that the behavior and inner experience of such stutterers is primarily determined by the nature of their personalities, not necessarily by a rigid and arbitrary progression of developmental stages. Some of these stutterers show this avoidance from the very beginning of the disorder. Most of them develop it very early. They tend to run away from other unpleasantnesses. Why should we expect them to do otherwise when confronted by stuttering? The fearful adult was a fearful child. This is not to say that this type (the most common type) of stuttering cannot appear as a terminal stage in the development of the disorder. We are certain that it can, but we feel that when it does, it represents the change in personality which stuttering itself can provoke. We would suspect, however, that even in such cases, there exists a basic personality structure which latently predisposes the person toward withdrawal and avoidance (Freund, 1966, p. 138).

Our own position is that the neurosis in stuttering represents the end result of a learning process. We do not feel that most stutterers begin as neurotics. Certainly, the research has failed to show that stutterers have basically different personalities from normal speakers even after years of stuttering, and our clinical experience has convinced us that at onset and for some years later, most young stutterers do not show the features that are said to characterize neurosis. When they do appear, the "neurotic symptoms" stem from communicative frustration and social penalty. They are learned defenses designed to minimize the misery. They occur as responses to conflict and trap situations involving communication. They are secondary to the experience of unpleasant interruptions in uttering words. At first, they do lessen the unpleasantness, but as they become automatized, they contribute to it.

We do not therefore generally view stuttering as a symptom of some other neurosis—except in a few individuals. In most of our cases the fears have been learned; the behaviors which are so conspicuously maladaptive were once useful in minimizing the stutterer's difficulties. Through generalization, reinforcement, and automatization they have undergone a morbid growth and change. They persist despite their punishing characteristics because they are continually reinforced by the consummation of communication. When we keep our eyes on what the stutterer does, and understand what he is feeling, we find it very hard to hang the label of primary neurosis around his neck. As Brutten and Shoemaker (1967) put it, "Learning theory has shifted away from the idea that individuals are neurotic or *have* neuroses and toward the idea that they have learned maladaptive stimulus-response relationships." Most of our stutterers have been pretty normal individuals—except when they had to say something.

RESEARCH ON NEUROSIS

The research on stuttering generally, though voluminous, leaves much to be desired when examined critically, but the research dealing with the neurotic nature of the disorder is especially vulnerable to questioning. One almost feels an urge to discard all the old studies and start all over. Deficiencies in design, lack of control groups, an inadequate number of assorted subjects, these and many other weaknesses make it difficult to discern the grains of truth in all the chaff. Nevertheless it is worth summarizing if only to help future researchers from making the same mistakes, and at the very least it demonstrates clearly that those who consider stuttering a neurosis and only a neurosis have very little solid foundation for their beliefs.

ARE STUTTERERS NEUROTIC?

McDowell (1928) found no major differences between stuttering children and their controls on three paper and pencil personality tests and teachers' judgments. Johnson (1932), using the Woodworth-House Mental Hygiene Inventory, found that stutterers as a group were not significantly different in childhood maladjustment problems from normals, and they had significantly less maladjustment than a comparison group of diagnosed psychoneurotics. Bender (1939) administered the Bernreuter to 249 adult stutterers and found them slightly poorer in social adjustment and speech attitudes than normals. Bearss (1950) examined college stutterers with the Rotter Incomplete Sentence Test and the Adam's Personal Audit but found no differences between his subjects and their controls. Brutten (1951) administered the Maslow Security Index to adult stutterers and their controls and found no significant differences. Boland (1952) used four scales and indices of anxiety and neuroticism and a test of speech anxiety. No differences were found in general anxiety level or neuroticism, but stutterers had more speech anxiety. Dahlstrom and Craven (1952) administered MMPI to four groups of college subjects: stutterers, normal speakers, normal speakers seeking counseling, and psychiatric patients. They found that, although the stutterers were within the test norms, they resembled the normal speaking students seeking counseling more than they did either of the other two groups. Several other similar MMPI studies by Pizzat (1949), Walnut (1954), and Thomas (1951) have shown the same tendency for stutterers to fall within the norms on most of the subscales of the test inventory. Certainly no marked tendency toward neuroticism has been shown by these MMPI investigations.

There are several studies in which the Bell Adjustment Inventory, the California Test of Personality, and other instruments whose validity is highly suspect were used, and we will list the authors here: Duncan (1949), Perkins (1946), Schultz (1947), Powers (1944), and Redwine (1959). Goodstein (1958) reviewed a number of the investigations of stutterers' personalities and concluded that they have not been shown to be severely maladjusted or to have unique personalities.

There have also been many investigations of stuttering using projective tests, especially the Rorschach and the TAT (Thematic Appreciation

Test). Meltzer (1944) used the Rorschach with 50 child stutterers and their controls and discovered a number of differences between the groups, chiefly in negativism, fantasy, withdrawal, depression. Krugman (1946) also tested 50 child stutterers and a control group of children having other emotional problems. Using the Rorschach, he found that both groups showed strong evidence of neuroticism and instability. The stutterers were characterized as having rigid personalities, great anxiety, and obsessive-compulsive traits. It should be noted, as Sheehan (1958) pointed out, that the latter conclusion is not supported by Krugman's statistics. Both of these studies must be viewed with caution, especially since Wilson (1951), and Christensen (1952) using the child stutterer's sibling as his control found no significant differences between siblings on the Rorschach or on the TAT insofar as neuroticism was concerned. Stroobant (1952) found no significant Rorschach signs of neuroticism in his New Zealand stutterers. Matsuoka (1964) in Japan administered the Rorschach to 20 fourth- to sixth-grade children and found that although they were "cautious, nervous, and anxious, their emotional control was not bad."

Adult stutterers, who according to Freund have already developed an expectancy neurosis, have also been subjected to projective testing. In 1944 Greene and Small found that "from 30 to 40 per cent of their stutterers showed Rorschach indications of marked emotional instability," but no data are provided. There are two studies by Pitrelli (1948) and Haney (1951) [which used no control group for their Rorschach investigations] that found indications of neurosis among stutterers, and one by Richardson (1944), which did use matched controls, but found no major significant differences between the groups. In one of the most careful studies yet performed, Andrews and Harris (1964) explored in various ways the characteristics of children who stuttered as compared with their controls. Among the many items which failed to distinguish significantly between the groups were the following: dependency, sensitivity, shyness, fears, enuresis, disturbing dreams, ability to form relationships with peers, mother-child relationships, and father-child relationships. If stuttering were indeed *only* a neurosis, surely some of these characteristics should have been shown to occur more frequently in the stutterers. Sheehan (1958) critically reviewed a large number of the projective investigations of stuttering and came to the conclusion that they failed to establish the neurotic theory of stuttering.

DO STUTTERERS SHOW EVIDENCE OF ORAL OR ANAL FIXATION?

We have been able to find only two studies which bear on the question of excessive orality. Meltzer (1933) found no Rorschach evidence to support Coriat's thesis, and Lowinger (1952), using the TAT, also found none in his study of institutionalized children who stuttered. Coriat cited the fact that stutterers generally had much more stuttering on the bilabial than on other sounds as evidence for his theory, but, as our review of the loci research has demonstrated, this is simply not true.

More work has concerned itself with excessive anality. Dickson (1954) used the Blacky Pictures Test (which shows dogs doing dirty deeds), a projective instrument of questionable validity, and found that more stutterers than nonstutterers had scores indicating anal-sadistic fixations. Carp (1962) also used the Blacky Test but failed to find excessive anal eroticism in the stutterers. The most extensive study was done by Keisman (1958). He used an Anal Trait Check List and an Anal Interest Picture Test (in which the time spent in looking at pictures of anal and non-anal activities was measured.) The "findings were largely negative." This then seems to be the only experimental evidence for and against oral and anal fixation theory, and it hardly seems impressive, especially considering the work of Barnes (1951) and Sewell and Mussen (1952) who found little experimental evidence to support the Freudian view of oral and anal fixation.

DO STUTTERERS SHOW MORE COMPULSIVITY, HOSTILITY, ANXIETY, AND GUILT THAN NORMAL SPEAKERS?

Using the Rosenzweig Picture Frustration Test, Madison and Norman (1952) found that their stutterers, as compared against the test norms but not against a matched control group, showed more intropunitiveness and need persistence and less extrapunitiveness. Quarrington, a year later (1953), repeated the study on 30 stutterers and their controls but failed to find any significant differences between the groups. Santostefano (1960) found more hostility and anxiety in his 11 stutterers, using the Rorschach, and free associations to neutral and emotion-toned words. Brutten (1957) discovered no differences between stutterers and nonstutterers using the Palmar Sweat Index of anxiety when they were silent, but the data showed a trend that stutterers had more anxiety over speech. Riley and White (1967) gave the Objective Analytic Anxiety Battery to 17 stutterers and controls and found that the stutterers had more anxiety than the controls but that it was well below the neurotic level.*

---

* There are, of course, many case studies and reports which describe the hostile, anxious, and guilty feelings of stutterers or attempt to trace them back to early conflicts. Since it is impossible to present an adequate picture of such material in summary, we merely list some but not all of these references: Aikins (1925), Fogerty (1930), Fuchs (1934), Spring (1935), Wedberg (1937), Latif (1938), Heilpern (1941), Rotter (1942), Despert (1942), Usher (1944), Gustavson (1944), Harle (1946), Maas (1946), Naidu (1946), Bakes (1947), Renen (1950), Wallen (1961), and Massengill (1965). We have reread all these studies and conclude that, although some stutterers could certainly be called neurotic, we cannot accept the statement that all of them are.

DO THE PARENTS OF STUTTERERS
CREATE THE SUBSOIL FOR NEUROSIS?

There are several studies indicating that the parents of stutterers show behaviors and attitudes which might generate the sorts of conflicts which would create neuroses in their children. Moncur (1952) interviewed the mothers of 48 stuttering children and their controls and found that the mothers were overdominating, overcritical, and tended to discipline their children excessively and to overcriticize them. Kinstler (1961) used the University of Southern California Maternal Attitude Scale to assess the attitudes of 30 mothers of male stuttering children and an equal group of mothers of normal speaking children. He found that the stuttering children's mothers rejected their children more covertly than the control mothers. Snyder, Henderson, Murphy, and O'Brien (1958), using the Sacks Sentence Completion Test in a study that is hard to evaluate, found that their sample of parents of stutterers felt slightly inadequate in interpersonal relationships, and had many fears. No control group was used. Abbott (1957) found evidence of overprotection but few other differences. Bloom (1958) compared mothers of child stutterers with their controls in terms of child training practices and found that the former showed differences in that they tended to lack empathy, were less concerned with cleanliness and neatness, and were more concerned with sex-role identification. La-Follette (1956) found the fathers of stutterers more anxious and submissive and less well adjusted than the control fathers. Goodstein and Dahlstrom (1956) found much the same for parents of child stutterers in an MMPI study. Darley (1955), in an intensive interview investigation, found that stutterers' mothers had high standards and social striving tendencies. This has also been reported by Johnson (1959) in his *Onset of Stuttering* research. Goldman and Shames (1964) studied goal-setting with the Rotter Level of Aspiration board and a speech task, and found that the fathers of stutterers tended to set higher goals than the fathers of nonstutterers although the mothers did not differ. Andrews and Harris (1964) using a variety of tests failed to find any major parental differences.

Several studies have concerned themselves with the question of whether or not parents of stutterers diagnose stuttering more readily than parents of normal speaking children. We will cite just three of these. Bloodstein, Jaeger, and Tureen (1952) had the parents of stutterers listen to a tape composed of segments of the speech of stutterers and nonstutterers. They made more diagnoses and more erroneous ones than did the parents of nonstutterers who served as controls. Berlin (1960) criticized the former study as tending to bias the judgments and, in a modified replication, failed to find that the parents of stutterers were more concerned about or more sensitive to nonfluencies than the control parents. Seligman (1966) in her evaluative review of the research concerning parents of stutterers concludes that "the hypothesis of an etiological relationship between the attitudes, personality, and practices of parents has not been sufficiently explored" to allow us to come to any firm beliefs that parents are indeed responsible for the stuttering. Our own independent review leads us to agree with Seligman.

One final topic should probably be included in this summary of the research. Both Barbara (1946) and Pitrelli (1948) found a remarkably low incidence of stuttering among institutionalized psychotics and some evidence that a previously observed stutter had disappeared when the individual developed the psychosis. Since neuroses have been known occasionally to mask or to serve as a defense against psychosis, the implication was that these findings corroborated the neurotic nature of stuttering. However, Freund (1955), in a very scholarly review of the literature, showed clearly that the incidence of stuttering was three times as great (3.2 per cent) in 149 veterans who were schizophrenic than "among the general population."

Despite the fact that we have scrutinized all of these investigations with some care, it is difficult to fit them all together into a coherent judgment. So many of them fail to fulfill basic criteria of good research. So many of them contradict each other. The case for stuttering as a neurosis and only a neurosis has not been made.

COMMENTARY

All the neuroses so far recorded can be understood as being the outcome of one or another (perhaps sometimes both) of two basic situations—the exposure of the organism to ambivalent stimuli or its exposure to noxious stimuli, in either case under conditions of confinement (Wolpe, 1952, p. 4).

The very fact that the research and clinical findings are often so different suggests that stuttering persons are definitely varied, somewhat in kind but mostly in degree. The needs and motives of the individual stutterer are so numerous, complicated, and different from those of many other stutterers that it is virtually impossible to categorize dynamics in patterns descriptive of these persons as a group (Murphy and Fitzsimons, 1960, p. 134).

At the *ego-protective level* of conflict, stuttering can serve unconsciously as a means for keeping the individual out of competitive endeavors which would pose threat of failure or threat of success. The stutterer can adjust his aspirations so as to keep within the zones of safety. This rather than the expression of forbidden impulses in the traditional Freudian sense, is probably the chief defensive function of stuttering (Sheehan, 1958, p. 137).

The stammerer unconsciously wishes to remain a suckling. The patient, owing to anxiety, unconsciously reverts to the suckling stage and so replaces consonants with clicks (Stein, 1949, p. 102).

Jimmy invariably went off to defecate at some point during his interviews, and I noticed that on his return his stammer became almost unnoticeable. Most certainly he did equate words with feces, so that once he had externalized his aggression, or "let out the bowels" as he expressed it, the symptom disappeared (Usher, 1944, p. 63).

Thus when a stutterer unconsciously senses that he may want to bite or suck when he is supposed to speak, a conflict ensues the result of which contains some elements of biting or sucking as well as attempts to block such expressions through amnesia, mutism, and articulatory spasms. It is possible that other elements stemming from more diffuse phobic and startle reactions may be contributory. The fixation in the speech apparatus may subserve libidinal and aggressive oral drives in their active and passive expressions. Secondarily these may be merged with onanistic, exhibitionistic, voyeuristic, and masochistic drives (Glauber, 1958, p. 94).

The expulsion and retention of words means the expulsion and retention of feces (Fenichel, 1945, p. 312).

He cannot take any substitutions for the original pleasures which were denied him. Time and experience do not touch or alter them. His early infantile wishes and hates and fears remain dynamic and force their way into expression as the symptoms of stuttering. . . . In general, stuttering is a symptom; it gives a disguised expression to repressed impulses in which both the repressed and repressing force may be recognized. It gives a peculiar kind of gratification corresponding to the impulses which have been repressed (Travis, 1940, p. 197).

It is our contention that these strong anal and sexual aggressions of antisocial quality grew out of the important training situations of infancy and early childhood. Because of the pain and anxiety meted out by the parents in temporal and spatial relation to the patient's expression of early instinctual drives, he repressed (drive-reduction by stopping thinking and feeling) these drives and the interpersonal relationships connected with them and henceforth carried them as unconscious, motivating forces. When these forces taxed the patient's repressing or inhibiting forces (fear and anxiety) to the limit, other forces were called into action. When these defenses in turn could not hold, a final stand was made through stuttering. Stuttering may be conceptualized then as a final defense or block against the threatening revelation through spoken words of unspeakable thoughts and feelings (Travis, 1957, p. 934).

A two-year-old boy was cured of his stuttering by the following method. Apparently, his condition was caused by regression, since during his suckling period he had been seriously ill and now had a poor appetite. It was arranged to allow him to return to this previous level by supplying him with candy suckers. After a few days this return was so complete that he had discarded his previously acquired habits of cleanliness but had ceased stuttering. Three months later he had acquired bladder and bowel control again, his appetite had improved, and his speech control became perfect [our translation] (Brunner, 1936, p. 362).

Since guilt conspicuously produces blocking in the speech of young children and guilt is an important dynamic in the advanced stutterer, it is likely that guilt feelings lie heavily in the background of the onset of stuttering (Sheehan, 1958, p. 135).

The stutterer's inhibitions, symptom, and character traits have flowed from traumatic experiences; of these, the first and most fateful was the nursing and early feeding situation. . . . The wish to become one with the phallic mother was countered by two fears: the fear of complete regression into passivity as a kind of inertia or death, and its opposite—the fear of getting enough satisfaction to be stimulated or maneuvered sooner or later into activity and final separation (Glauber, 1958, pp. 162–163).

As a result of conflicting tendencies, for approach and for avoidance, for self-exposure and self-concealment, stuttering has an expressive aspect. Stuttering patterns themselves are the result of a long process of shaping, of continual modification through the irregular reinforcement of tricks and their eventual incorporation into the pattern. Yet the pattern is not the chance product of random instrumental learning. All through his life the stutterer has been exercising choice in his selection of tricks or grimaces to cope with his fear. The choices are necessarily projective of the dynamics of the chooser and reflective of the interpersonal relationship out of which they emerge. Some stutterers are active and aggressive in their patterns; others are meek and acquiescent, nice guys finishing last verbally (Sheehan, 1968, p. 81).

BIBLIOGRAPHY

Abbott, J. A., "Repressed Hostility as a Factor in Adult Stuttering," *Journal of Speech Disorders*, XII (1947), 28–30.

Abbott, T. B., "A Study of Observable Mother-Child Relationships in Stuttering and Non-Stuttering Groups," *Dissertation Abstracts*, XVII (1957), 1148–49.

Aikins, A., "Casting out the Stuttering Devil," *Journal of Abnormal Social Psychology*, XVIII (1925), 137–52.

Andrews, G., and M. Harris, *The Syndrome of Stuttering*. London: Heinemann, 1964.

Bakes, F., "Case of a Stutterer." In A. Burton, and R. Harris, *Case Histories in Clinical and Abnormal Psychology*. New York: Harper, 1947.

Barbara, D. A., "A Psychosomatic Approach to the Problem of Stuttering in Psychotics," *American Journal of Psychiatry*, CIII (1946), 188–95.

———. (ed.), *New Directions in Stuttering: Theory and Practice*. Springfield, Ill.: Thomas, 1965.

———. *Stuttering: A Psychodynamic Approach to Its Understanding and Treatment*. New York: Julian, 1954.

Barnes, M. L., "A Study of the Attitudes of Parents and Teachers Toward Children who Stutter." Master's thesis, Ohio State University, 1951.

Bearss, L. M., "An Investigation of Conflict in Stutterers and Nonstutterers." Master's thesis, Purdue University, 1950.

Bender, J. M., *The Personality Structure of Stuttering.* New York: Pitman, 1939.

Berlin, C. I., "Parents' Diagnoses of Stuttering," *Journal of Speech and Hearing Research,* III (December, 1960), 372–79.

Berlinsky, S. L., "A Comparison of Stutterers and Nonstutterers in Four Conditions of Experimentally Induced Anxiety," *Dissertation Abstracts,* XIV (1954), 719.

Bloodstein, O., W. Jaeger, and O. Tureen, "A Study of the Diagnosis of Stuttering by Parents of Stutterers and Nonstutterers," *Journal of Speech and Hearing Disorders,* XVII (1952), 308–15.

Bloom, J., "Child Training and Stuttering." Doctoral dissertation, University of Michigan, 1958.

Boland, J. L., "A Comparison of Stutterers and Nonstutterers on Several Measures of Anxiety," *Speech Monographs,* XX (1952), 144.

Brutten, E. J., "A Colorimetric Anxiety Measure of Stuttering and Expectancy Adaptation," *Dissertation Abstracts,* XVII (1957), 2707–8.

Brunner, M., "Beeinflussung des Stotterns," *Zeitschrift für Psychoanalysis Padag.,* X (1936), 360–65.

Brutten, E. J. "Anxiety as a Personality Trait Among Stutterers." Master's thesis, Brooklyn College, 1951.

Brutten, E. J., and D. J. Shoemaker, *The Modification of Stuttering.* Englewood Cliffs, N. J.: Prentice-Hall, 1967.

Burtscher, H. T., Jr., "The Operation of Frustration in the Transition to and the Development of Secondary Stuttering," *Speech Monographs,* XIX (1952), 191 (abstract).

Carp, F. M., "Psychosexual Development of Stutterers," *Journal of Projective Techniques and Personality Assessment,* XXVI (1962), 388–91.

Christensen, A. H., "A Quantitative Study of Personality Dynamics of Stuttering and Nonstuttering Siblings," *Speech Monographs,* XIX (1952), 144–45.

Coriat, I. H., "The Oral-Erotic Components of Stammering," *International Journal of Psychoanalysis,* VIII (1927), 56–69.

———. "The Nature and Analytical Treatment of Stuttering," *Proceedings of the American Speech Correction Association,* I (1931), 151–56.

———. "The Psychoanalytic Concept of Stammering," *Nervous Child,* II (1943), 167–71.

Dahlstrom, W. G., and Craven, D. D., "The Minnesota Multiphasic Personality Inventory and Stuttering Phenomena in Young Adults," *American Psychologist,* VII (1952), 341 (abstract).

Darley, F. L., "The Relationship of Parental Attitudes and Adjustments to the Development of Stuttering." In W. Johnson (ed.), *Stuttering in Children and Adults.* Minneapolis: University of Minnesota Press, 1955.

Despert, J. L., "A Therapeutic Approach to the Problem of Stuttering in Children," *Nervous Child,* II (1942), 134–47.

———. "Psychosomatic Study of Fifty Stuttering Children," *American Journal of Orthopsychiatry,* XVI (1946), 100–113.

Dickson, S., "An Application of the Blacky Test to a Study of the Psychosexual Development of Stutterers." Master's thesis, Brooklyn College, 1954.

Dollard, J., and N. E. Miller, *Personality and Psychotherapy*. New York: McGraw-Hill, 1950.

Douglass, E., and B. Quarrington, "Differentiation of Interiorized and Exteriorized Secondary Stuttering," *Journal of Speech and Hearing Disorders,* XVII (1952), 377–85.

Duncan, M. H., "Home Adjustment of Stutterers Versus Nonstutterers," *Journal of Speech and Hearing Disorders,* XIV (1949), 255–59.

Eysenck, H. J., and S. Rachman, *The Causes and Cure of Neuroses*. London: Routledge and Kegan Paul, 1965.

Fenichel, O., *The Psychoanalytic Theory of Neurosis*. New York: Norton, 1945.

Fogerty, E., *Stammering*. New York: Dutton, 1930.

Freund, H., *Psychopathology and the Problems of Stuttering*. Springfield, Ill.: Thomas, 1966.

———. "Psychosis and Stuttering," *Journal of Nervous and Mental Diseases,* CXXII (1955), 161–72.

———. "Über Inneres Stottern," *Zeitschrift Ohrenheilkunde,* LXIX (1935), 146–48.

Fuchs, E., "Zur Psychoanalyse des Stotterns," *International Journal of Psychoanalysis,* XX (1934), 375–89.

Glauber, I. P., "Psychoanalytic Concepts of the Stutterer," *Nervous Child,* II (1943), 172–80.

———. "The Nature of Stuttering," *Social Casework,* XXXIV (1954), 95–103.

———. "The Psychoanalysis of Stuttering." In J. Eisenson (ed.), *Stuttering: A Symposium*. New York: Harper, 1958.

Goldman, R., and G. Shames, "A Study of Goal-Setting Behavior of Parents of Stutterers and Parents of Nonstutterers," *Journal of Speech and Hearing Disorders,* XXIX (1964), 192–94.

Goodstein, L. D., "Functional Speech Disorders and Personality: A Survey of the Research," *Journal of Speech and Hearing Research,* I (1958), 359–76.

———. "MMPI Profiles of Stutterers' Parents: A Follow-Up Study," *Journal of Speech and Hearing Disorders,* XXI (1956), 430–35.

Goodstein, L. D., and W. Dahlstrom, "MMPI Difference Between Parents of Stuttering and Nonstuttering Children," *Journal of Consulting Psychology,* XX (1956), 365–70.

Greene, J. S., and S. M. Small, "Psychosomatic Factors in Stuttering," *Medical Clinics of North America,* XXVIII (1944), 615–28.

Gustafson, C. G., "A Talisman and a Convalescence," *Quarterly Journal of Speech,* XXX (1944), 1165–1471.

Haney, H. R., "Motives Implied by the Act of Stuttering as Revealed by Prolonged Experimental Projection," *Speech Monographs,* XVIII (1951), 129.

Harle, M., "Dynamic Interpretation and Treatment of Acute Stuttering in a Young Child," *American Journal of Orthopsychiatry,* XV (1946), 156–62.

Heilpern, E., "A Case of Stuttering," *Psychoanalytic Quarterly,* I (1941), 95–115.

Johnson, W., "The Influence of Stuttering on the Personality," *University of Iowa Studies in Child Welfare,* V (1932), 1–140.

———. *The Onset of Stuttering*. Minneapolis: University of Minnesota Press, 1959.

Keisman, I. B., "Stuttering and Anal Fixation." Doctoral dissertation, New York University, 1958.

Kinstler, D. B., "Covert and Overt Maternal Rejection in Stuttering," *Journal of Speech and Hearing Disorders*, XXVI (1961), 145–55.

Krasnogorski, N. I., "The Conditioned Reflexes and Childrens' Neuroses," *American Journal of Diseases of Children*, XXX (1925), 756–68.

Krugman, M., "Psychosomatic Study of Fifty Stuttering Children," *Journal of Orthopsychiatry*, XVI (1946), 127–33.

LaFollette, A. C., "Parental Environment of Stuttering Children," *Journal of Speech and Hearing Disorders*, XXI (1956), 202–7.

Latif, I., "Some Aetiological Factors in the Pathology of Stammering," *British Journal of Medical Psychology*, XVII (1938), 307–18.

Liddell, H. S., "The Challenge of Pavlovian Conditioning and Experimental Neuroses in Animals." In J. Wolpe, A. Salter, and L. J. Reyna, *The Conditioning Therapies*. New York: Holt, 1964.

Lowinger, L., "The Psychodynamics of Stuttering: An Evaluation of the Factors of Aggression and Guilt Feelings in a Group of Institutionalized Children." Doctoral dissertation, New York University, 1952.

Maas, O., "On the Aetiology of Stuttering," *Journal of Mental Science*, XCII (1946), 357–63.

Madison, L., and R. A. Norman, "Comparison of the Performance of Stutterers and Nonstutterers on the Rosenzweig Picture Frustration Test," *Journal of Clinical Psychology*, VIII (1952), 179–83.

Massengill, R., "Phobias Present in Three Stuttering Cases," *Perceptual and Motor Skills*, XX (1965), 579–80.

Masserman, J. H., *Behavior and Neurosis*. Chicago: University of Chicago Press, 1943.

Matsuoka, T., ["Psychological Study of Young Stutterers"], convention address, Japanese Psychology Association, 1964. Abstracted in G. Kamiyama, *A Handbook for the Study of Stuttering*. 1967.

McDowell, E., *Educational and Emotional Adjustment of Stuttering Children*. Columbia University Teachers College Contributions to Education, No. 314, 1928.

Meltzer, H., "Personality Differences Between Stuttering and Nonstuttering Children as Indicated by the Rorschach Test," *Journal of Psychology*, XVII (1933), 39–59.

Miller, N. E., and J. Dollard, *Social Learning and Imitation*. New Haven: Yale University Press, 1941.

Moller, H., "Stuttering, Predelinquent, and Adjusted Boys: A Comparative Analysis of Personality Characteristics as Measured by the Wisc and the Rorschach Test." Doctoral dissertation, Boston University, 1960.

Moncur, J. P., "Parental Domination in Stuttering," *Journal of Speech Disorders*, XVII (1952), 155–65.

Mower, O. H., *Learning Theory and Personality Dynamics*. New York: Ronald Press, 1950.

———. "Stuttering as Simultaneous Admission and Denial," *Journal of Communication Disorders*, I (1967), 46–50.

Murphy, A. T., "An Electroencephalographic Study of Frustration in Stutterers." Doctoral dissertation, University of Southern California, 1952.

Murphy, A. T., and R. M. Fitzsimons, *Stuttering and Personality Dynamics*. New York: Ronald, 1960.

Nadoleczny, M., ["Stuttering as a Manifestation of a Spastic Coordination Neurosis"], *Archives of Psychiatry* LXXXII (1927), 235–46.

Naidu, P. S., and S. K. Ahmad, "Some Excerpts from a Clinical Record of a Case of Stammering," *Indian Journal of Psychology,* XXI (1946), 69–72.

Perkins, D., "An Item by Item Compilation and Comparison of the Scores of 75 Young Adult Stutterers on the California Test of Personality." Master's thesis, University of Illinois, 1946.

Pitrelli, F. R., "Psychosomatic and Rorschach Aspects of Stuttering," *Psychiatry Quarterly,* XXII (1948), 175–94.

Pizzat, F. L., "A Personality Study of College Stutterers." Master's thesis, University of Pittsburgh, 1949.

Powers, M. R., "Personality Traits of Junior High School Stutterers as Revealed by the California Test of Personality." Master's thesis, University of Illinois, 1944.

Quarrington, B., "The Performance of Stutterers on the Rosenzweig Picture Frustration Test," *Journal of Clinical Psychology,* IX (1953), 189–92.

Redwine, G. W., "An Experimental Study of the Relationship Between Self-Concepts of Fourth and Eighth Grade Stuttering and Nonstuttering Boys," *Speech Monographs,* XXVI (1959), 140–41 (abstract).

Renen, S. B. V., "Tongue Troubles," *Journal of Logopaedics* (South Africa), I (1950), 16–19.

Richardson, L. H., "A Personality Study of Stutterers and Nonstutterers," *Journal of Speech Disorders,* IX (1944), 152–60.

Riley, G. D., and H. White, "Anxiety Among Adults Who Stutter," convention address, A. S. H. A., 1967.

Rotter, J. B., "A Working Hypothesis as to the Nature and Treatment of Stuttering," *Journal of Speech Disorders,* VII (1942), 263–88.

―――. "The Nature and Treatment of Stuttering: A Clinical Approach," *Journal of Abnormal and Social Psychology,* XXXIX (April 1944), 150–73.

Santostefano, S., "Anxiety and Hostility in Stuttering," *Journal of Speech and Hearing Research,* III (1960), 337–47.

Schultz, D. A., "A Study of Nondirective Counseling as Applied to Adult Stutterers," *Journal of Speech Disorders,* XII (1947), 421–27.

Seaman, R., "A Study of the Responses of Stutterers to the Items of the Rosenzweig Picture Frustration Study." Master's thesis, Brooklyn College, 1956.

Seligman, J., "The Personality, Attitudes and Behavior of Parents of Children Who Stutter: An Annotated Bibliography," *Journal of Ontario Speech and Hearing Association,* II (1966), 35–106.

Sewell, W., and P. Mussen, "The Effects of Feeding, Weaning, and Scheduling Procedures on Childhood Adjustment and the Formation of Oral Symptoms," *Child Development,* XXXIII (1952), 185–91.

Sheehan, J. G., "An Integration of Psychotherapy and Speech Therapy Through a Conflict Theory of Stuttering," *Journal of Speech and Hearing Disorders,* XIX (1954), 474–82.

―――. "Conflict Theory of Stuttering." In J. Eisenson (ed.), *Stuttering: A Symposium.* New York: Harper, 1958.

―――. "Stuttering as Self-Role Conflict." In H. H. Gregory, *Learning Theory and Stuttering Therapy.* Evanston: Northwestern University Press, 1968.

————. "Projective Studies of Stuttering," *Journal of Speech and Hearing Disorders*, XXIII (1958), 18–25.

————. "Theory and Treatment of Stuttering as an Approach-Avoidance Conflict," *Journal of Psychology*, XXXVI (1953), 27–49.

Sheehan, J. G., P. Cortese, and R. Hadley, "Guilt, Shame, and Tension in Graphic Projections of Stuttering," *Journal of Speech and Hearing Disorders*, XXVII (1962), 129–39.

Snyder, M. A., D. Henderson, M. Murphy, and R. O'Brien, "The Personality Structure of Stuttering as Compared to that of Parents of Stutterers," *Logos*, II (1958), 97–105.

Spring, W. J., "Words and Masses: A Pictorial Contribution to the Psychology of Stammering," *Psychoanalysis Quarterly*, IV (1935), 244–58.

Stein, L., *The Infancy of Speech and the Speech of Infancy*. London: Methuen, 1949.

————. *Speech and Voice*. London: Methuen, 1942.

Stroobant, R. E., "A Psychological Study of Some Stammering Children," *New Zealand Speech Therapists Journal*, VII (1952), 8–13.

Thomas, L., "A Personality Study of a Group of Stutterers Based on the Minnesota Multiphasic Personality Inventory." Master's thesis, University of Oregon, 1951.

Travis, L. E., "The Need for Stuttering," *Journal of Speech Disorders*, V (1940), 193–202.

————. "The Unspeakable Feelings of People with Special Reference to Stuttering." In L. E. Travis (ed.), *Handbook of Speech Pathology*. New York: Appleton-Century-Crofts, 1957.

Travis, L. E., and L. D. Sutherland, "Psychotherapy in Speech Correction." In L. E. Travis (ed.), *Handbook of Speech Pathology*. New York: Appleton-Century-Crofts, 1957.

Usher, R. D., "A Case of Stuttering," *International Journal of Psychoanalysis*, XXV (1944), 61–70.

Wallen, V., "Primary Stuttering in a 28 Year Old Adult," *Journal of Speech and Hearing Disorders*, XXVI (1961), 394–95.

Walnut, F., "A Personality Inventory Item Analysis of Individuals who Stutter and Individuals who Have Other Handicaps," *Journal of Speech and Hearing Disorders*, XIX (1954), 220–27.

Watson, J. B., and P. Rayner, "Conditioned Emotional Reactions," *Journal of Experimental Psychology*, III (1920), 1–14.

Wedberg, C. F., *The Stutterer Speaks*. Redlands, Cal.: Valley of Fine Arts Press, 1937.

Wilson, D. M., "A Study of the Personalities of Stuttering Children and Their Parents as Revealed Through Projection Tests," *Speech Monographs*, XVIII (1951), 133.

Wolpe, J., "Objective Psychotherapy of the Neuroses," *South African Medical Journal*, XXVI (1952), 825–29.

————. *Psychotherapy by Reciprocal Inhibition*. Stanford: Stanford University Press, 1958.

Wolpe, J. A., A Salter, and L. J. Reyna, *The Conditioning Therapies*. New York: Holt, 1964.

Wright, B. A., *Physical Disability: A Psychological Approach*. New York: Harper, 1960.

twelve

STUTTERING
AS LEARNED BEHAVIOR

Almost all the current theories of stuttering have an ancient history. By knowing something about how these theories developed, one gets a perspective which can be acquired in no other way. We see concepts born, revised, and reborn. Our predecessors were eloquent in convincing themselves and their contemporaries of explanations which are at best only partial truths and at worst biased absurdities. We see also that many of our present beliefs, at least in germinal form, were formulated and even discarded long ago. We find concepts concerning stuttering as a learned response recurring again and again. It is a humbling experience to search through those old dusty books. Few who have done so can ever be very sure of the validity of their own beliefs. Some scholar two centuries hence, if by chance he comes across a tattered copy of this present book, will assuredly smile at our quaint benightedness—though not (we hope) at our hunger to understand.

At present we seem to be at the crest of a wave of explanations of stuttering based on learning theory. Two earlier major waves, those of organicity and neurosis, have swept in and spent their energies on our theoretical shores, and far out on the horizon we discern the gathering force of servotheory. There will be other waves and these will repeat themselves too. Fortunately each one brings us some treasure as well as junk. So let us look back at the precursors of the present flood of learning theory.

Perhaps it was Amman (1700) who first stated flatly that stuttering was a bad habit. Indeed he called "haesitantia" a vicious one, claiming that there was nothing organically wrong with the tongue but that it had fallen into evil ways. In his therapy Amman sought to break the bad habit by training his stutterers to speak loudly and slowly, memorizing set passages and reciting them to friends. It was almost another hundred years before Erasmus Darwin (1800), the grandfather of the stuttering Charles Darwin of evolution fame, attributed the disorder to emotionally conditioned interruptions of motoric speech, and suggested continual practice on the difficult sounds and learning to begin the plosives with loose contacts. In 1818 a Dr. Joseph Frank, recommended that stutterers receive a good flogging for their exhibitions of abnormality. In the early decades of the nineteenth century, there were many workers interested in solving the puzzle of stuttering, and although the writers of that period usually attributed the cause of the abnormality to some debility of one or another of the "speech organs," they all felt that their stutterers required training to break the bad habits thereby engendered. One of the practitioners of that time was Madame Leigh (1825), who believed that the disorder was due to an abnormal tongue thrust habit and trained her patients to speak with the tonguetip up against the palate and used a pad of cotton to help it do so. And there was Arnott (1828) who sought to prevent the "spasm of the glottis" by teaching his stutterers to prefix each word with an "*e* vowel." And we find McCormac in 1828 saying that since stutterers habitually spoke with empty lungs, they should be trained to inhale deeply and exhale forcibly on each word. According to an old book by Potter (1882), Palmer in 1829

> divided speech defects into two classes, organic and functional; the latter (including stuttering) being chiefly due to irregular muscle action, which being established from habit, becomes independent of the original cause and closely resembles chorea in its nature and phenomena. His treatment was one of moral discipline, with varied details for each case (p. 48).

In this brief sampling of the literature, we find the basic rationale for the retraining of improper breathing, incorrect articulation, or inadequate voice, according to the bias of the particular author.

By the middle of the century, at about the time of our Civil War, the belief that stuttering was a bad habit had attained widespread acceptance especially in Britain and the United States. Alexander Melville Bell (1853), the inventor of Visible Speech and the father of Alexander Graham Bell of telephone fame, wrote several books dealing with stuttering. At first, Bell found it very difficult to get others to believe in his view that stuttering was a learned response. He writes, "The popular impression is that the impediment is 'organic,' or altogether 'in the nerves,' and its eradication beyond the reach of art." Bell was outraged by the surgical mutilations of his time and spoke his mind. He insisted that since speech is learned, so must be its defects:

Speaking is an artificial process—an acquirement, not a natural instinct—and its defects can only be amended by the same means through which its exercise is first obtained—by imitative education. . . . The impediment has been shown to be a habit; it is therefore beyond the province either of medical or surgical treatment, and within that, exclusively, of the educator (p. 47).

As Bell's belief that stuttering was only a bad habit took hold others besides physicians began to treat it. A large number of laymen, usually former stutterers, set up treatment centers in their own homes and conducted a private practice. Among the best of these were the Hunts, father and son, who were evidently highly successful practitioners. A fascinating article in Fraser's Magazine by "A Minute Philosopher" (who was probably Charles Kingsley, the famous orator and preacher, who himself had stuttered severely) describes the Hunt method as one in which the stutterer was trained "naturally and without dodge or trick to speak consciously as other men spoke unconsciously." The abnormal behaviors of the lips, tongue, jaw, and breath were compared with the normal behaviors and the latter were then strongly reinforced in a kindly environment.

Among these practitioners, however, were many ruthless charlatans who used all sorts of tricks and speech-exercise rituals based on distraction and suggestion to prey on their victims. Their secret methods of cure were jealously guarded, with the stutterers being sworn to "eternal secrecy" before being accepted into one of their "stammering institutes." For our purposes here, it is enough to say that these persons all felt that stuttering was a bad habit which could be extinguished by penalizing it and replacing it with strongly reinforced normal speech. Ignoring the fact that every stutterer can speak normally under certain conditions, they believed that by getting completely fluent speech and practicing it often enough and strongly enough, the old bad habit of stuttering would be weakened and finally broken. To achieve this fluency, they used rhythmic speech, breath control, a lalling form of utterance, syllable tapping, a cork between the teeth, abnormal inflections, and a host of other devices and routines. Some of these techniques are still being advocated today (Andrews and Harris, 1964; Beech, 1967; Goldiamond, 1965) and essentially for the same reasons—to create a nucleus of stutter-free speech which can then be strengthened.

There were also some early beginnings to the modern learning-theory concept that stuttering is due to approach-avoidance conflicts. Mendelssohn in 1729 attributed the disorder to a conflict between ideas and emotions. Wyneken (1868) writes: "Stammering consists of a temporary clumsiness in the managing of the voice, a clumsiness which can be conditioned by various influences." He also has this to say about the conflicts in speaking:

Should I attempt to give an explanation, then I would say that, with reference to the muscles which are active in speech, the will is more or less bound, and that by doubt. The stutterer is thus a doubter of speech. If he dares the word which seems difficult to him, then however his will is partially paralyzed by doubt, which, in a manner, can also be called a will, and one which is directly opposed to the will proper. The muscles which underlie respiration, phonation, and articulation often are not sure, if I may express myself thus, whom they should obey, and as a consequence thereof do not fulfill their functions with the necessary synergy, and stuttering occurs. The relation is similar as when somebody, for example, wants to venture a jump, but in the very moment in which he leaps doubts that he will succeed. Often he can no longer stop the leap, but also does not jump with sufficient assurance (l'aplomb nécessaire), and so does not reach his goal. A striking analogue to the influence of doubt upon speech we find in the influence of doubt upon sexual potency. Many people, says Niemayer, are impotent only because they doubt their sexual potency; when the doubt is overcome: then there is nothing the matter with them (pp. 20–21).

A similar point of view is expressed by Denhardt (1890) in these words:

> If we examine the mental processes during stuttering, we see that the disturbance typifies the struggle between two opposing forces. The volition which tries to convert the thought into speech is pitted against the belief that we are unable to accomplish what we intended. One drives, the other restrains. The will to speak initiates the impulse toward movement; at the same time fear prevents it. From their conflict and the desire of the stutterer to gain a victory for his desire to speak, result the total characteristics of stuttering. Finally the will to speak wins out and produces the word which had been withheld by the stutterer's lack of faith in his own expressive ability (pp. 176–177).

An early example of the modern desensitization and counterconditioning sort of therapy advocated today by Wolpe (1958) and Eysenck and Rachman (1965) is found in the writing of Sandow (1898). Sandow believed that each spasmodic moment of stuttering was triggered by "psychic" stimuli, usually those invested with emotion. He insisted that through relaxation and calming procedures, these stimuli would become unable to produce the stuttering paroxysms and that this was the way stuttering should be extinguished. A quotation illustrating the importance of this use of relaxation as a counterconditioner may make his position clear:

> Every stutterer should treat himself—or if very young should be treated—as one afflicted with serious neurasthenia. . . . With every movement of the body he should keep this serious manner of treatment in mind. He should act with extreme slowness and self-comfort, and with as much nonchalance and indifference as possible. . . . Not any kind of slowness in the use of arms and legs is meant hereby for there is more than one meaning to "slowness." One person walks slowly because an ambling person in front of him is blocking the way. Another walks that way because he is too sleepy to want to, or be able to do otherwise. A comfortable slowness similar to this

latter one of quiet inner satisfaction must become second nature to the patient (p. 35).

As we enter the present century, we find a growing emphasis on stuttering as learned behavior, although during its first three decades, due to the influence of Freud, the most commonly held theory of stuttering, at least in this country, was that it was a neurosis. As late as 1936, Blanton made a survey of all the important American authorities on stuttering and found only one (Bluemel) who believed that stuttering was learned. But other voices had also made themselves heard. Dunlap (1932) made no bones about his certainty that stuttering was a habit. He felt that it stemmed from parental corrections, interruptions, or verbal conflicts. He had no patience with corrective speech exercises which merely tried to reinforce normal speech, saying:

> Since every stammerer has a habit of correct speech, along with his stammering habit, manifesting one habit in some circumstances and the other habit in other circumstances, we can understand why no cases can be remedied by the procedure so often advised by persons who had not worked with stammerers, who say, "All you need to do is to form the habit of correct speech. . . ." In order to extend the patient's habit of correct speech to the situations in which he now stammers, the stammer must be attacked directly (p. 273).

And Dunlap did attack it directly through the voluntary practice of stuttering—his *beta*-hypothesis. "The patient is instructed also that when the critic commands 'again' he is to say the word over (or to say the initial syllable again, if stopped on a syllable) in the same way as that in which he said it before, or in a way as near as possible to the erroneous way." After using this negative practice several times, the therapist then commands "right!" and the stutterer then attempts to say the word without stuttering. This use of the moment of reactive inhibition anticipates such present day practices as cancellation.

Bluemel (1935), who had previously discarded his earlier organic theory of stuttering as a transient auditory aphasia, outlined a learning theory of stuttering based on Pavlovian conditioned inhibition. He held that since speech had been learned, it could be considered a conditioned reflex. By applying to stuttering the principles of conditioned inhibition derived from Pavlov's experiments, he sketched how the disorder could be generated and maintained. Bluemel also distinguished between "pure or primary stammering," which was the result of conditioned inhibition, and "secondary stammering" which also included many habituated strategies for coping with the interruptions. With a little stretching, he may be considered to have been the person who first discovered the two-factor theory of stuttering. As McDearmon (1966) has pointed out in his review of Bluemel's contribution, his writings did much to lay the groundwork for the favorable reception that modern learning theory approaches to stuttering have had in this country.

Finally, we should certainly mention two European workers, Hoepfner (1912) and Froeschels (1943; 1955; 1964), who described how stuttering may develop out of normal childhood disfluency through a learning process and who opposed the organicists and the psychoanalysts who had dominated the field. It is probably difficult for any contemporary student of stuttering to appreciate the contributions of all these men. All of them met powerful opposition. The author remembers well how viciously he was criticized when he published a paper (Van Riper, 1937a) showing how many of the most abnormal behaviors of stuttering were learned instrumental responses used to avoid, minimize, or escape from expected or experienced speech interruptions. At that time everyone spoke of "stuttering spasms." All breathing abnormalities were viewed as neurological dysfunctions. If a stutterer said, "um-um-um-uh-er-no" the breakdown began with that first "um." If he jerked his head to time the moment of the speech attempt, that head jerk was part of the neurological spasm. The idea that these reactions were only the habituated residues of behaviors once deliberately used to cope with the fear or experience of speech interruptions was heresy. Other correspondents were less abusive but just as certain that only ignorance or stupidity could lead anyone to believe that these behaviors were something more than symbolic symptoms of a deep seated neurosis. Symptomatic therapy (the unlearning of these coping behaviors) was viewed as completely inadequate and probably dangerous since conversions to more abnormal reactions would assuredly result.

MODERN CONCEPTS
OF STUTTERING
AS LEARNED BEHAVIOR

Most of the current thinking about stuttering reflects the influence of learning theory. Few writers today deny that learning plays some part in determining the patterns of behavior shown by advanced stutterers. The different varieties of stuttering reactions, the changes that occur as the disorder develops, the role of situational and verbal cues in its precipitation, all these and many other features of the problem testify to the influence of learning.

There is much disagreement, however, about the exact role that learning plays. Is the original stuttering learned, and, if so, how is it learned? How is stuttering maintained? How is it shaped? How can it be unlearned? There are different answers to these questions, and consensus is far away. We find explanations of stuttering based on classical conditioning, operant conditioning, cognitive learning theory, and many combinations of these.

This situation with regard to stuttering merely reflects the confused state of current learning theory which has been in great flux. The drive reduction concepts of Hull (1951) have been under attack. The views of Tolman and Guthrie and the Gestaltists refuse to roll over and stay dead. Learning theorists such as Mowrer revise their thinking so often that it is difficult to discern their current concepts. Attempts to translate the Freudian concepts of conflict into behavior theory as illustrated by Dollard and Miller (1950) have added further complications. All theoretical positions are under severe challenge and most of them seem vulnerable. Controversy is rampant among psychologists as evidenced by the criticisms of Chomsky (1959) and Breger and McGaugh (1965) and the countering stout defense by Wiest (1967). No learning theory yet seems to account for all the facts of learning, so we should not be surprised to find different explanations for how stuttering is learned, shaped, and maintained. At the present time most of the learning theories of stuttering are based on classical conditioning, operant conditioning, or both despite evidence that neither has been shown to be entirely acceptable. Let us first consider the operant point of view.

STUTTERING AS OPERANT BEHAVIOR

Most of the operant explanations are based on the assumption that stuttering results from the reinforcement of normal disfluencies. Thus Flanagan, Goldiamond, and Azrin (1959) say:

> Stuttering has often been considered an emotional blocking; it can, however, be regarded as a unit of verbal behavior; that is, breaks, pauses, repetitions, and other nonfluencies can be considered operant responses, having in common with other operants the characteristic of being controllable by ensuing consequences. For the chronic stutterer, such nonfluencies may have immediately been followed by consequences which did not occur in connection with regular speech, thereby becoming isolated as response units. Some consequences, such as attention on the part of the listener, noninterruption, and the like, may increase the likelihood of occurrence—that is, may be reinforcing (p. 979).

It should be stated that this position is not held exclusively by operant theorists. Wendell Johnson, Froeschels, and many others have also felt that stuttering was the problem child of the family of normal disfluencies. And Bloodstein, Alper, and Zisk (1965) state that: ". . . stuttering as a clinical disorder is simply an exaggeration or extension of certain kinds of disfluency to be heard in the speech of normal children" (p. 63).

Even though stuttering disfluencies are largely confined to syllabic repetitions or phonemic prolongations, so that other forms of disfluency are less prominent, the crucial point made by those who hold the operant view is that all children and all adults occasionally emit these behaviors. The stutterer emits too many of them because somehow they have been rewarded and reinforced. Of all the possible types of disfluency, why must these particular ones somehow be singled out to receive special reinforcement that finally predominate in stuttering? No other explanation of the change in distribution of types of disfluencies is consistent with the operant view. But why should the syllabic repetitions and phonemic prolongations be reinforced so exclusively? This is a question which evidently has not been considered by operant conditioners although it is a vital one. Indeed no systematic theory of stuttering based specifically on operant conditioning has yet been formulated.* Laboratory demonstrations that the frequencies of stuttering behavior may be increased or decreased by operant strategies, and a few pilot investigations in the application of operant conditioning principles to actual stuttering therapy, compose the major bulk of the literature.

Nevertheless, the basic assumption on which these advocates of operant explanations usually seem to base their reasoning is that the core behavior of stuttering originally consisted of the same kind of syllabic repetitions and phonemic prolongations which all children (and all adults) experience occasionally. We must remember that this is an assumption. The only research we know which bears on the subject is that of Stromsta (1965), who showed that sonograms of the original syllabic repetitions of children who were still stuttering ten years later were markedly different from those of children who had "outgrown" the disorder. Admittedly this research is hardly crucial and we urgently need longitudinal studies in which the specific "stuttering" behaviors of children who do or do not become stutterers can be repeatedly compared.

Actually the operant framework does not require that the original reinforcement had to be a consequence of normal disfluency. All that it demands is that broken words occur, that they are emitted. If emitted, a behavior can be shaped into another form. Operant behaviorists are not particularly concerned about the causes of behaviors, although occasionally they may speculate a bit, as this quotation from Shames and Sherrick (1963) illustrates:

> The conditions surrounding the original emission and early development of nonfluencies in the speech of infants are still quite obscure and in need of detailed observation. It is possible that the repetitions observed in later speech may be related to the vocal behavior emitted by infants during their early speech development (babbling and chaining of syllables). . . . It is also possible that nonfluency in speech is a characteristic of the human organism because of its physiological limitations (p. 5).

* Theory construction has been deliberately eschewed by most adherents of operant conditioning. They seem to feel that their behavioral science is in its early stages and prefer to stick to observables. Theoretical constructs are not observable. The closest approach to an operant theory of behavior is in B. F. Skinner's book *Verbal Behavior* (1957).

Thus Shames and Sherrick (1963) apply operant conditioning principles to stuttering and suggest that when childhood disfluencies are emitted but have no important consequences, the child is and will remain a normal speaker no matter how many syllabic repetitions he exhibits or what kind they are. On the other hand, these authors state that if the normal disfluencies produce desired consequences (gaining parental attention, permitting the child to speak without interruption, etc.) they will increase in frequency until they become a major feature of his communication. Then, if they get punished through rejection or frustration, the child will start doing things to avoid or escape them, and whatever he does (if it leads to less unpleasantness) will also increase. It may be the use of a stalling trick or a sudden head-jerk or anything else. There are gaps in the reasoning here but some of them can be filled. On the one hand listener reactions (attention, concern, etc.) are so positively reinforcing that they create the stuttering problem by increasing the normal disfluencies. On the other hand, listener reactions are so punishing that successful efforts to escape them are negatively reinforced. This could be true if the child's listeners changed their behavior from attending to rejecting, or from concern to punishment as soon as the frequency of stutterings increased beyond a certain cut-off point. This may indeed take place, although we have no evidence that it does.

Adherents of the operant position are not particularly concerned about the antecedents of behavior. All they require is that a specified behavior be emitted and subjected to contingent reinforcement. If it increases or decreases as its consequences are reinforcing or punishing, respectively, the behavior is to be considered an operant. It operates, has effects upon, the environment. According to Shames and Sherrick, disfluency of any kind, normal or abnormal, can be considered an operant because it can be increased or decreased, or shaped into varied forms by differential reinforcement. These authors make a strong case for shaping when they point out that the adult stutterer shows a markedly different form of stuttering than he did when he was a child. What changed his stuttering? According to the operant conditioners, specific reinforcements which followed (were contingent upon) the deliberate or chance variations in the disfluent behavior were the agents which caused the modification.

Let us give some oversimplified illustrations. If a stutterer happens to shut his eyes in a block, he may thereby shut out the impatient or mocking looks on the listener's face that have been punishing him. Thus this negative reinforcement (the termination of punishment) is contingent on the eye-closing since it follows it, so that eye-closing is strengthened and maintained. Or, if a stuttering child hungers for a parent's attention and gets it whenever he repeats a syllable several times, then repeating syllables receives positive reinforcement. Even if these reinforcements occur only occasionally they can maintain the stuttering. This is an explanation for the shaping of stuttering that comes as the disorder passes through its developmental stages; it is also an explanation for its maintenance.

WHY DO PUNISHED
BEHAVIORS PERSIST?

But the stuttering gets punished more and more as it grows in severity and frequency, and punishments (contingent aversive stimuli) usually weaken a response. Why doesn't the stuttering then diminish or get suppressed? The operant therapists explain that most of the so-called secondary symptoms are instrumental responses used to cope with the aversive stimuli given by the listener. The postponement tricks which eventually become habitual are intermittently reinforced because, occasionally by using them, the stutterer can escape the listener's punishment. An avoidance trick enables the stutterer to avoid listener rejection. A head-jerk that terminates a long prolongation would be strongly reinforced because it *ends* the listener's shocked expression, the punishment. So, through enough negative reinforcements, the head-jerk becomes stronger and stronger. It may occur not once but many times if the punishing listener's look continues. As Ayllon and Azrin (1965) state:

> It appears that human behavior can be maintained by punishment if the punisher has been given discriminative or conditioned reinforcing properties. These results provide an experimental basis for interpreting clinical phenomena such as "masochism" wherein an individual seeks out punishment and does nothing to avoid it (p. 418).

Thus, even though stuttering gets punished by the listener, the things (all his avoidance and struggle behaviors) that the stutterer does to try to escape that punishment—and they are by far the greatest part of the abnormality—get strengthened. Every time we do something that enables us to escape punishment, that behavior will be reinforced and maintained. No person likes aversive stimuli whether they be electric shocks or the shocked expressions on a listener's face.

The same sort of reasoning may apply to the punishing characteristics of the stuttering itself quite apart from any listener reaction. The presence of repetitions and prolongations and gaps in the forward flow of speech, when they continue long enough to produce communicative frustration, and when there are too many of them, can be viewed as punishing. They are unpleasant to the speaker as well as to the listener. If the stutterer in responding to this unpleasant experience, suddenly exhales and manages to emit the word on the end of his breath that sudden exhalation coincides with the escape from unpleasantness. It will therefore be strengthened by negative reinforcement. If a long tremor of the lips is terminated by a sudden lip protrusion, the lip protrusion will be similarly reinforced, and when tremors appear in the future, the stutterer will be likely to stick out his lips again . . . and again. When stutterers are asked why they do these bizarre things, they answer, "because sometimes they work." As all students of conditioning know, intermittent reinforcement produces responses that are more resistant to extinction than continuous reinforcement. It is not necessary therefore for the attempt on the end of the breath or the lip protrusion or any other such behavior to coincide each time with the final emission of a stuttered word. It is sufficient that they do so occasionally. The author of this text well remembers how one of his own most abnormal behaviors developed. When he was in college, an instructor in psychology who had befriended him, noticed his laryngeal fixation and suggested that he should open his constricted throat passage by raising his head whenever such a blocking occurred. Although the technique failed more often than it succeeded, there were a few times when the head-lifting did coincide with release. Within a few months this deliberate head-lifting had turned into a compulsive head-jerking, and the author was unable to inhibit it no matter how hard he tried. It persisted for years and finally became the major feature of his stuttering. Moreover, the jerking spread to other structures, to the arms and even the trunk. We remember only too vividly the experience of trying to ask a cab driver in a strange city to take us to a hotel and thrashing around there in the back seat to such an extent that the driver took us instead to a hospital because he thought his fare was having an epileptic seizure. Only a desperate written message on a card there in the hospital let us go free. Despite this traumatic experience which should certainly have taught us that head or body jerks were ineffective, they continued to persist. There were enough times when they "did work," or we thought they did. Intermittent reinforcement is powerful.

We must also point out, however, that conjoined with this escape from punishment is the ability to continue talking, a positive reinforcement added to the negative reinforcement we have been illustrating. We not only get relief but also reward for using these "secondary symptoms." After all the purpose of talking is to communicate a message. Stutterers desire the consummation of communication with an intensity that normal speakers can hardly fathom. Deprivation creates drive. Only the desert wanderer knows the wonder of water. The stutterer wants badly to complete the message he is sending. Anything that seems to further that end will be positively reinforcing. Thus the head-jerk that coincided with the final utterance of the word not only ends his frustration, but it also enables him to continue. Reinforcement is both negative and positive. This double dose of relief and reward is sufficient to instate a host of inappropriate behaviors and to maintain them at high emission levels. This, and other learning theory explanations of stuttering, explains clearly why confirmed stutterers show such a wide variability of behaviors. The set of instrumental responses that happens to get reinforced differs from one stutterer to the next. We all cope with our troubles in different ways. Stutterers experiment with different strategies of avoidance and escape. Certain ones receive the double-barrelled reinforcement we have mentioned, and these become the major features of the stuttering he exhibits. It is in this way that different stuttering patterns are shaped. It is in this way that stuttering grows. Escape from punishment and communicative progress, in our opinion, are sufficiently reinforcing to account for most of what Wingate called the accessory features of stuttering, but we find it very difficult to explain the core behavior of stuttering in these terms. We can do so with a lot of stretching but we are not happy with the result. A temporally distorted word requires some other explanation.

It should be strongly stated that these applications of conditioning principles to stuttering do not rest on a very substantial foundation of research. As we shall see in the section on the research that has been done with stutterers, the results are far from substantiating these attractive explanations of how the disorder is created, developed, and maintained. Indeed the experimental foundation is most insecure, probably because it is fairly new, and hastily built. It has been clearly demonstrated that the frequency of stuttering behaviors can be manipulated in a controlled laboratory situation by arranging their consequences and perhaps their antecedents, but this is far from sufficient evidence that the same or similar consequences or antecedents are responsible for the acquisition of all the features of the disorder. A theory that explains only selected portions of an assembly of related phenomena is not an adequate theory, particularly when the evidence for it is so meager and has been gathered under conditions that differ so much from the conditions surrounding the phenomena the theory seeks to explain.

THE EXPERIMENTAL PRODUCTION
OF "STUTTERING"

If stuttering is only learned behavior—nothing else—then we ought to be able to demonstrate not only how it is shaped or maintained but also how it can be originated (or "instated," to use the jargon.) The evidence here is insubstantial and unsatisfactory. It is difficult and even dangerous to do such experiments. We have enough stutterers without trying to produce them in the laboratory. Nevertheless, the attempt has been made. Moore (1938) administered severe electric shocks to 18 stutterers and their normal speaking controls as the subjects uttered nonsense syllables according to a predetermined set of intervals. He found that both groups of subjects showed similarly disintegrated breathing during speaking. Moore also demonstrated that these breathing disruptions could be conditioned, for they appeared later on when the subjects listened silently to a recording of the syllables.

In an unpublished study, Van Riper in 1954 administered a very severe shock for failure to choose the correct word from three possibilities in the utterance of consecutive sentences such as this: "The (1. boy; 2. girl; 3. child) was playing in the (1. yard; 2. grass; 3. snow.)" Without foreknowledge of which word was correct, and with a series of very strong shocks as a penalty for not completing the sentence within a set time, two subjects were run, a man and a woman, both highly fluent students and individuals who were fond of the author. To our surprise, despite the approach- avoidance conflicts, which were very evident, and the many severe shocks and profound emotional upheaval experienced by the subjects, no stuttering appeared. Then, appalled by what he was doing to his friends, this author said, "Here, let me share the shock. I can't stand to have you take it alone." And then suddenly real stuttering, uncontrollable repetitions and blockages, appeared as a consequence of the shocks. What is even more painful to recount, this behavior intermittently persisted for months in the man. Three years later, the woman reported she was having an occasional runaway repetition or complete blockage. We never ran another subject and could not account for the result until long afterward we read the research of Brady (1958) in which the executive monkeys got the ulcers rather than the monkeys who got the shocks.

During a complicated serial motor task performed by his normal speaking subjects, Hill (1954) paired a red light with a shock until the light became a conditioned stimulus, and it was then administered while the subjects were speaking. He reported the occurrence of repetitions and prolongations indistinguishable from stuttering.

These three reports can probably best be explained through the principles of classical conditioning, but we also have one in which strictly operant procedures were used. Flanagan, Goldiamond, and Azrin (1959) administered a persistent shock to three normal speaking subjects who had previously been trained to depress a key for each nonfluency while reading. During the experimental condition, the subjects could free themselves from the continuous shock by depressing the key, and it was found that their nonfluencies increased markedly and persisted for a short time even when the shock was removed. They disappeared, however, as soon as the subjects left the laboratory. According to the authors, "Stuttering was defined as any hesitation, stoppage, repetition, or prolongation in the rhythmic flow or vocal behavior" and, from their brief report, it is difficult to be certain that stuttering rather than normal disfluency was the behavior that was "instated." The study evidently showed that an increase in frequency of disfluencies of all types occurred when negative reinforcement was employed. It did not show, however, for example, that the number of syllable repetitions per word increased or that the prolongations became longer, or that coarticulation failure occurred within the syllables, or that airflow or voice was interrupted. It is even possible that the only behaviors which increased were deliberately faked disfluencies which the subjects used to stop the continuous shock.

These four reports of the deliberate creation of stuttering-like behaviors do not seem sufficiently applicable to explain the usual onset of stuttering. Any hard evidence that stuttering *originates* through operant conditioning procedures is lacking. The view that *all* of the behaviors shown by the adult stutterer are maintained and shaped by their consequences has also not been satisfactorily established. As our review of the research will show, punishment of normal or abnormal disfluencies does not always decrease them, nor does the positive reinforcement of fluency always make a stutterer more fluent. Sometimes it makes him worse.

It is true that some, but not all, of our research shows that certain stuttering behaviors can be brought under stimulus and experimenter control to a certain degree in the laboratory, but even the most effective punishments used in the Minnesota experiments by Siegel, Martin and others never seemed to have suppressed it or extinguished it completely. Carryover to normal communicative situations outside the laboratory has also been very disappointing despite the use of tokens and wrist straps and the like. No objective long-term follow-up reports seem at present to be available although there are some anecdotal claims of successful transfer. Moreover we were not at all impressed with those operant studies which use rhythmic and rate controlled forms of speech as a replacement for the stuttering response. *If operant conditioning is truly effective, we should be able to reinstate normal speech and extinguish stuttering without having to use these hoary old methods which for hundreds of years failed our ancient predecessors.* In half an hour any therapist can get a stutterer to speak without stuttering temporarily by using rhythmic speech or relaxation or suggestion or any of a hundred other such procedures. Sometimes the fluency may last a half hour or even more if the suggestion is very effective or the stutterer very suggestible. To use the precarious fluency achieved by such procedures as a proof that stuttering is nothing more than an instrumental response controlled by discriminative stimuli seems at worst sophistry or at best naiveté

This criticism may have been too vehement and may therefore have given the erroneous impression that we feel operant conditioning plays no part in the stuttering problem. Quite the contrary, we are convinced that most of the so-called "secondary" symptoms of stuttering, the most abnormal features of the disorder in the confirmed stutterer, are probably *maintained* by the positive reinforcement of communicative consummation and by the negative reinforcement of decreased frustration. We are not so sure that these behaviors were originally learned in this way, but once they occurred or were deliberately used in the search for relief, the chances are that they persist because of their consequences. Operant conditioning explains only a part of the problem but it does explain a very important part.

RESPONDENT LEARNING THEORY: CLASSICAL CONDITIONING

Some learning theorists attribute the core behavior of stuttering to the disruptive effects of negative emotion on the sequencing of speech. As they see it, strong emotions such as those accompanying the expectation of imminent

unpleasantness, punishment, or frustration are disintegrative, and they produce breakdown not only in the formulation of messages but also in their
motoric expression. For example, if one is consumed with fear or anxiety,
it is difficult to organize the flow of thought sufficiently to produce fluent
speech. Also, if the fear is great enough, it tends to disrupt the intricate
coordination patterns required for fluency so that broken speech results. In
the stutterer any stimulus previously associated with the emotions that
originally produced such breakdown would tend to create fear and also to
disrupt speech. In this view stuttering is learned in the same way that dogs
learn to stop eating and to jump spasmodically when a tone is presented
which was previously paired with an electric shock. If this is its origin, stuttering has been classically conditioned. Brutten and Shoemaker (1967) describe the learning process in this way:

> . . . disintegration created by negative emotion is fundamental to any dis-
> cussion of that specific form of fluency failure termed stuttering. In this light,
> stuttering is not seen as an instrumental response that depends on reinforce-
> ment for acquisition or maintenance, but as a fluency failure caused by the
> cognitive and motoric disorganization associated with negative emotion.
> Whatever else may be involved in stuttering, the speaker is engaged in the
> performance of a motor act that requires fine coordination and this per-
> formance is disrupted. The disorganization is seen as part of the generalized
> autonomic response complex which in essence defines negative emotion. . . .
> This learning to respond with negative emotion to stimuli takes place
> through classical conditioning. In essence, then, it is hypothesized that
> when an individual stutters, he is experiencing learned negative emotion
> (autonomic activity) which is disrupting to his normally fluent speech be-
> havior (p. 30).

This explanation—that the basic behaviors of stuttering are produced
by emotion that has been conditioned to certain stimuli—differs from the
operant point of view in several important ways. First of all, this account
does not assume that the original stuttering behavior was normal disfluency,* so it does not have to explain *why* the syllabic repetitions and phonemic prolongations received so much more reinforcement than the other
types of normal disfluency. Secondly, this theory of stuttering states that
the original fluency breaks consist of disorganized forms of previously integrated behaviors, a concept which we will remember was held by Bluemel.†
Thirdly, this classical conditioning theory of stuttering considers the antecedents of stuttering to be as important as its consequences. Certain stimuli
produce emotional upheaval and that upheaval disrupts speech. When neutral stimuli are paired with those that originally produced the emotional

---

* It assumes instead that the disfluent behaviors of nonstutterers are not "normal,"
which makes the distinction between stutterers and nonstutterers imprecise.

† Bluemel (1957) explained the early onset of "stammering" as being due to the fact
that in childhood speech was not yet thoroughly integrated and was therefore more
vulnerable to emotional stress.

upset, these become the antecedents of stuttering. The stuttering is the by-product of this emotional learning. Thus Brutten and Shoemaker (1967) state: "We have taken the position that stuttering is that form of fluency failure which results from conditioned negative emotion."

This is respondent rather than operant learning. It is based on the association of stimuli with other stimuli. To cite some oversimplified examples: One of the children we studied shortly after the onset of stuttering was reported to have stuttered first at mealtime in a summer cabin. On the table was a lighted kerosene lamp. The boy had just begun to say "Mummy, I . . ." when he knocked over the lamp and set fire to the cabin.

The parental report seemed pretty clear that immediately afterward, when he tried to talk, especially to his mother, and most often at mealtimes, the first word of each utterance showed very frequent syllabic repetitions, and that complete blocking often occurred especially when he used the words "Mummy" and "I." (Let us say immediately that this report is hardly typical of the onset histories we have seen, and that we use it here only to illustrate the respondent learning explanation.) The occasions on which these words were appropriately uttered contained stimuli which were similar, or had been paired with those which originally resulted in broken speech because they triggered a discharge of negative emotion which had come to have the power to break it.

It is apparent that this view of the nature of stuttering has an ancient history and that there is a decided folklore flavor to it. "He began to stutter when he was scared by a horse." "He began to stutter when a tramp came to the door." Every speech therapist has heard such tales, but those of us who have investigated many of these accounts usually find that others had recognized stuttering in the child long before the alleged traumatizing incident occurred and so we have become a bit cynical and suspicious of such evidence. We have, however, found reason to believe that some few of these accounts were indeed true and that some stuttering problems did apparently arise in this way.

In general, this belief that stuttering is the by-product of conditioned negative emotion rests on the assumption that the original moments of stuttering were produced by unpleasant emotional upheaval, and that they represent disruptions and disorganizations of normal speech. Is this assumption true? Do the first stutterings always occur under conditions of emotional stress? Do the first stutterings always show the same sort of features characteristic of other stress-produced disorganization? Do these repetitions and prolongations of a syllable or sound really deserve the term "disintegrated behaviors?" In the beginning stutterer, they do not appear to be highly random or chaotic. An extensive review of the research and our own clinical experiences make us reject the adverb "always." As Johnson (1959) has shown in his monumental study of the onset of stuttering, most stuttering does not originate in situations involving emotional trauma, nor does it begin suddenly, nor does it involve marked disruptions in verbal behavior.

Rather it seems, in most instances, to be discovered first in fairly normal communicative situations, to show a gradual course of developmental increase and initially to be characterized by rather stereotyped syllabic repetitions. Brutten and Shoemaker have pointed to breathing abnormalities, especially the sharp inhalation characteristic of startle, as evidence of emotionally produced disruption, but we have not found these to be characteristic of most beginning stutterers. Most of the literature dealing with beginning stutterers indicates that the initial behaviors do not show the profound disorganizations that characterize stress responses. They are not accompanied by great emotional upheaval. Beginning stuttering most often is reverberatory and fixative. It does not show the picture of startle or panicky awareness, nor is it random struggle.

Because information about the beginning stutterer is sparse, those theorists who attribute the core behavior solely to emotional disruption have again assembled data from adult stutterers to support their hypothesis. Most of them have punished or threatened to punish stutterers on certain words or for each moment of stuttering, using electric shock, or noxious noise, or simple verbal responses such as "No" or "Wrong!" * Unfortunately, even these adult studies have failed to show conclusively that threatened punishment (which should produce emotional disruption) consistently increases stutterings or disfluencies. Some researchers find that it does; others that it has no effect; still others that punishment (or its expectation) decreases disfluencies. Some of the confusion may be due to differences in research design or to the difficulty in creating in the laboratory the appropriate kinds of punishment to which adult stutterers are especially vulnerable. When we think of how many children have been punished during the act of speaking and how many children have had to speak in the throes of profound emotion, we wonder why so few stutterers have been produced. If originally stuttering is created by trying to talk under the influence of negative emotion, all of us should be stutterers.

We feel that the real contribution of classical conditioning theory as it is applied to stuttering lies in its ability to explain the development of the disorder. The spread and generalization of situational and word fears is probably due to the linking of antecedent stimuli. The intricate avoidance strategies employed deliberately by the confirmed stutterer are triggered by conditioned stimuli which were previously associated with negative emotion. We are not so sure that the basic disruptions in the speech of stutterers are always necessarily the product of emotional upheaval. Stuttering can occur when no anxiety or other evidence of negative emotion seems to be present, not only in the beginning stutterer but also in the adult at times. To restrict the term stuttering to that class of fluency failure created by conditioned negative emotion may be convenient to the theorists but it fails to account for a large part of the problem.

---

* A summary of this research is provided in the last section of this chapter.

TWO-FACTOR THEORIES OF HOW
STUTTERING BEHAVIOR IS LEARNED

For purposes of clear exposition in describing the application of classical conditioning to stuttering, we have neglected to state that few theorists today believe that everything the stutterer does and feels can be explained with classical conditioning concepts. The stereotyped avoidance and struggle reactions, which Wingate (1964) called the accessory symptoms of stuttering, are not considered by any modern writer as breakdown phenomena. The stutterer who characteristically says, "ah . . . ah . . . ah . . . um" prior to making a speech attempt is not caught in the throes of panic-produced disintegration. He is deliberately postponing an expected unpleasantness. The typical stuttering patterns in the adult seem to be too individualized and too organized to fit such an hypothesis. Accordingly, Brutten and Shoemaker (1967), applied Mowrer's (1950) two-factor learning theory to stuttering. In their formulation, they combine both the operant and classical kinds of conditioning. They feel that the core behavior, the disruption of the motor sequences of speech into repetitions and prolongations, are precipitated by classically conditioned negative emotions as described in our last section. They also feel that the stutterer learns various methods for coping with the threat or experience of broken speech and that these reactions of avoidance and escape are instrumental responses which have been conditioned through their reinforcing consequences. Brutten and Shoemaker say, "We have proposed that the stutterer may evidence two classes of learned behavior. The first class includes the conditioned negative emotion that tends to disrupt fluent speech. This conditioned emotionality may lead to the second class, escape or avoidance behavior (p. 62)." In various other statements they make clear that in their view the onset and development of involuntary stuttering behaviors can be accounted for best by the classical conditioning of negative emotion, whereas the voluntary coping reactions with which the stutterer tries to solve his problem are instrumentally conditioned. About the latter, they write: "Although these learned instrumental responses are not found among all stutterers, in many they are more prevalent and more dramatic than the repetitions and prolongations that define stuttering. These instrumental responses are often nonverbal behaviors such as facial tics, body twitches, or leg movements (p. 61)." In their therapy, Brutten and Shoemaker use classical conditioning procedures, such as counter conditioning (reciprocal inhibition) or deconditioning to weaken the conditioned negative emotion, and massing or negative practice to weaken the instrumental behaviors through nonreinforcement. They feel, however, that the basic target should be the classically conditioned negative emotion, since if this is eliminated, much of the utility served by the instrumental responses would be lost. When the latter continue to be demonstrated, Brutten and Shoemaker conveniently attribute their persistence to the past history of intermittent reinforcement.

All of the theories of stuttering which are based on learning theory fit exactly into the templates of classical or operant conditioning or even two-factor theory. One of these other theories is that tentatively formulated by Wischner (1947; 1950; 1952). Wischner applied the Hullian concepts of drive-reduction to account for the maintenance of stuttering behaviors, the main drive being that of anxiety. Wischner adopts Johnson's position that stuttering begins when the child, because of parental disapproval or other penalties, begins to react to his normal disfluencies with tension, anxiety, and avoidance. Wischner however, in contradistinction to Johnson, states that the stutterer is not trying to avoid the now noxious normal disfluencies but instead to avoid "the original consequences which attended the original nonfluent behavior," the feelings of anxiety, hurt, and shame. Certain situational or verbal cues come to precipitate these learned anxieties, and the person takes steps to reduce them by various avoidance behaviors. "This anxiety possesses drive properties and motivates the child to activity designed to avoid the noxious stimulation." Since the avoidance behaviors do keep the original disfluencies out of the stutterer's mouth (even though they may appear to the listener to be much more abnormal) the learned anxiety-tension connected with these disfluencies does not arise. It is in this way that the stutterer's avoidance behaviors are actually able to lessen anxiety while speaking. Through anxiety reduction, these avoidance reactions are strongly reinforced and thereby developed and maintained.

Certainly, avoidance behaviors do occasionally avoid unpleasantness. They are successful often enough. The stutterer who substitutes the non-feared word "youth" instead of "boy" terminates the specific fear that was connected with the latter word. Or, if the stutterer utters "um-um-um-er-um" before a word colored black by learned anxiety, sometimes, if he postpones long enough, that specific anxiety goes down, and he experiences no stuttering whatsoever. Any behavior that reduces the anxiety drive gets strongly reinforced. The performance of these stuttering rituals thus becomes a major feature of stuttering. Like whistling in the dark as you pass a graveyard, if nothing evil happens, you are more likely to whistle the next time you pass that place—and, if the fear is greater, to whistle louder and longer. Each successful avoidance strengthens the probability that it will be used again.

But these anticipatory struggle and avoidance behaviors are themselves punished by listeners. Why then do they persist? Wischner answers this question by saying that the punishment occurs after the anxiety reduction,

since the listener's punishment is usually perceived after the utterance is
completed. He also uses the concepts of anxiety confirmation and secondary
gains to explain why stuttering behaviors persist. With regard to the latter,
he writes:

> Clinical experience reveals a wide variety of material benefits that may
> accrue to the stutterer without his necessarily being aware of them. Thus
> there may be "considerate" teachers who excuse Jimmie from recitation. Or
> Bill may receive a medical discharge from the Army on the basis of his
> speech with a disability pension attached. All of these may well serve to
> reinforce stuttering behavior. It seems important from a therapeutic stand-
> point to investigate very carefully the possibility of secondary gain in each
> stuttering case. To accept the stutterer's negative reply at face value to the
> question, "Does your stuttering bring any rewards?" is inadequate, since the
> stutterer very often is not directly aware of the benefits that he might be
> deriving from his speech behavior (1950; p. 332).

Wischner says that the punishment doesn't occur until after the anxiety reduction has occurred. We doubt this. The social punishments may come
later, as Wischner says, but an equally strong punisher, frustration, comes
immediately.

SHEEHAN'S APPROACH-AVOIDANCE
CONFLICT THEORY

Like most of the other explanations of stuttering in terms of learning theory, Sheehan's theory (1958) is an application of an earlier formulation, in
this instance the approach-avoidance conflict theory of Dollard and Miller
(1950). Unresolved conflict is always unpleasant. Ambivalence, indecision,
uncertainty are noxious emotional states. They are as unpleasant as pain,
hunger, or other human miseries. There are various kinds of conflict. The
child in a candy shop, torn between buying a sucker or a chocolate, has an
approach-approach conflict. He wants both but must choose. A fisherman
suddenly confronted by a mother bear with cubs wonders whether to lie
down in the water, to run upstream, or downstream, or cross the river to the
other side. He is in an *avoidance-avoidance* conflict—and he isn't particularly happy. Some of the most unpleasant conflicts in life are *approach-
avoidance* conflicts—like going to the dentist. One is caught in a tug of war
between opposing needs and drives. The conflict is only resolved by certain
behaviors which permit one urge to become stronger than the other and
these resolving behaviors are thereby strongly reinforced. Anything we do
that reduces our unpleasantness is reinforced. One of the main unpleasant
features of conflict is the tension and the oscillation or fixation which occur
when the opposing forces are about equal. You find that the closer you
come to the dentist's office, the stronger is the opposing urge to run the

other way and so you find yourself in the uneasy miserable balance of conflicting forces. In Sheehan's words:

> Caught as he is in a double approach-avoidance conflict, the stutterer is caught between two choices, each one of which threatens the bitter along with the sweet. He can speak, thus achieving his aim of communication, but at the cost of the shame and guilt he has learned to attach to his stuttering. Or he can remain silent, abandon communication, and suffer the frustration and guilt that such a retreat carries with it (1958; p. 126).

Thus Sheehan claims that in stuttering we have double approach-avoidance conflicts. Not only is there the approach-avoidance conflict in which there is a desire to speak and at the same time a desire not to speak, but also another one going on at the same time: the desire to be silent and the fear of silence (silence being equated with death and impotence).

Considering the onset of stuttering, Sheehan (1958) maintains that when an individual experiences guilt, he also experiences the conflicting needs to express himself and to be silent. This Sheehan would also call an approach-avoidance conflict. It is created by opposing needs, and it leads to oscillations and fixations in behavior. In speech these become the repetitions and prolongations found in stuttering. In other words, since the verbal expression of guilt is the focus of the conflict, the turmoil of the inner self is revealed in the verbal nonfluencies of the child. Since the child feels rejected, he believes that he has done something wrong, and this reaction leads to an unhappy choice: either he must believe his parents are mean and unjust (which decreases his security) or else he must justify their rejection by doing something that deserves their rejection. Stuttering may be that thing.

This tug of war between opposing forces, according to Sheehan, shows up on various levels: (1) the word level (saying sounds or words which have been feared, or are hard to pronounce as "statistics," or carry unpleasant meanings); (2) the situation level, where communicative situations are such that you both desire to enter or avoid them; (3) the level of emotional expression in which opposing desires to express hate and love, etc., are involved; (the level of interpersonal relationships, e.g., wanting to impress the boss and fearing he may reject you; (5) the ego-protective conflicts that result in the oscillations and fixations of speech. The more of these conflicts that are involved in any moment of stuttering, the harder and longer one stutters. The more equal the approach-avoidance drives in a speaking task, the more likely one will fixate or oscillate, i.e., stutter.

Sheehan's basic treatment is to bring the therapist's force to bear toward strengthening the approach grandient and weakening the avoidance one. His is basically a classical conditioning therapy since he holds that the stutterer should experience the stimuli (which originally produced the conflict or were associated with it) in a therapeutic situation where no conflict would occur. Speak even though you do stutter. Enter the feared situations even though you fear them. Accept the challenge even though you fear you'll fail. Say the dirty word or the feared word. And do all of these in group therapy with other stutterers or in the presence of an accepting therapist so you won't feel the miseries of conflict. Experience the buzzer without the shock. Test the reality; it isn't as bad as you think. Decrease all avoidance behaviors at all levels. Learn to live with a minimum of ambivalence.

Sheehan sets up two principal hypotheses: (1) the conflict hypothesis—that the stutterer blocks or stops or repeats whenever the conflicting approach and avoidance tendencies (on any level) reach a precarious equilibrium, and (2) the fear reduction hypothesis—that the stuttering itself reduces the fear of the occurrence of stuttering sufficiently to permit the release from the blocked word, thus resolving the conflict momentarily and so enabling the stutterer to continue.

SUMMARY

Although the theoretical positions of Sheehan and Wischner, based on familiar Hullian concepts, are very attractive, they have found limited acceptance. The research cited in their support, consisting mainly of projective drawings, is not impressive. They have not shown that stuttering can be produced in the fashion they claim it is produced. Also, if stuttering is reinforced every time it occurs, repeated readings of the same material should increase not decrease their frequency of occurrence. As Beech and Fransella (1968) point out, their position that the stuttering reduces the fear that triggers it is not convincing even when we take into consideration the possibility that the punishment may come later than the relief, a proposition that has not been substantiated. Approach-avoidance conflicts doubtless play some part in stuttering, but many fractured words occur without such conflicts being evident. Both of these writers fail to provide satisfactory accounts of the onset, development, sex ratio, loci, and many other basic features of the disorder. One feels that they have crammed the poor stutterer into the Procrustean beds of their theoretical models so very hard that, though a good portion of his trunk is encompassed therein, his head and limbs are missing.

COGNITIVE LEARNING THEORIES
OF STUTTERING

Not all those who feel that stuttering behaviors are learned attribute all of that learning to the various associative relationships between stimuli and responses. The same is true of many psychologists concerned with learning. Although they do not deny that habits may be acquired through classical or operant conditioning, they feel that these models do not account adequately for all the intricate and complex kinds of learning found in human beings, or for that matter even in the lower animals. Tolman (1951) showed long ago, for example, that a rat running a maze seems to be learning a kind of map of the terrain rather than a set of serial turning habits. Latent learning, one-trial insightful learning, exploratory behavior, and a good many other problems in the acquisition of responses present considerable difficulty for the S-R conditioning theorists. Pavlov himself noted these and attempted to solve them by positing a second signal system—the use of overt or covert language—for the control of human behavior, and many behaviorists today are investigating the possibility of conditioning language themes as ways of reconciling their theory with more of the facts. Most cognitive learning theorists organize their positions on the concepts of perception and information theory and the organization of cognition consisting of models, maps, systems, strategies, or programs, and the like. This text cannot possibly explore these old and new developments in detail, but explanatory concepts such as Miller, Galanter, and Pribam's (1960) TOTE hypothesis, Festinger's (1957) cognitive dissonance theory, and Feigenbaum's (1959) EPAM all seem to indicate that sooner or later we will have a cognitive learning theory for stuttering.

At present there is no comprehensive cognitive theory of stuttering. The closest attempt is that by Smith (1966). He bases his preliminary theoretical formulation on Festinger's (1957) belief that behavior is always directed toward a reduction of cognitive dissonance. Cognitive dissonance is present when there is an incompatibility between opinons, beliefs, or attitudes; or between expected performance and actual performance, or between stored information (expectations) and incoming stimuli, or between goals and plans. The brain as a computer is inherently programmed to seek always a reduction in cognitive dissonance by varying the output of the system until the incongruity no longer exists. The relationship of this view to information theory is obvious, and Miller, Galanter, and Pribam (1960) even go so far as to describe a possible brain mechanism which could account for this reduction of error signalling in the form of two feedback loops which comprise a feedback comparator system. Smith, in applying this theoretical construct to stuttering, does not seem to us to be very successful. He employs the concept of the GIAL (General Incongruity Adaptation Level) developed by Driver and Streufert (1965) who state: "Organisms with past experiences rich in general incongruity would develop high GIAL's and those with very predictable peaceful pasts would evolve very low GIAL's (p. 50)." A brief excerpt from Smith's work may communicate its disappointing flavor:

> Let it be assumed that the parents have begun calling attention to the child's speech through pressure to speak more fluently or to stop "stuttering." The incongruity created by the pressure may represent an overload which

could produce one of the radical shifts in the GIAL. . . . However, if the child has responded to the pressure of his parents by trying to speak as they would prefer, the incongruity thereby induced by his parents may not be resolved through a new, higher GIAL because he may not be developmentally able to speak more fluently. Conscious efforts to control speech may only compound the difficulty. Therefore the incongruity from the environment persists or even intensifies, and, even though the GIAL may be rising, it does not resolve the conflict. For that reason, the child may find himself in a dilemma: he cannot adjust to the incongruity coming from his parents through a higher GIAL (General Incongruity Adaptation Level) because his efforts to control his speech fail, which can create even more incongruity which would require still more change in the GIAL (p. 21).

Two other cognitive learning theories of stuttering, although they have rarely been viewed as such, are those by Emil Froeschels and Wendell Johnson. When their writings are closely examined, it seems apparent that both of these men base their explanation of the disorder on misperception. Froeschels, for example, in several articles stresses the role of the misperception that speaking is difficult. He says that this wrong belief leads a child to respond to his physiological stuttering (normal disfluency) by struggle and avoidance, thereby creating the real disorder. Froeschels (1952) writes:

> The child, believing in speech difficulty, and perhaps being asked not to iterate (repeat), will try to overcome the "difficulty" by using more muscular energy. In this way the iterations will be spoken with strongly contracted muscles, and the single iterations will therefore proceed more slowly than the iterations without pressure. . . . As time goes on, new signs and symptoms are developed. It is the author's opinion that every stage in the development of the clinical picture is caused by the patient's belief in his inability to speak normally (p. 113).

Froeschels also makes the point that all of the accessory struggling movements are those which can be made voluntarily, and he seems to say that initially at least they are deliberately used as strategies to cope with the illusory inability.

Although Johnson shifted his theoretical beliefs several times during his productive lifetime—indeed all the way from the cerebral dominance theory to an interactionist position—he is best known for his semantogenic theory, a representative account of which is found in his book *People in Quandaries* (1946). Johnson's basic thesis was that stuttering is the result of misperception and misevaluation, that it has its onset in the parent's misjudging the child's normal disfluencies as being abnormal and unacceptable. Again, once the stutterer has interiorized these misevaluations, has labeled them inappropriately, and has begun to think about them in a language which is full of semantic errors, he adopts various strategies of avoidance to lessen his distress. Even Johnson's therapy uses a cognitive approach.

RESEARCH ON LEARNING THEORY AND STUTTERING

Since most of the research bears directly or obliquely on respondent or operant views of stuttering, we shall organize it about these topics. The crucial questions concern the way it is first learned, how it is maintained, how it is shaped during the course of its development, and the procedures by which its frequency may be increased or decreased.

DOES STUTTERING ORIGINATE UNDER CONDITIONS OF NEGATIVE EMOTION?

Our own investigations of onset were reported in Chapter IV and indicated that only rarely did the first stutterings appear in emotionally loaded situations. The only other significant research is that done at Iowa. In a comprehensive interview investigation of the onset of stuttering in 246 children, Johnson (1959) found only a very few instances in which its onset was reported by the parents to have occurred in association with "illness or injury, shock or frights, as a consequence of imitation, or under any other unusual or memorable, or dramatic circumstances." Indeed most of the parents interviewed found it difficult to recall the circumstances under which the disorder first appeared. This is sparse evidence indeed.

DOES NEGATIVE EMOTION INCREASE NORMAL DISFLUENCIES?

In an attempt to bypass the great difficulties involved in deeply investigating the onset of stuttering, and using the doubtful assumption that normal disfluencies are equivalent to stuttering, some workers have sought to determine whether punishment or other unpleasant stresses will increase the number of disfluencies in normal speakers. Savoye (1954) had her normal speakers read aloud, then repeatedly introduced a tone followed, after an interval, by a shock while they were speaking. They had more fluency failures during the 10 seconds immediately following the tone than during a 10 second period midway between shocks. Bilger and Speaks (1959) paired a green light with a 100 dB tone to punish disfluencies of normal speakers along with noncontingent delayed auditory feedback. More disfluencies occurred during the conditioned tone—but not with the DAF. Stassi (1961) reported that normal speakers became more disfluent under contingent punishment of disfluencies with the word "wrong" than they did when the word "right" was used.

Brookshire and Martin (1967) used "wrong," "no" and "uh-uh" paired with normal spearkers' disfluencies and found a temporary suppression of the latter which varied somewhat depending on which "punishing" word was used. Siegel and Martin (1965a) found no significant differences when shock was made contingent on disfluency in two experiments, but in a third study using oral reading they found that random shock slightly increased disfluencies although unexpected contingent shocks significantly reduced them. These investigators then used nonshock "punishments" (Siegel and Martin, 1965b and 1966)—the words "right" and "wrong," and a buzzer. These contingencies, including the buzzer, decreased the normal disfluencies. The word "right" did not increase them. Brookshire (1968) used bursts of randomly presented aversive noise as normal speakers read aloud one day and aversive noise contingent upon disfluencies the other day, the order of conditions being counterbalanced. The subjects who received the contingent noise after having experienced the random noise did not show the usual decrease in disfluencies. In a somewhat similar study, Brookshire and Eveslage (1969) used contingent random noise and contingent "No!" whenever their normal speakers were disfluent. The random noise increased disfluency and the "No" decreased it. Siegel and Martin (1968) used verbal punishment of spontaneous speech and found a similar decrease in disfluency and also a slowing down in rate—the subjects probably became more careful in how they talked. There have been other experiments of this sort but their pertinence depends on the assumed equivalence of normal disfluencies to those of stuttering, an assumption which we do not feel has been validated.

IS STUTTERING LINKED
TO ANTECEDENT STIMULI?

There exists ample evidence to show that, at least in the adult, stuttering does not occur randomly but instead is associated with certain antecedent stimuli. Johnson and Sinn (1937) eliminated 98 per cent of the subjects' stutterings by having them omit those words on which they had stuttered on a previous reading. Johnson and Knott (1937) had their stutterers read the same passage after an interval of time and found that 72 per cent of the moments of stuttering occurred on the same words previously stuttered in the first reading. Berwick (1955) showed that the frequency of stuttering was greater when the subjects spoke to photographs of preselected listeners evaluated as "difficult" than when they spoke to those evaluated as "easy listeners." Connett (1955) attempted, through suggestion, to increase the perception of the consonant /t/ as a difficult sound and found a slight but not significant increase in the frequency of stuttering on words beginning with this sound in adaptation readings.

The research on the relationship between expectancy and subsequent stuttering has already been reviewed. To summarize it briefly in this context: the studies of Knott, Johnson, and Webster (1937), Johnson and Inness (1939), Johnson and Ainsworth (1938), Milisen (1938), Van Riper (1936), Van Riper and Milisen (1939), Dixon (1947), and such recent ones as those by Brutten and Gray (1961), Brutten (1963), and Martin and Haroldson (1967), and others show very clearly that a substantial positive relationship between expectancy and subsequent stuttering has been demonstrated at least for adults. The research also shows, however, that *expectancy is not always followed by stuttering* and that stuttering can occur even when no expectancy is subjectively experienced. After all, all expectancy *proves* is that the stutterer knows the conditions under which stuttering has occurred in the past. Nevertheless, in general, the loci, the frequency and the severity of stuttering seem to be somewhat predictable on the basis of the conditions preceding utterance, thus providing some evidence that those conditions are related to the occurrence of stuttering.

EMOTIONAL AROUSAL
AS AN ANTECEDENT CONDITION

Respondent learning is generally viewed as involving emotional arousal triggered by antecedent stimuli. We shall cite only a few of the more pertinent studies here. Van Riper (1936) showed that breathing records indicative of emotion appeared during the anticipatory period prior to the utterance of a stuttered word. Bearss (1951) shocked her stutterers randomly and found a decrease in stuttering frequency. Lingwall (1967) failed to find any significant correspondence between GSR indications of emotion during the period of word exposure and the occurrence of stuttering on that word. Sixty-eight per cent of abnormal GSRs to exposed words resulted in no stuttering. When no GSRs whatsoever occurred, 18 per cent of the words still showed stuttering. However, stutterers showed more GSR activity in speaking than did the controls. This may well indicate that the galvanic skin response measures generalized or speech anxiety but not specific word fear, a conclusion supported partly by Boland's (1953) research. Gray and Karmen (1967) found subgroups of stutterers differing in nonverbal anxiety as related to adaptation. Steer and Johnson (1936) found a correlation of only .36 between desire to avoid stuttering and frequency of stuttering. Shumak (1955) did a somewhat similar study and found an r of .52. Goss (1956) concluded that expectancy probably operates on a time gradient since short intervals between word exposure and the signal to speak produced less stuttering than longer intervals. Two interesting researches explored what happens when expectancy rather than the occurrence of stuttering is punished. Curlee and Perkins (1968) administered shock during signalled expectancy and found that the subsequent stuttering decreased.

This result might possibly be explained by the punishment's suppressing effect on the covert rehearsal behavior of the preparatory set to stutter if such preparatory rehearsals of anticipated stuttering help to make it inevitable. This explanation could possibly be extended to cover most of the punishment research since most subjects soon learned to expect shock or disapproval as well as stuttering. Daly and Frick (1968) also shocked stutterers when they signalled expectancy of stuttering but found only a "moderate" decrease in the later stutterings on the same material.

If the expectancy period prior to stuttering is characterized by certain covert rehearsal behaviors such as those described by Van Riper (1936) and others, this might be viewed as oblique evidence for classical conditioning. In this regard we should also mention the research of Wendahl and Cole (1961), which is frequently cited as demonstrating that the normal speech of stutterers prior to stuttering is easily distinguished from that of normal speakers and can be identified as that of a stutterer. They prepared taped segments in which the "actual" stuttering behavior was removed by clipping and paired these with other similar segments from the speech of normal speakers. They found that listeners could identify the samples from the stutterers with ease. However, Young (1964) used Wendahl and Cole's original taped segments with a slightly different procedure and with other listeners, and failed to corroborate the earlier findings.

THE CONSISTENCY EFFECT

Learning theorists have also pointed to the consistency effect (the tendency of stuttering to occur repeatedly in the same situations and on the same words) as supporting the position that stuttering is learned behavior. They argue that this consistency implies the presence of specific cues to which the stuttering response has been conditioned. Golub (1951) reported a much more rapid rate of adaptation on words presented singly but repeatedly when the same words rather than different words were used. Bloodstein (1961a) observed 14 children between the ages of three and six years (and we must remember that this age range may include fully developed stutterers) as they repeated short sentences. He found some consistency (from 50 to 100 per cent) in all of his subjects and concluded that this must indicate the presence of subliminal fear reactions to the words on which the stuttering occurred. This inference, which is all it is, was not supported by the later research of Neeley and Timmons (1967), and much of the consistency effect, which Williams, Silverman, and Kools (1969) and others have shown occurs also in the disfluencies of normal speakers, can be explained in other ways, namely, in terms of information load, coordination difficulty, prosodic variables, uncertainty, and word positional effects.

Another facet of consistency which might support the learning hypothesis is the observation that the stuttering behaviors of an individual stutterer often are stereotyped, which is a characteristic of other well-learned responses. Van Riper (1936) revealed that the breathing abnormalities of adult stutterers, though varying from stutterer to stutterer, were remarkably typical for the individual when repeatedly stuttering on the same word. Although Prins and Lohr (1969) found little commonality or consistency in the stuttering behaviors of individual stutterers in a frame by frame analysis of photographed moments of stuttering, they did not, unfortunately, compare the stutterings on the same syllable or words. In any event, the consistency of adult stuttering behaviors can hardly be considered crucial evidence in support of the belief that stuttering, particularly the *original* stuttering was produced by conditioned negative emotion.

STIMULUS GENERALIZATION AS EVIDENCE THAT STUTTERING IS LEARNED

Stimulus generalization of the antecedent cues also seems to point in the direction of respondent learning. Fierman (1955) and Johnson, Larson, and Knott (1937) showed that a colored border associated with an adaptation reading passage in which stuttering occurred seemed to precipitate more stutterings than an equivalent sheet without the distinctive border. Johnson and Millsapps (1937) showed some tendency for stuttering to be linked to inkblots representing previously stuttered but deleted words. Brutten and Gray (1961) demonstrated that, by inserting words (which had previously been stuttered upon several times) into lists of words that had been fluently spoken, less stuttering occurred on the previously stuttered words. These authors attributed the decrease to the generalization of positive emotion to adjacent words and seem to feel that their view of stuttering as a stimulus contingent response had been supported by the results, an interpretation which seems less than secure.

Better evidence for stimulus generalization is found in a study by Peters and Simonson (1960). Using a memory drum to expose word-pairs to be memorized by their stutterers, these investigators selected words of high and low "stuttering potential" as rated by the individual subjects, then arranged them so that the first member of the pair of words to be exposed was always a word of low stuttering potential while the second member of the pair was, in half the instances, another word of low stuttering potential and in the other half, a word of high potential. The results of this verbal memory task showed that stuttering occurred more frequently on words learned in association with words of high stuttering potential than those with low potential. Associative learning through stimulus contiguity seemed to have taken place. This would also support the respondent learning hypothesis.

This brief review shows clearly that much still needs to be done in investigating the period antecedent to the moment of stuttering. Clinical reports seem almost unanimous in their positing a noxious state of emotional arousal antecedent to overt stuttering in the adult stutterer though not in the young one. The research, however, is very thin and often not to the point. If stuttering is learned through the processes of classical conditioning, all the evidence assuredly is not yet in.

DOES PUNISHMENT INCREASE
OR DECREASE STUTTERING?

The literature is rife with case reports indicating that rejection and other penalties increase the frequency and severity of stuttering, and the first experimental approach to the question was applied by Van Riper (1937b). Finding it impossible, in a pilot experiment, to administer an electric shock so that it would be truly contingent upon stuttering,* he instead gave a sample shock then threatened to give another shock for each moment of stuttering which occurred during an adaptation reading. The subject was told that the shocks would be given at the end of the reading, but actually were not administered. A reversal of the adaptation effect and an increase in stuttering was found during the reading in which shock was threatened.

Frick (1952) had stutterers read single words, comparing the frequency of stutterings under four conditions: 1. no shock or threat; 2. contingent shock; 3. threatened shock per stuttering moment which was actually administered at the conclusion of the reading; 4. shock administered after every word whether stuttered or not. Frick found no decrease in stutterings in any condition, but the combined shock conditions showed more stuttering than the control condition. Shock, contingent or threatened, did not suppress stuttering. The stuttering subjects of Frederick (1955) read a word list orally while receiving a steady shock and had the shock intensity increased contingent on stuttering. More stuttering occurred in the contingent condition, and the more anxious the subjects were before the readings, the more effective the punishment was in increasing stuttering. Hansen (1955) had an audience signal favorable reactions to fluency and unfavorable reactions to stuttering. A slight increase in stuttering occurred during the latter condition. Webster (1968) had two subjects differentially define two classes of stuttering behavior as "voluntary" and "involuntary." Using the word "wrong" as the contingent punishment, he found that the "involuntary" stuttering behaviors increased while the "voluntary" ones decreased in one of the subjects. This has been cited as supporting the Brutten-Shoemaker (1967) point of view that two classes of stuttering behaviors

---

* Webster (1968) has shown that it is very difficult to apply punishment contingently; that often it is applied during the fluent utterance of the word following the stuttered word. We should remember this.

occur, one as a result of respondent learning and the other as a result of operant learning.

Another group of studies apparently reveals that contingent punishment neither increases or decreases stuttering. Timmons (1966), using an experimental and a control group of stutterers, gave the first group the word "wrong" as a punishment contingent upon stuttering in the middle series of repeated readings of the same material. The controls received no "punishing" word. No significant increases or decreases in stuttering were found. Daly and Cooper (1967) studied adaptation readings in which shock was administered first during, and then after each moment of stuttering, and then in a third condition no shock was given. Differences among conditions were not significant. Stevens (1963) gave a sample shock prior to the stutterers' readings and found no significant change as a result of making it contingent on the stuttering moment. Gross (1968) gave his subjects coins—then took them away as punishment for moments of stuttering with 30 stutterers. Some reduction in the frequency of stuttering resulted. To cite another study which should make us cautious, Cady and Robbins (1968) used three words contingent upon stuttering: "wrong," "right," and the neutral word "tree." All three words produced decreases both in the stutterers' stutterings and in the disfluencies of the control subjects, and there were no significant differences between their effects. Why should "tree" decrease stuttering? According to the operant conditioners, all three words must have been punishing since they produced a response decrement. A more meaningful explanation is probably that they called attention to stuttering. As alerting devices they may simply have eliminated some of the minor stutterings. Or perhaps all these words, including "tree" interrupted the preparatory sets to stutter or served as distractors. In this connection it is interesting that Siegel and Martin for example had found that the most dramatic drop in frequency of disfluencies came when their subjects were simply instructed to try not to repeat words.

Finally, another group of studies indicates that stuttering is reduced as a result of contingent punishment (which would fit the operant view of the disorder.) Flanagan, Goldiamond, and Azrin (1958) had three stutterers read for about 30 minutes until adaptation had occurred and a baserate seemed stabilized. Then a 105 dB tone was presented continuously through earphones except that each stuttering moment turned off the sound for five seconds (negative reinforcement). All three subjects showed an increase in stuttering. When the contingent tone was omitted, the frequency of stuttering decreased to the baseline rate. Then the noxious tone of one second-duration was administered contingent upon each stuttering moment, and the stuttering decreased, one subject becoming entirely free there in the laboratory. In a similar study, Goldiamond (1965), using delayed auditory feedback as a "punishment" instead of the loud tone, showed that when a short pulse of DAF was made contingent upon stuttering, stuttering decreased. Escape from continuous DAF however did not produce the expected increase in stuttering but instead produced a slower rate and increased fluency—which is about what we would expect from our knowledge of the fluency-facilitating effects of DAF. In an attempt to replicate Flanagan, Goldiamond, and Azrin's research, Biggs and Sheehan (1969) used a 108 dB high frequency tone as an aversive stimulus in three conditions: presented contingently with a moment of stuttering, presented randomly, and stopping it when stuttering occurred. Since they found that stuttering decreased under all three conditions they attributed the decrease mainly to distraction.

Several studies from the University of Minnesota have also dealt with punishing stuttering. Using three stutterers, Martin and Siegel (1966b) studied the effects of administering contingent shock for different types of stuttering behavior (nose-wrinkling, tongue-protrusion, etc.) and found that these specific stuttering behaviors decreased but returned to baseline as soon as the contingent shock was removed. However, at the same time, an increase in prolongations occurred. In another experiment (Martin and Siegel, 1966a) with two male stutterers these authors simultaneously "punished" stuttering by the words "not good" and rewarded fluency by the word "good." Both of these contingencies increased the fluency, and when they were no longer used, more stuttering occurred. A nylon strap used as a discriminative stimulus was shown to have some effectiveness. Brady (1967) shocked his subjects contingently for each moment of stuttering while reading a 1000 word passage and found that there was less stuttering in this condition than when no shock was employed. Quist and Martin (1967) used the word "wrong" as a consequence for any repetition and prolongation in one stutterer and for "uh" or prolonged "n" sounds in two others after baselines had been established. They reported reductions in frequency of stuttering under these contingencies. The responses returned to base rates when the contingencies were removed, but let's not forget the Cady and Robbins

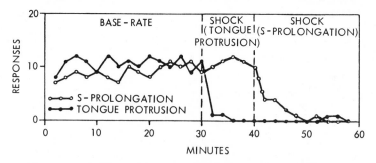

Figure 13. Number of tongue protrusions and S-prolongations emitted by subject O each two minutes during session B. *(Reproduced by permission from Houghton-Mifflin Co., publishers of Sloane, H. N. and B. D. Macaulay (eds.) Operant Procedures in Remedial Speech and Language Training. Chapter 16 by R. Martin "The Experimental Manipulation of Stuttering Behaviors.")*

(1968) use of the word "tree." Ryan (1964) alternated positive and negative reinforcement contingencies in a hierarchic therapy situation using oral reading and found a marked decrease in stuttering which was maintained later in unreinforced reading. Gross and Holland (1965) showed a decrease in stuttering when shock was made contingent on stuttering, but they found too that shocking *the listener* for each stuttered moment produced a similar reduction in stuttering. Haroldson, Martin, and Starr (1968) used a "time out" or silence period as a punishing consequence for stuttering and found a marked decrease in four stutterers, but Adams (1970), reviewing the same data, concluded that the instability of the base rates make their findings very doubtful. Starkweather (1970) suspected that the contradictory results of these punishment studies might reflect two tendencies of opposite direction: the unpleasantness of the shock or reprimand which would tend to increase involuntary stuttering behaviors and the contingent feature which would tend to decrease them. By varying the intensity of the shock and making it either contingent or noncontingent, he showed that there was an interaction of these two factors. There are other studies but these are representative enough to demonstrate that the case for explaining stuttering in terms of either operant or classical conditioning is still far from being substantiated.

DOES POSITIVE REINFORCEMENT INCREASE STUTTERING?

Although various writers have speculated that attention or parental concern or other kinds of neurotic profit may be the rewards which cause stuttering to be maintained or to grow, there is very little evidence to substantiate this hypothesis. Van Riper (1957) gives a clinical report in which a male stutterer was rewarded for quotas of stuttering by being kissed by an attractive girl. This resulted in an immediate and dramatic decrease in stuttering. In another case report, a very hostile boy was rewarded for stuttering moments by being contingently allowed to give Van Riper a severe electric shock, a procedure which also almost completely eliminated the stuttering. Stevens (1963) found no significant increase in stutterings when verbal approval was made contingent on stuttering. Gross (1968) rewarded (paid his subjects money for each moment of stuttering and found that the frequency of stuttering declined rather than increased.

DOES NEGATIVE REINFORCEMENT FOR STUTTERING INCREASE IT?

Negative reinforcement is the contingent cessation of unpleasant or noxious stimulation. This type of reward has shown up in some of the experiments previously cited. Flanagan, Goldiamond, and Azrin (1958), **Goldiamond**

(1965), and others have shown that the contingent removal of noxious stimulation will increase the frequency of stuttering.

IS STUTTERING SELF-REINFORCING?

Theorists have always had difficulty in explaining why stuttering—presumably an unpleasant experience not only to the listener but to the stutterer himself—persists. Various explanations have been offered. Wischner (1952) suggests several possibilities beside the old one of secondary gains such as attention-getting: 1. the unpleasant tension built up during prior expectancy ceases once the feared word has been spoken. (If you are terribly afraid the bear will bite you, *that specific fear* disappears once the bear does bite.) 2. If stuttering is, as Johnson suggested, an avoidance of normal disfluency which has been colored by unpleasant parental concern, the successful avoidance (even though the behavior is abnormal) is more rewarding than were the normal disfluency to have occurred. Even though the stuttering behavior gets punished, the reward precedes it and so has more effect. Sheehan (1953) attributes the persistence of stuttering to negative reinforcement. Stutterers are caught in unpleasant double approach-avoidance conflicts on various levels; the stuttering behavior immediately precedes the resolution of the conflict and so it is reinforced. Since most of these conflicts are solved by reducing the avoidance by the actual stuttering, the fear reduction that occurs during the stuttering reinforces the behavior.

The pertinent research in support of these views is very scanty. Sheehan and Voas (1954) found that masseter action current records showed a buildup in tension that peaked just before the stuttering ended. Shrum (1967) however failed to corroborate this peaking in his electromyographic study, finding instead that the tension often persisted even after the word was spoken. Wischner (1952) [unconvincingly to us at least] interpreted a series of projective drawings done by his stutterers just before, during, and after a moment of stuttering to indicate that tension, anxiety, and stress built up before and during the block but subsided when it was completed. Sheehan, Cortese, and Hadley (1962) in a similar study also had their stutterers "draw" their own behavior before, during, and after a moment of stuttering. They found self-pictures which they "interpreted" as indicating that tension-reduction did occur following the blockage in some but not all stutterers, and that often the release was followed by the increased unpleasantness of guilt and shame. These few conflicting and rather dubious studies are hardly enough to allow us to feel confident in the adequacy of such explanations. If stuttering is self-reinforcing we will probably have to look elsewhere for the reinforcement.

Another possible reinforcement might be that of communicative drive-reduction. Presumably when a stutterer begins to say a sentence he wants to complete it. The basic drive in speaking is to communicate a message to a listener. When, for any reason, that communicative progress is blocked, any behaviors that end that block will be strongly reinforced. Sheehan, for example, in another study (1951), found that stuttering decreased much more rapidly in adaptation readings when the stutterer had to repeat any stuttered word *until it was spoken normally* than when he merely stuttered on it and went on. Van Riper (1957) devised his cancellation technique in therapy to use this kind of nonreinforcement of abnormality. Haroldson, Martin, and Starr (1968) also showed that contingent "time-outs" from talking reduced stuttering.

THE ADAPTATION EFFECT AS EVIDENCE THAT STUTTERING IS LEARNED

The well known adaptation effect (that stuttering decreases with repeated readings or speakings of the same words) has been variously interpreted by those who believe that stuttering is learned behavior. Johnson (1959) explained it as extinction due to anxiety reduction, i.e., the stutterer expects to have more stuttering than he actually experiences, and so the anxiety subsides. Dixon (1947) had her subjects rank three situations in terms of anticipated difficulty and then had them do adaptation readings in each. The amount of adaptation varied directly with the anticipated difficulty. Shulman (1955) found that greater adaptation occurred when the audience was increased. Wischner (1947) asked his stutterers to read a passage silently several times and to indicate feared words. An adaptation curve for these expectancies was similar to that for overt stuttering. Others, however, have discovered the same adaptation curves for normal speakers' nonfluencies and presumably they have no fears of stuttering.

Using an independent measure of emotion, the Palmar Sweat Index (PSI), Brutten (1957) showed that although both stutterers and normal speakers adapted in successive readings, the former showed a marked decline in palmar sweating whereas the normal speakers did not. However, Gray and Brutten (1965) discovered that adaptation could take place even when the (PSI) was not declining so that they attributed the decline in frequency of stuttering to reactive inhibition rather than to extinction. In an excellent view of adaptation research, Wingate (1966) demonstrates very clearly that there are marked differences between the features of adaptation in stutterers and those of extinction of learned responses. The curves are different, those of normal extinction being gradual whereas those of stuttering decline precipitously. He also argued that if stuttering is an old response it should extinguish more slowly than it does. He points out that extinction usually tends to generalize and stuttering adaptation evidently does not. The spontaneous recovery of most learned responses seldom is complete while stuttering returns to pre-adaptation levels. Moreover, Newman (1963) found that certain stutterers did not show the adaptation effect at all, and Rousey

(1958) found little adaptation in long periods of talking. We find it very difficult to conclude that the research on adaptation strongly supports the position that stuttering is nothing more than learned behavior. In our view the adaptation effect in stuttering is merely a special case of stimulus habituation.

CONCLUSIONS

When each of these studies is subjected to the critical analysis they require many more questions are raised than are answered. Why do these investigations of punishment and stuttering yield such disparate results? How important is the problem of the definition of stuttering? What was punished, the core behavior, or the associated struggle and avoidance reactions? Perhaps both normal and abnormal disfluencies were punished? Was the punishment truly contingent or contiguous? Were the punishments truly punishing? Are there other explanations for the reduction of stuttering under punishment? Subjects differ in vulnerability and attitude toward shock; electrode contacts shift; the utterance of the word "wrong!" can be spoken in many ways, and in the laboratory situation it may possess little real unpleasantness. Are these punishments anything like the ones usually encountered by the stutterer in the outside world? Was he merely playing the experimenter's game? Can we be sure that these stimuli were not merely alerting devices, or, on the other hand, distractors? How truly stable were the base rates? Why did punishment produce only limited decreases in stuttering and have such temporary and restricted effects? Was the noxious noise effective because of its lingering masking effects? Did not DAF or its residual effects facilitate fluency quite apart from its presumed punishing characteristics? How representative of the general stuttering population were the subjects? What controls were made for possible experimenter bias? How important was the role of awareness? Did the fear of punishment wipe out the fear of stuttering?

This author has asked these and many other similar questions about each experiment, and his conclusion is to him a disappointing one. It is this: the research has not yet established that stuttering behavior can be entirely explained by present learning theory, neither its origin nor its maintenance. Neither classical nor operant conditioning nor their combination (as in Brutten and Shoemaker's two-factor theory) are completely explanatory. Each of these accounts for some of the phenomena of stuttering but not for all. No one today would deny that stutterers learn to use various behaviors in coping with their stigmatized and frustrating speech difficulties. Fifty years ago all stuttering behaviors were thought to be unlearned spasmodic disintegration (an era this author remembers well), but that era has long passed and rightly so. Stuttering behavior is not simply convulsive seizure activity. Let us say again that much of it is learned. We are convinced that much of the behavior which goes under the name of stuttering is learned behavior. We can account for its variability of symptoms and its consistency of patterning in no other way. We have watched it being learned. We have taught different kinds of stuttering. We have extinguished stuttering behaviors of many varieties. Our own experiments in therapy have been based on learning theory, and we know that stuttering behavior can be modified by applying its principles. We are convinced that proper scheduling of appropriate reinforcements and punishments can alter the frequency with which certain avoidance and struggle behaviors are emitted. However, let us make it very clear that we are also convinced that though both respondent and operant learning are involved in stuttering, the core behavior (especially in its form at onset) requires some other explanation. Our questions still remain: does learning theory account for the genesis or the complete phenomenology of stuttering? Does it adequately explain how children begin to stutter? Does it account for all the behaviors? We really regret that we cannot give these questions affirmative answers on the basis of the explanations presently offered, or the research that is available. We wish we could.

COMMENTARY

. . . stuttering is an extremely difficult kind of behavior to describe in learning theory concepts. It is very intermittent, it varies a great deal from one individual to another, and it appears to be a type of sequential behavior consisting of many stimuli and many responses rather than an isolated event. We have a very hard time in the field of speech pathology in agreeing on single instances of stuttering. Experimental studies of learning, on the other hand, tend to involve rather simple behaviors in situations where the important variables are fairly easy to control. To explain stuttering in traditional S-R terms is to oversimplify it. As I said earlier, I feel quite strongly that the problem called stuttering involves a great deal of what is referred to as learning, but I do not believe that the psychology of learning has yet developed concepts that can give more than a rough approximation of the learning involved in stuttering (Luper, 1968, p. 88).

One might also question whether drive-reduction operates in the simple and direct manner suggested by Wischner. Is it possible that fluencies, which are generally greater in number than nonfluencies, might also be increased by drive reduction? Alternatively, if drive reduction operates differentially in favor of stuttering, it is difficult to see why the stutterer should not become, at some stage, completely incapacitated (Beech and Fransella, 1968, p. 68).

I have covered a great deal of ground here, perhaps too much for the creation of a clear picture. The major points I have made are as follows: *First, the effectiveness of punishment as a controller of instrumental be-*

havior varies with a wide variety of known parameters. Some of these are: (a) intensity of the punishment stimulus, (b) whether the response being punished is an instrumental one or a consummatory one, (c) whether the response is instinctive or reflexive, (d) whether it was established originally by reward or by punishment, (e) whether or not the punishment is closely associated in time with the punished response, (f) the temporal arrangements of reward and punishment, (g) the strength of the response to be punished, (h) the familiarity of the subject with the punishment being used, (i) whether or not a reward alternative is offered during the behavior-suppression period induced by punishment, (j) whether a distinctive, incompatible avoidance response is strengthened by omission of punishment, (k) the age of the subject, and (l) the strain and species of the subject (Solomon, 1964, p. 250).

In the long run, punishment, unlike reinforcement, works to the disadvantage of both the punished organism and the punishing agency. The aversive stimuli which are needed generate emotions, including predispositions to escape or retaliate, and disabling anxieties (Skinner, 1953, p. 183).

(1) For all subjects the introduction of response contingent shock resulted in an almost total reduction of stuttering behaviors; removal of shock was followed by a return to base rate frequency.
(2) When the response was defined in terms of a specific behavior, it proved possible to manipulate independently two such behaviors emitted by the same subject.
(3) For two subjects the frequency of stuttering behaviors was increased or decreased without occasioning any systematic change in word output rate; for the third subject a reliable inverse relationship obtained between stuttering frequency and word output rate.
(4) For one subject stuttering behavior was brought under the discriminative stimulus control of a plain, nylon wristband; for another subject the same discriminative stimulus control was conditioned to a blue light (Martin and Siegel, 1966a, pp. 351–352).

In the experiments cited above, stuttering suppression under punishment was achieved in controlled laboratory situations. With the exception of a study reported by Martin and Siegel (1966b), no attempts have been made to assess carry-over of the decreased stuttering frequency in situations outside the laboratory. In our efforts to devise systematic carryover procedures, it has become apparent that the use of shock, loud tone, or delayed feedback as the aversive stimulus has certain disadvantages. Generation, presentation, and control of the stimuli require complex and relatively cumbersome instrumentation. This necessitates that the subject be returned periodically to the laboratory situation in order to strengthen the association between the primary punisher and a discriminative stimulus or a secondary punisher.

In an effort to circumvent certain of these mechanical problems, we decided to explore the use of time-out from positive reinforcement as a potential means of bringing stuttering under experimental control in a laboratory situation, and subsequently extending this control into a variety of stimulus environments (Haroldson, Martin and Starr, 1968, p. 560).

The data presented suggest that the stuttering response is an operant which occurs in the context of another operant, namely, verbal behavior. Although one cannot stutter without talking, neither can one limp without walking, and limping can be controlled separately from walking. . . . The way in which stuttering responses reacted to operant controls in this study cannot be distinguished from reactions of other operant behaviors, and suggests that they are in this class of behaviors.

When termination of a noxious stimulus was made contingent upon stuttering, response rate rose. When onset of a noxious stimulus was made contingent upon stuttering, response suppression occurred, displaying compensation upon cessation of such consequences (Flanagan, Goldiamond and Azrin, 1958, p. 176).

A conception of stuttering as instrumental-escape learning offers these advantages: (a) it is not embarrassed in its account of the role of disapproval in stuttering, since it need not formulate disapproval of speech pattern as a necessary nor the critical factor in stuttering, (b) it provides a theoretical position consistent with widely employed treatment procedures which aim to help the individual modify his stuttering responses and control his fears, and (c) it allows for a variety of dynamics underlying the tension surrounding the speech act. It also allows consideration of the still very real possibility that some stutterers may be inferior in terms of neuromotor function; that is, in some individuals more than others, fine coordinative acts (such as those involved in speech) might be more difficult to learn, might be more susceptible to the pressures of situational stresses, and blocks thus more readily occur (Wingate, 1959, p. 334).

It is well known that anxiety has a disruptive effect on finely coordinated behavior, and speech is an instance of finely coordinated behavior, par excellence. Speech disturbance may be a purely automatic generalized consequence of anxiety in the same way that general changes in muscular coordination or attention span, for example, are brought about by anxiety. . . . Except in extreme instances, the speech disturbances occur largely outside of awareness of either speaker or listener, which means that they are unlikely to be the target of deliberate social control or individual control (Mahl, 1961, p. 179).

. . . when an individual stutters, he is experiencing learned negative emotion (autonomic activity) which is disrupting to his normally fluent speech behavior. This position is supported by the research which has shown that noxious stimuli are capable of disrupting the speech behavior of non-stutterers and that the fluency failures that result are not distinguishable from the universal characteristics of stuttering (Brutten and Shoemaker, 1967, p. 30).

If an individual becomes disfluent as a result of punishment, and there is a persistence of this disfluency in response to specific word and situation cues, then it is possible that there may be some application of the results found in this study to the understanding of the onset and development of stuttering (Stassi, 1961, p. 361).

An interesting parallel to the experiment by Hamilton and Krechevsky took place in my own speech last Friday. I had been talking very well, having on the average of 30-50 spasms a day, 90 per cent of which were handled with the stop-go and the rest of which were slight prolongations much different from the old type of spasms which composed my former pattern of stuttering.

On Friday noon, Moore made an appointment with me to take part in an experiment which involved a large number of severe electric shocks. I have always been afraid of electric shocks, and I did do some worrying about the experiment, and didn't look forward to it with any pleasure. Just prior to the experiment, I went up to see Moore and I was talking without any of the old spasms, although I was having some spasms when I did talk to him, however, they were very short in duration. I certainly was very much afraid of those shocks and hated them terribly when they came, although Moore declared that the shocks given me were of minimum intensity—they did not seem like that to me, however.

The shocks were applied to me after a certain word in a series of words and I began to become tense and expectant two words previous to this certain word. My muscles would contract, I would seem to stop breathing and would continue in this state until a few seconds after the shocks which were given about once every forty-five seconds. (During all this time I was not allowed to talk.)

During the last fourth of the experiment, when this certain word was voiced, there was no shock. During this post-period after the word I was tensed until about thirty to forty-five seconds after the shock for fear of being shocked at an unprecedented time—none occurred, but that didn't relieve any emotion on the next omitted shock.

At the end of the experiment, perspiration was running down my body in streams and the room wasn't any too warm.

When Moore took off the electrodes and pneumographs, I began to talk about my relief at the experiment being finished. He then asked me questions concerning my feelings during the experiment, which I have previously stated above.

During the fifteen minutes, while talking to Moore, I had all of my old spasm patterns. The new way to stutter, which I had adopted, was entirely forgotten. (It might be interesting to note that while I am writing this, I can feel those same reactions that I had in the experiment—my hand is very shaky and I am breathing quickly.) Every spasm I had, and there were a very great number of them, was forced and all my old old reactions were unconsciously used.

After I left the laboratory, I began to realize how I had been stuttering and began to "catch hold" of myself. During the next two or three hours, my anticipation of spasms was increased 75 per cent, my handling of spasms was very poorly done, and all my old reactions were trying and trying to become predominate.

Now, two days afterwards, I still find my anticipations very high, my old spasm pattern is still a conflicting element in using my new spasm pattern, but the old fears, etc. are slowly being driven out again (McCall, 1936).

. . . certain of the overt nonfluent or struggle behaviors emitted during stuttering are susceptible to experimental manipulation in much the same way as other operant behaviors. This does not necessarily mean, of course, that stuttering behaviors are instated originally by means of instrumental, operant conditioning. It is possible, and indeed probable, that the early acquisition and development of stuttering behaviors involve both classical and instrumental conditioning (Martin, 1968, pp. 342–343).

The susceptibility of an organic function to modification through learning does not indicate that the original behavior was learned. Certain reflexive or autonomic functions of the organism are modifiable through learning (Wingate, 1966, p. 149).

To summarize: The "law of effect," or reinforcement, conceived as a *"law of learning"* occupies a very dubious status. Like the principles of conditioning, it appears to be an unlikely candidate as an explanatory principle of learning. As a strong law of learning it has already been rejected by many of the theorists who previously relied on it. As an empirical "law of *performance*" it is noncontroversial, but usually so generally stated as to be of little explanatory value (Breger and McGaugh, 1965, p. 397).

The notions of "stimulus," "response," and "reinforcement" are relatively well defined with respect to the bar-pressing experiments and others similarly restricted. Before we can extend them to real-life behavior, however, certain difficulties must be faced. We must decide, first of all, whether any physical event to which the organism is capable of reacting is to be called a stimulus on a given occasion, or only one to which the organism in fact reacts; and correspondingly, we must decide whether any part of behavior is to be called a response, or only one connected with stimuli in lawful ways. Questions of this sort pose something of a dilemma for the experimental psychologist (Chomsky, 1959, p. 30).

Arrayed against the reflex theorists are the pessimists who think that living organisms are complicated, devious, poorly designed for research purposes. They maintain that the effect an event will have upon behavior depends upon how the event is represented in the organism's picture of itself and its universe. They are quite sure that any correlation between stimulation and response must be mediated by an organized representation of the environment, a system of concepts and relations within which the organism is located. A human being—and probably other animals as well—builds up an internal representation, a schema, a simulacrum, a cognitive map (Miller, Galanter, and Pribam, 1960, p. 7).

The central hypothesis of the theory is that the presence of dissonance gives rise to pressure to reduce that dissonance, and that the strength of this pressure is a direct function of the magnitude of the existing dissonance. There are three major ways in which the dissonance may be reduced. The person may change one or more of the cognitions involved in dissonant relations; and he may decrease the subjective importance of the cognitions which are involved in the dissonant relations. Dissonance is conceived as a motivating state comparable to other drive states (Festinger and Bramel, 1962, p. 256).

Learning goes on in part through automatic processes with little rational direction from the learner and in part through processes in which the learner perceives relationships and acts with knowledge (Hilgard and Atkinson, 1967, p. 303).

BIBLIOGRAPHY

Adams, M. R., "Some Comments on 'Time-Out' as Punishment for Stuttering," *Journal of Speech and Hearing Research,* XIII (1970), 218–20.

Adams, M. R., and E. J. Brutten, "Auditory Extinction and Reinforcement Procedures for Modifying Stuttering and Instating Fluency," convention address, A.S.H.A., 1967.

Amman, J. O. C., *A Dissertation on Speech* (1700). Reprinted 1965, New York: Stechert-Hafner.

Andrews, G., and M. Harris, *The Syndrome of Stuttering.* London: Heinemann, 1964.

Appelt, A., *The Real Cause of Stammering and Its Permanent Cure.* London: Methuen, 1912.

Arnott, N., *Elements of Physics.* Edinburgh: Adams, 1828.

Ayllon, T., and N. H. Azrin, "The Measurement and Reinforcement of Behavior of Psychotics," *Journal of Experimental Analysis of Behavior,* VIII (1965), 357–83.

Bearss, M., "An Investigation of Penalty on the Expectancy and Frequency of Stuttering," Master's thesis, Purdue University, 1951.

Beasley, B., *Stammering: Its Treatment.* London: Hamilton, 1879.

Beech, H. R., "Stuttering and Stammering," *Psychology Today,* I (1967), 49–51; 61.

Beech, H. R., and F. Fransella, *Research and Experiment in Stuttering.* New York: Pergamon, 1968.

Bell, A. M., *Observations on Defects of Speech, the Cure of Stammering, and the Principles of Elocution.* London: Hamilton-Adams, 1853.

Berwick, N. H., "Stuttering in Response to Photographs of Certain Selected Listeners." In W. Johnson (ed.), *Stuttering in Children and Adults.* Minneapolis: University of Minnesota Press, 1955.

Biggs, B., and J. Sheehan, "Punishment or Distraction? Operant Conditioning Revisited," *Journal of Abnormal Psychology,* LXXIV (1969), 256–62.

Bilger, R. C., and C. E. Speaks, "Operant Control of Nonfluent Speech in Normal Talking," *Asha,* III (1959), 97 (abstract).

Blanton, S., "The Treatment of Stuttering," *Proceedings of the American Speech Correction Association,* Vol. 6, No. 1 (1936), 24–31.

Bloodstein, O., "The Development of Stuttering," *Journal of Speech and Hearing Disorders,* XXV (1960), 219–37; 366–76; 26 (1961), 67–82.

Bloodstein, O., J. Alper, and P. Zisk, "Stuttering as an Outgrowth of Normal Disfluency." In D. E. Barbara (ed.), *New Directions in Stuttering: Theory and Practice.* Springfield, Ill.: Thomas, 1965.

Bluemel, C. S., *Stammering and Allied Disorders.* New York: Macmillan, 1935.

———. "Stammering and Inhibition," *Journal of Speech Disorders,* V (1940), 305–8.

———. *The Riddle of Stuttering.* Danville, Ill.: Interstate, 1957.

Boland, J. L. "A Comparison of Stutterers and Nonstutterers on Several Measures of Anxiety," *Speech Monographs,* XX (1953), 144 (abstract).

Boomer, D. S., and D. W. Goodrich, "Speech Disturbance and Judged Anxiety," *Journal of Consulting Psychology,* XXV (1961), 160–64.

Brady, J. V., "Ulcers in Executive Monkeys," *Scientific American,* CXCIX (1958), 539–40.

Brady, W., *The Effect of Electric Shock on the Frequency of Stuttering.* Master's thesis, Pennsylvania State College, 1967.

Breger, L., and J. L. McGaugh, "Critique and Reformulation of 'Learning Theory' Approaches to Psychotherapy and Neurosis," *Psychological Bulletin,* LXIII (1965), 338–58.

Brookshire, R. H., "Simple and Interactive Effects on Random and Response Contingent Aversive Stimuli upon Disfluencies of Normal Speakers," convention address, A.S.H.A., 1968.

Brookshire, R. H., and R. A. Eveslage, "Verbal Punishment of Disfluency Following Augmentation of Disfluency by Random Delivery of Aversive Stimuli," *Journal of Speech and Hearing Research,* XII (1969), 383–88.

Brookshire, R. H., and R. R. Martin, "The Differential Effect of Three Verbal Punishers on the Disfluencies of Normal Speakers," *Journal of Speech and Hearing Research,* X (1967), 496–505.

Brutten, E. J., "Fluency and Disfluency," *Asha,* III (1963), 781 (abstract).

———. "A Colorimetric Anxiety Measure of Stuttering and Expectancy Adaptation," *Dissertation Abstracts,* XVIII (1957), 2707–8.

———. "Palmar Sweat Investigation of Disfluency and Expectancy Adaptation," *Journal of Speech and Hearing Research,* VI (1963), 40–48.

Brutten, E. J., and B. B. Gray, "Effects of Word Cue Removal on Adaptation and Adjacency: A Clinical Paradigm," *Journal of Speech and Hearing Disorders,* XXVI (1961), 385–389.

Brutten, E. J., and D. J. Shoemaker, *The Modification of Stuttering.* Englewood Cliffs, N. J.: Prentice-Hall, 1967.

Cady, B., and C. J. Robbins, "The Effect of the Verbally Presented Words 'Wrong,' 'Right' and 'Tree' on the Disfluency Rates of Stutterers and Nonstutterers," convention address, A.S.H.A., 1968.

Chomsky, N., "Review of B. F. Skinner, 'Verbal Behavior,'" *Language,* XXXV (1959), 26–58.

Connett, M. H., "Experimentally Induced Changes in the Relative Frequency of Stuttering on a Specified Speech Sound." In W. Johnson (ed.), *Stuttering in Children and Adults.* Minneapolis: University of Minnesota Press, 1955.

Curlee, R. F., and W. H. Perkins, "The Effect of Punishment of Expectancy to Stutter on the Frequencies of Subsequent Expectancies and Stuttering," *Journal of Speech and Hearing Research,* XI (1968), 787–95.

Daly, D. A., and E. B. Cooper, "Rate of Stuttering Adaptation Under Two Electroshock Conditions," *Behaviour Research and Therapy,* V (1967), 49–54.

Daly, D. A., and J. V. Frick, "Frequency of Stuttering Under Three Punishment (Electroshock) Conditions," convention address, A.S.H.A., 1968.

Darwin, E., *Zoonomia*. London: 1800.

Denhardt, R., *Das Stottern eine Psychose*. Leipzig, 1890.

Dixon, C. C., "The Amount and Rate of Adaptation of Stuttering in Different Oral Reading Conditions." Master's thesis, State University of Iowa, 1947.

Dollard, J., and N. E. Miller, *Personality and Psychotherapy*. New York: McGraw-Hill, 1950.

Donahue, I., "Change in Stuttering Frequency Under Specified Conditions." Master's thesis, State University of Iowa, 1941.

Driver, M., and S. Steufert, *The 'General Incongruity Adaptation Level' (GIAL) Hypothesis: An Analysis and Integration of Cognitive Approaches to Motivation*. Lafayette, Ind.: Purdue University Institute for Research in the Behavioral, Economic and Management Sciences, 1965.

Dunlap, K., "The Technique of Negative Practice," *American Journal of Psychology*, LV (1932), 270–73.

Eveslage, R. A., and R. H. Brookshire, "Verbal Punishment of Disfluency Following Augmentation of Disfluency by Random Delivery of Aversive Stimuli," convention address A.S.H.A., 1968.

Eysenck, H. J., and S. Rachman, *The Causes and Cures of Neuroses*. London: Routledge and Kegan Paul, 1965.

Feigenbaum, E. A., "An Information Processing Theory of Verbal Learning," RAND Report P-1817, Santa Monica, Cal.: RAND Corporation, 1959.

Festinger, L.: *A Theory of Cognitive Dissonance*. Evanston, Ill.: Row, Peterson Co., 1957.

Festinger, L., and D. Bramel, "The Reactions of Humans to Cognitive Dissonance." In A. J. Bachrach (ed.), *Experimental Foundations of Clinical Psychology*. New York: Basic Books, 1962.

Fierman, E. Y., "The Role of Cues in Stuttering Adaptation." In W. Johnson (ed.), *Stuttering in Children and Adults*. Minneapolis: University of Minnesota Press, 1955.

Flanagan, B., I. Goldiamond, and N. H. Azrin, "Instatement of Stuttering in Normally Fluent Individuals Through Operant Procedures," *Science*, CXXX (1959), 979–81.

———. "Operant Stuttering: The Control of Stuttering Behavior Through Response Contingent Consequences," *Journal of Experimental Analysis of Behavior*, I (1958), 173–77.

Frederick, C. H., "An Investigation of Learning Theory and Reinforcement as Related to Stuttering Behavior." Doctoral dissertation, University of California, Los Angeles, 1955.

Frick, J. V., "An Exploratory Study of the Effect of Punishment (Electric Shock) Upon Stuttering Behavior," *Speech Monographs*, XIX (1952), 146–47.

Froeschels, E., "Core of Stuttering," *Acta-Oto-Laryngologica*, XLV (1955), 115–19.

———. "Pathology and Therapy of Stuttering," *Nervous Child*, II (1943), 148–61.

———. *Selected Papers (1940–1964)*. Amsterdam: North-Holland, 1964.

Froeschels, E., "The Significance of Symptomatology for the Understanding of the Essence of Stuttering," *Folia Phoniatrica*, IV (1952), 217–30.

Goldiamond, I., "Stuttering and Fluency as Manipulatable Operant Response Classes." In L. Krasner and L. P. Ullman (eds.), *Research in Behavior Modification*. New York: Holt, 1965.

Golub, A. J., "The Influence of Constant and Varying Word Stimuli on Stuttering Adaptation." Master's thesis, State University of Iowa, 1951.

Goss, A. E., "Stuttering Behavior and Anxiety as a Function of Experimental Training," *Journal of Speech and Hearing Disorders,* XXI (1956), 343–51.

Gray, B. B., "Theoretical Approximations of Stuttering Adaptation," *Behavior Research and Therapy,* III (1965a), 171–85.

———. "Theoretical Approximations of Stuttering Adaptation: Statement of Predictive Accuracy," *Behaviour Research and Therapy,* III (1965b), 221–27.

Gray, B. B., and E. J. Brutten, "The Relationship Between Anxiety, Fatigue, and Spontaneous Recovery in Stuttering," *Behaviour Research and Therapy,* III (1965), 251–59.

Gray, B. B., and J. L. Karmen, "The Relationship Between Nonverbal Anxiety and Stuttering Adaptation," *British Journal of Communication Disorders,* 1 (1967), 141–51.

Gregory, H. H. (ed.), *Learning Theory and Stuttering Therapy.* Evanston: Northwestern University Press, 1968.

Gross, M. S., "The Effects of Punishment and Reinforcement on the Disfluencies of Stutterers," convention address, A.S.H.A., 1968.

Gross, M. S., and H. L. Holland, "The Effects of Response Contingent Electroshock Upon Stuttering," *Asha,* VII (1965), 376 (abstract).

Guthrie, E. R., *The Psychology of Learning.* New York: Harper, 1935.

Hall, J., *The Psychology of Learning.* New York: Lippincott, 1966.

Halvorson, J., "The Effects on Stuttering Frequency of Pairing Punishment (Response Cost) with Reinforcement." Doctoral dissertation, University of Minnesota, 1968.

Hansen, H. P., "The Effect of Measured Audience Reaction on Stuttering Behavior Patterns." Doctoral dissertation, University of Wisconsin, 1955.

Haroldson, S., R. Martin, and C. D. Starr, "Time-out as Punishment for Stuttering," *Journal of Speech and Hearing Research,* XI (1968), 560–66.

Hilgard, E. R., and R. C. Atkinson, *Introduction to Psychology.* New York: Harcourt, 1967.

Hill, H., "An Experimental Study of Disorganization of Speech and Manual Responses in Normal Subjects," *Journal of Speech and Hearing Disorders,* XIX (1954), 295–305.

Hoepfner, T., "Stottern als assoziative Aphasie," *Zeitschrift für Pathopsychologie,* I (1912), 448–553.

Hull, C. L., *Essentials of Behavior.* New Haven: Yale University Press, 1951.

Hunt, J., *Stammering and Stuttering, Their Nature and Treatment* (original Ed., 1861). Reprinted, New York: Hafner, 1967.

Johnson, W., *People in Quandaries.* New York: Harper, 1946.

———. *The Onset of Stuttering.* Minneapolis: University of Minnesota Press, 1959.

Johnson, W., and S. Ainsworth, "Studies in the Psychology of Stuttering: X. Constancy of Loci of Expectancy of Stuttering," *Journal of Speech Disorders.* III (1938), 101–4.

Johnson, W., and M. Inness, "A Statistical Analysis of the Adaptation and Consistency Effects in Relation to Stuttering," *Journal of Speech Disorders,* IV (1939), 79–86.

Johnson, W., and J. R. Knott, "Certain Objective Cues Related to the Precipita-
    tion of the Moment of Stuttering," *Journal of Speech Disorders,* II (1937),
    17–19.
Johnson, W., R. P. Larson, and J. R. Knott, "Studies in the Psychology of Stutter-
    ing: III. Certain Objective Cues Related to the Precipitation of the Moment
    of Stuttering," *Journal of Speech Disorders,* II (1937), 105–9.
Johnson, W., and L. S. Millsapps, "Studies in the Psychology of Stuttering: VI.
    The Role of Cues Representative of Past Stuttering in the Distribution of
    Stuttering Moments During Oral Reading," *Journal of Speech Disorders,* II
    (1937), 101–4.
Johnson, W., and A. Sinn, "Studies in the Psychology of Stuttering: V. Frequency
    of Stuttering with Expectation of Stuttering Controlled," *Journal of Speech
    Disorders,* II (1937), 98–100.
Kingsley, C., "Irrationale of Speech," *Frazer's Magazine,* London, 1859.
Klingbeil, G. M., "Stuttering and Stammering," *Journal of Speech Disorders,* IV
    (1939), 115–32.
Knott, J. R., W. Johnson, and M. J. Webster, "A Quantitative Evaluation of
    Expectation of Stuttering in Relation to the Occurrence of Stuttering," *Jour-
    nal of Speech Disorders,* III (1937), 20–22.
"Leigh, Mme.," in J. Hunt, *Stammering and Stuttering* (original ed., 1861). Re-
    printed, New York: Hafner, 1967.
Lingwall, J. B., "Galvanic Skin Responses of Stutterers and Nonstutterers to Iso-
    lated Word Stimuli," convention address, A.S.H.A., 1967.
Lohr, F. E., "Visible Manifestation of Stuttered Speech," convention address,
    A.S.H.A., 1969.
Luper, H. L., "A Study of the Relationship Between Stuttering Adaptation and
    Improvement During Speech Therapy." Master's thesis, Ohio State University,
    1950.
————. "An Appraisal of Learning Theory Concepts in Understanding and
    Treating Stuttering." In H. H. Gregory (ed.), *Learning Theory and Stuttering
    Therapy.* Evanston: Northwestern University Press, 1968.
————. "The Consistency of Selected Aspects of Behavior in the Repetitions of
    Stuttered Words." Doctoral dissertation, Ohio State University, 1954.
Mahl, G. F., "Measures of Two Expressive Aspects of a Patient's Speech in Two
    Psychotherapeutic Interviews." In L. A. Gottschalk (ed.), *Comparative Psy-
    cholinguistic Analysis of Two Psychotherapeutic Interviews.* New York: Inter-
    national Universities Press, 1961.
Martin, R., "The Experimental Manipulation of Stuttering Behaviors." In H. W.
    Sloane and B. D. Macaulay (eds.), *Operant Procedures in Remedial Speech
    and Language Training.* Boston: Houghton-Mifflin, 1968.
Martin, R. R., and S. K. Haroldson, "The Relationship Between Anticipation and
    Consistency of Stuttered Words," *Journal of Speech and Hearing Research,* X
    (1967), 323–27.
Martin, R. R., and G. M. Siegel, "The Effects of Simultaneously Punishing Stutter-
    ing and Rewarding Fluency," *Journal of Speech and Hearing Research,* IX
    (1966a), 466–75.
————. "The Effects of Response Contingent Shock on Stuttering," *Journal of
    Speech and Hearing Research,* IX (1966b), 340–52.

————. "The Effects of a Neutral Stimulus (Buzzer) on Motor Responses and Disfluencies in Normal Speakers," *Journal of Speech and Hearing Research,* XII (1969), 73–82.

McCall, J., Personal Communication, 1936.

McDearmon, J., "C. S. Bluemel and the Learning Theory Approach to Stuttering," *Western Speech,* XXX (1966), 106–11.

Milisen, R., "Frequency of Stuttering with Anticipation of Stuttering Controlled," *Journal of Speech Disorders,* III (1938), 207–14.

Miller, G. A., E. Galanter, and K. H. Pribam, *Plans and the Structure of Behavior.* New York: Holt, 1960.

Miller, N. E., and J. Dollard, *Social Learning and Imitation.* New Haven: Yale University Press, 1941.

Moore, W. E., "A Conditioned Reflex Study of Stuttering," *Journal of Speech Disorders,* III (1938), 163–183.

Mowrer, O. H., *Learning Theory and Personality Dynamics.* New York: Ronald Press, 1950.

Neelley, J. N., and R. J. Timmons, "Adaptation and Consistency in the Disfluent Speech Behavior of Young Stutterers and Nonstutterers," *Journal of Speech and Hearing Research,* X (1967), 250–56.

Newman, P. W., "Adaptation Performances of Individual Stutterers: Implications for Research," *Journal of Speech and Hearing Research,* VI (1963), 293–94.

Owen, T. V., and M. G. Stemmermann, "Electric Convulsive Therapy in Stammering," *American Journal of Psychiatry,* CIV (1947), 410–13.

Peters, R. W., and W. E. Simonson, "Generalization of Stuttering Behavior Through Associative Learning," *Journal of Speech and Hearing Research,* III (1960), 9–14.

Potter, S. O. L., *Speech and Its Defects.* Philadelphia: Blakeston, 1882.

Prins, D., and F. E. Lohr, "Behavioral Dimensions of Stuttered Speech," convention address, A.S.H.A., 1969.

Quist, R. W., and R. R. Martin, "The Effect of Response Contingent Verbal Punishment on Stuttering," *Journal of Speech and Hearing Research,* X (1967), 795–800.

Rezzozi, T. E., and M. R. Adams, "A Study of the Disfluency of Prosody of Stuttering Adaptation," convention address, A.S.H.A., 1968.

Rousey, C., "Stuttering Severity During Prolonged Spontaneous Speech," *Journal of Speech and Hearing Research,* I (1958), 40–47.

Rubin, M., "A Study of the Consistency and Adaptation Effects in Ten to Thirteen-Year-Old Stutterers." Master's thesis, Brooklyn College, 1957.

Ryan, B., "The Construction and Evaluation of a Program for Modifying Stuttering Behavior." Doctoral dissertation, University of Pittsburgh, 1964.

Sandow, L., *Mechanik des Stotterns.* Nordhansen: Edler, 1898.

Savoye, A. L., "The Effect of the Skinner-Estes Operant Conditioning Paradigm upon the Production of Nonfluencies in Normal Speakers." Master's thesis, University of Pittsburgh, 1959.

Shames, G. H., D. B. Egolf, and R. C. Rhodes, "Experimental Programs in Stuttering Therapy," *Journal of Speech and Hearing Disorders,* XXXIV (1969), 30–47.

Shames, G. H., and C. E. Sherrick, "Discussion of Nonfluency and Stuttering as

Operant Behavior," *Journal of Speech and Hearing Disorders,* XXVIII (1963), 3–18.

Sheehan, J. G., "Conflict Theory of Stuttering." In J. Eisenson (ed.), *Stuttering: A Symposium.* New York: Harper, 1958.

―――. "The Modification of Stuttering Through Non-reinforcement," *Journal of Abnormal and Social Psychology,* XLVI (1951), 51–63.

Sheehan, J. G., "Theory and Treatment of Stuttering as an Approach-Avoidance Conflict, *Journal of Psychology,* XXXVI (1953), 27–49.

Sheehan, J. G., P. Cortese, and R. Hadley, "Guilt, Shame, and Tension in Graphic Projections of Stuttering," *Journal of Speech and Hearing Disorders,* XXVII (1962), 129–39.

Sheehan, J. G., and R. B. Voas, "Tension Patterns During Stuttering in Relation to Conflict, Anxiety Binding, and Reinforcement," *Speech Monographs,* XXI (1954), 272–79.

Shrum, W. F., "A Study of the Speaking Behavior of Stutterers and Nonstutterers by Means of Multichannel Electromyography," convention address, A.S.H.A., 1967.

Shulman, E., "Factors Influencing the Variability of Stuttering." In Johnson, W. (ed.), *Stuttering in Children and Adults.* Minneapolis: University of Minnesota Press, 1955.

Shumak, I. C., "A Speech Situation Rating Sheet for Stuttering." In W. Johnson (ed.), *Stuttering in Children and Adults,* Minneapolis: University of Minnesota Press, 1955.

Siegel, G. M., and R. R. Martin, "Experimental Modification of Disfluency in Normal Speakers," *Journal of Speech and Hearing Research,* VIII (1965a), 235–44.

―――. "Verbal Punishment of Disfluencies in Normal Speakers," *Journal of Speech and Hearing Research,* VIII (1965b), 245–51.

―――. "Punishment of Disfluencies in Normal Speakers," *Journal of Speech and Hearing Research,* IX (1966), 208–18.

―――. "The Effects of Verbal Stimuli on Disfluencies During Spontaneous Speech," *Journal of Speech and Hearing Research,* XI (1968), 358–64.

―――. "Verbal Punishment of Disfluencies During Normal Speech," *Language and Speech,* X (1967), 244–51.

Skinner, B. F., *Science and Human Behavior.* New York: Macmillan, 1953.

―――. *Verbal Behavior.* New York: Appleton, 1957.

Smith, R. W., "A Cognitive Motivation Approach to Stuttering: An Initial Formulation." Master's thesis, Purdue University, 1966.

Solomon, R. L., "Punishment," *American Psychologist,* XIX (1964), 239–53.

Starkweather, C. W., *The Simple, Main, and Integrative Effects of Contingent and Noncontingent Shock of High and Low Intensities on Stuttering Repetitions.* Doctoral dissertation, Southern Illinois University, 1970.

Stassi, E. J., "Disfluency of Normal Speakers and Reinforcement," *Journal of Speech and Hearing Research,* IV (1961), 358–61.

Steer, M. D., and W. Johnson, "An Objective Study of the Relationship Between Psychological Factors and the Severity of Stuttering," *Journal of Abnormal and Social Psychology,* XXXI (1936), 36–46.

Stevens, M. M., "The Effect of Positive and Negative Reinforcement on Specific

Disfluency Responses of Normal Speaking College Males." Doctoral dissertation, State University of Iowa, 1963.

Stromsta, C., "A Spectrographic Study of Dysfluencies Labeled as Stuttering by Parents," *De Therapia Vocis et Loquellae*, I (1965), 317–20.

Timmons, R. J., "A Study of Adaptation and Consistency in a Response-Contingent Punishment Situation." Doctoral dissertation, University of Kansas, 1966.

Tolman, E. C., *Collected Papers in Psychology*. Berkeley, Cal.: University of California Press, 1951.

Van Riper, C., "Effect of Devices for Minimizing Stuttering on the Creation of Symptoms," *Journal of Abnormal and Social Psychology*, XXXII (1937a), 63–65.

——. "The Effect of Penalty Upon the Frequency of Stuttering." *Journal of Genetic Psychology*, L (1937b), 193–95.

——. "The Growth of the Stuttering Spasm," *Quarterly Journal of Speech*, XXIII (1937c), 70–73.

——. "Study of the Thoracic Breathing of Stutterers During Expectancy of Occurrence of Stuttering," *Journal of Speech Disorders*, I (1936), 61–72.

——. "Symptomatic Therapy for Stuttering." In L. E. Travis (ed.), *Handbook of Speech Pathology*. New York: Appleton, 1957.

Van Riper, C., and C. J. Hull, "The Quantitative Measurement of the Effect of Certain Situations on Stuttering." In W. Johnson (ed.), *Stuttering in Children and Adults*. Minneapolis: University of Minnesota Press, 1955.

Van Riper, C., and R. L. Milisen, "A Study of the Predicted Duration of the Stutterers' Blocks as Related to their Actual Duration," *Journal of Speech Disorders*, IV (1939), 339–45.

Webster, L. M., "A Methodological Investigation of the Contingent Stimulation of Stuttering Moments," convention address, A.S.H.A., 1968.

Wendahl, R. W., and J. Cole, "Identification of Stuttering During Relatively Fluent Speech," *Journal of Speech and Hearing Research*, IV (1961), 281–86.

Wiest, W. M., "Some Recent Criticisms of Behaviorism and Learning Theory," *Psychological Bulletin*, LXVII (1967), 214–25.

Williams, D. E., F. H. Silverman, and J. A. Kools, "Disfluency Behavior of Elementary School Stutterers and Nonstutterers: The Adaptation Effect," *Journal of Speech and Hearing Research*, XI (1968), 622–30.

——. "Disfluency Behavior of Elementary School Stutterers and Nonstutterers: The Consistency Effect," *Journal of Speech and Hearing Research*, XII (1969), 301–7.

Wingate, M. E., "A Standard Definition of Stuttering," *Journal of Speech and Hearing Disorders*, XXIX (1964), 484–89.

——. "Calling Attention to Stuttering," *Journal of Speech and Hearing Research*, II (1959), 326–35.

——. "Stuttering Adaptation and Learning: I. The Relevance of Adaptation Studies to Stuttering as 'Learned Behavior,'" *Journal of Speech and Hearing Disorders*, XXXI (1966), 148–56.

Wischner, G. J., "Experimental Approach to Expectancy and Anxiety in Stuttering Behavior," *Journal of Speech and Hearing Disorders*, XVII (1952), 139–54.

——. "Stuttering as Learned Behavior: A Program of Research." Doctoral dissertation, University of Iowa, 1947.

————. "Stuttering Behavior and Learning," *Journal of Speech and Hearing Disorders,* XV (1950), 324–35.

Wolpe, J., "Experimental Neuroses as Learned Behavior," *British Journal of Psychology,* XLIII (1952), 1–9.

————. "Learning Theory and Abnormal Fixations," *Psychological Review,* LX (1953), 111–16.

————. *Psychotherapy by Reciprocal Inhibition.* Stanford: Stanford University Press, 1958.

Wyneken, C., "Über das Stottern und dessen Heilung," *Zeitschrift für rationelle Medizin,* XXXI (1868), 1–29.

Young, M. A., "Identification of Stutterers from Recorded Samples of Their 'Fluent' Speech," *Journal of Speech and Hearing Research,* VII (1964), 302–3.

thirteen

ORGANICITY IN STUTTERING

There is something about the sight of an adult in the throes of a severe moment of stuttering which immediately suggests that there must be something organically wrong with him. As he gasps, forces, and jerks, his bizarre spasmodic behavior seems so utterly inappropriate to the task of saying one little word that it is very difficult to believe that he could possibly possess a normal speaking mechanism. This impression, of course, is not given so readily by most beginning young stutterers, but even they have so many broken words, under conditions which hardly seem stressful, that one wonders whether there may not be something basically defective about them too. All of us stumble occasionally in our walking, especially if there is an unexpected doorsill to trip over, but if someone stumbles often and when striding over what appears to be a smooth surface we might infer some fundamental difficulty in coordination. Even though such a person demonstrates that he can at times walk normally, the more often he stumbles, the more sure we are that there is something organically wrong. Indeed, one of the first signs of myasthenia gravis or muscular dystrophy may be this intermittent difficulty in locomotion.

Throughout the centuries this belief in the organic nature of stuttering has persisted—probably because of these first intuitive impressions. For more than a thousand years of recorded history, the tongue was felt to be the villain. Aristotle (384 B.C.) * attributed the disorder to tonguetie or tongue weakness: "the tongue is too sluggish to keep pace with the imagination." Celsus, the most famous of Roman physicians, who lived at the same time as Christ, insisted on gargling and massaging the tongue to strengthen it. Galen (A.D. 200) felt that the tongue was too cold and wet and so lacked strength. In the sixth century, Aetius of Amica recommended cutting the lingual frenum. De Chauliac (1336) felt that a person stuttered because of transitory convulsions and paralysis of the tongue. Mercurialis (1584) described two types of stutterers, those with too wet and those with too dry a tongue, and treated them accordingly with blistering substances or gargles. Francis Bacon (1627) thawed the stiff tongues of stutterers with hot wine, thereby producing more fluency as one might expect.

These older beliefs concerning the tongue as the culprit began to fade with the beginning of the nineteenth century, although some treatments persisted for a time—Itard's ivory fork, Madame Leigh's secret pad of cotton placed under the tonguetip, and the infamous surgical operations of Dieffenbach (1841), which divided or excised chunks from the tongue. By midcentury, this ancient belief in a defective tongue had pretty well subsided, but the quest for organicity had not. Let us trace some of the other theories of organic causation.

Structures other than the tongue were also blamed for stuttering. Hahn (1736) and Morgagni (1761) felt that the hyoid bone was the culprit. Yearsley (1841) attributed the difficulty in speaking to a narrowed airway caused by enlarged tonsils and uvula, and he removed these structures, as many other surgeons have since, in seeking the cure for stuttering. Velpeau, a contemporary of Dieffenbach, and also a tongue slitter, insisted that stuttering was due to an overly small mouth cavity caused by a palate which was too low.

Since even casual observation reveals that the tongues and other oral structures are no different in stutterers than in normal speakers, we find in the early 1800's some of the old writers beginning to speak of malfunctioning rather than defective organs. Thus Bertrand (1828) views the disorder as a "spasmodic nervous affection" and Serre d'Alais (1829) and Arnott (1829) found its source in a chronic "spasm of the glottis." Serre d'Alais described two types of stutterers, those with choretic and those with tetanic spasms and thus laid the foundation for the concepts of clonic and tonic varieties of stuttering still current today. This view of stuttering as a form of chorea (St. Vitis Dance) became very popular during the first half of the nineteenth century, because it superficially explained the intermittent na-

---

* In preparing this historical account, we read as many of the original references as we were able to procure. For the remainder, we have relied primarily on the following sources: Haase (1846), Hunt (1870), Potter (1882), Appelt (1911), Bluemel (1913), Klingbeil (1939), Froeschels (1943b), Larson (1949), and Freund (1966).

ture, the repetitive form, the spasmodic behaviors, and the tremors. It enabled the physicians of the day to throw away the outworn and patently false belief in defective organs but retain the concept of organicity. Moreover, the concept of localized spasm had ancient authority behind it. Avicenna (1037), the most famous of Arabian physicians, from whom many of the medieval European physicians procured their medical knowledge, attributed stuttering to brain lesions which in turn were the cause of the spasms of the epiglottis which produced the stuttering symptoms.

As one might expect from the common appearance of breathing abnormalities in stutterers, many of the older writers located the source of stuttering in the respiratory apparatus or its neurological governors. Thus Sir Charles Bell (1832) speaks of stuttering as a partial chorea resulting in respiratory incoordinations. Becquerel (1847) ascribed the disorder to deficiencies in the nervous centers governing thoracic breathing that caused a premature escape of air. Coen (1875) believed that stutterers were sub-breathers and that the breath spasms were the result of pathological changes in the respiratory apparatus. His remedy was to have the stutterer bare his chest, stand against a wall, and do breathing exercises. Many other writers held similar views and even as recently as 1930 Twitmeyer held that an abnormal state of neurological imbalance, created originally by emotion, produced the breathing abnormalities which triggered stuttering.

Another group of writers attributed stuttering to biochemical differences. Hippocrates (370 B.C.), the father of medicine, believed that stuttering was caused by an accumulation of "black bile," and he applied varices (substances which scarred or blistered the skin) which, by creating skin ulcers, would allow the evil (pus) to drain away. During the Middle Ages, the use of leeches and bloodletting for the relief of stuttering was also based on the belief that there was something wrong with the composition of the blood or "humours." Since the science of biochemistry appeared relatively recently, most of the organic theories that focus on differences in body fluids do not belong in this history. The research bearing on biochemical differences between stutterers and nonstutterers will be reviewed in a later section of this chapter.

In the nineteenth century a few writers began to ascribe stuttering to a malfunctioning or damaged brain. According to Hunt (1870), Rullier (1821) felt that "the cerebral irradiation which follows thought and puts the vocal and articulating organs in action gushes forth so impetuously and rapidly, that it outruns the degree of motility possessed by the muscles concerned, which are thus, as it were, left behind." Hence the latter are thrown into that convulsive and spasmodic state which characterizes stuttering. This quaint description may apply more to cluttering than to stuttering, but it shows the sort of medical thinking current only 150 years ago. Voisin (1821) and Astrie (1824) also believed that stuttering was due to disordered brain function, but their treatment of the disorder consisted of pressing the thumb against the cheek while talking and the use of Itard's fork under the tongue. Lichtinger (1844) distinguished between cerebral and spinal stuttering, and in his work we find the beginnings of the view of defective cortical inhibition of the lower brain centers. Rosenthal (1861) located the cause of the breathing abnormalities shown by stutterers in the malfunctioning of the medulla oblongata caused by psychic shocks during childhood. Kussmaul (1877) defined stuttering as a syllabic dysarthria produced by a lack of coordination of voice, respiration, and articulation, due to neurological deficits. He viewed it as a form of aphasia. Of the three Gutzmanns who wrote extensively on stuttering, H. Gutzmann, Senior, in his book *Das Stottern* (1898), which became the classical work on stuttering of his age, promulgated the concept that there was a deficiency in the cerebral cortex which impaired syllabic coordination and thus produced the clonic and tonic spasms. Gutzmann also collected a series of cases of aphasic stuttering to support his position of cerebral etiology. In this country Swift (1932) attributed stuttering to lesions in the cuneus (a wedge shaped convolution at the base of the occipital lobe of the cortex), which impaired the visual imagery of stutterers and so produced the blockages. Bluemel (1913), however, felt that it was the auditory imagery of stutterers which was deficient, and he defined the disorder as a transient auditory aphasia or amnesia. The stutterer had difficulty speaking because he had temporarily lost the auditory image of the word. Bluemel later dropped this explanation when it was pointed out how frequently stutterers could substitute synonyms, a fact that demolished his theory and led subsequently to his revised theory based on conditioned inhibition.

Most noteworthy of the later neurological explanations of stuttering was the cerebral dominance theory first espoused by Orton (1927) and developed by Travis (1931) and Bryngelson (1935).* Since all of the muscles used to produce speech are paired structures, and those on the right side receive motor impulses originating in the left hemisphere of the cortex while those on the left side from the right hemisphere, and both streams of impulses must be synchronized to produce smooth movement, it was hypothesized that this synchronization could only be achieved if one of the cortical hemispheres had a sufficient margin of dominance to enable it to impose its timing patterns over the other and thereby achieve the desired synchronization. These authors believed that stutterers had lower margins of cerebral dominance than normal speakers and that the thalamic static of accompanying emotion could further reduce that margin. When this occurred, dysynchronies ensued and neurological blockages and spasms resulted. It was an ingenious theory and stimulated much research, some of which seemed to support it, but it fell from grace primarily because homolateral motor tracts were discovered, because both right- and left-handed subjects seemed to have left hemisphere dominance, because the basic research was

---

* According to Kistler (1930) both Sachs and Stier as early as 1911 hypothesized that the battle for predominant control of speech between the right and left hemispheres was the cause of stuttering.

challenged, and because the presumed shift of handedness which had been thought to account for the reduced margin of dominance was not corroborated. One of the basic problems of the theory was that it was untestable except in terms of peripheral laterality. Some recent research which we will review in a later section indicates that a revision of the theory may again find some acceptance.

At about the same time, other organic concepts of the nature of stuttering were presented. Seeking some explanation for the sex ratio, the strong hereditary factor, the apparently poor diadochokinesis of stutterers, and certain biochemical differences brought out in the research of Kopp (1934), Robert West introduced the concepts of spasmophemia and dysphemia. "Stuttering," he said (1943), "is a manifestation of a fundamental atypia, or divergence from human norms, that, though not often interfering with the performance of the basic animal functions of the organism, often, however, interferes with the peculiarly human function of speech. This atypia is not usually adequate to produce stuttering without the complicity of certain contributory factors." West's view of the dysphemic atypia was that it was either a mild or latent epileptiform disorder called pyknolepsy which could be precipitated by various kinds of stress, or a mild "form of subclinical cerebral palsy."

In Europe, Szondi (1932) investigated 100 stutterers, using a variety of neurological and serological tests, and concluded that they were constitutionally different in that 20 per cent showed signs of brain pathology and a high proportion demonstrated other evidences of neurovascular difficulties. Seeman, in a series of publications (1934; 1947; 1959) developed the concept that stuttering was the result of disturbed functioning in the striopallidar system rather than in the cortical centers. He felt that in stutterers there was a basic imbalance in the functioning of the sympathetic and parasympathetic parts of the autonomic nervous system, the sympathetic being overactivated. He writes (Seeman, 1966):

> An attack of stuttering develops as a result of dynamic functional deviations of the striopallidum, the normal activity of which is impaired by acute affective and emotional influences of the subcortical region and thus the coordination of speech movements is impaired. It may thus be said that a paroxysm of stuttering is objectively characterized by an orthosympathetic reaction (p. 430).

As this quotation indicates, Seeman's theory should really not be included in the category of organic theories since the disturbed functioning of the autonomic nervous system is seen as the result of strong emotional experiences. We have seen fit to mention it here primarily because its emphasis on the striopallidum offers another site for organic etiology. Moreover, in his emphasis on hereditary factors, Seeman often seems to be implying some sort of organic predisposition.

Another organic theory was advocated by Weiss (1950;), who held that stuttering always stemmed from cluttering and that the latter was an inherited state of language imbalance based perhaps upon submicroscopic lesions in the striopallidum, as Seeman maintained, or upon delayed maturation of the nervous system. A related point of view |is| that of Karlin (1947) who theorized that stuttering was due to delayed myelinization of the nerve sheathes.

As we review this historical material, we are impressed by the ludicrousness of some of the beliefs that were stated so positively by the greatest authorities of the past, and we become highly aware of the limits of our own present information concerning the organicity of stuttering. We simply do not have the basic understanding of how motoric speech is organized and programmed in time. None of our predecessors' organic theories make much sense today, and those that are still current are more speculative than substantiated. Nevertheless, the continuing quest for an acceptable, organically based theory of stuttering is impressive. The sex ratio, the hereditary features, the disordered timing, and other aspects of stuttering impel certain workers in each generation to stage a new assault on what is basically wrong with the stutterer. It seems too early now to discard entirely the possibility that an organic factor is present, as our review of the research will probably demonstrate. We are currently in one of the oscillatory swings of theory in which stuttering is thought to be completely without organicity. We should perhaps be warned by some of the newer work on schizophrenia, long considered to be a functional disorder, which indicates that organic factors may indeed be very important in its genesis and maintenance. All the evidence is not in, and we should withhold judgment. We were born too soon to be sure that stuttering is merely learned or neurotic behavior. All the determinants of behavior are not environmentally produced. We may yet find the outlines of a constitutional predisposition to stutter.

The research on hereditary factors. Many of the early writings on the hereditary causes of stuttering reported the familial history in fairly general terms. Stutterers were interviewed to determine how many of their immediate ancestors or siblings stuttered. No control groups were used. Only the unanimity of their findings make them worth mentioning here. Mygind (1898) reported that 42 per cent of his stutterers had stutterers in their families. Makuen (1914) reported that 39 per cent of 1000 stutterers had relatives who stuttered. Scripture and Glogau (1916) found that 25 per cent of their stutterers had stuttering relatives. Bryant (1917) gives a figure of 50 per cent for an incredible 20,000 patients; Tromner in Germany (1929) raised the ante to 80 per cent. In England, Boome and Richardson (1932) found 34 per cent of 522 of their cases had stuttering "heredity." Bryngelson and Clark (1933) reported 75 per cent of the 127 stuttering Minnesota children they personally examined had stuttering in their immediate families. Abe (1934) lists 24 per cent of 225 stuttering Japanese soldiers as reporting familial incidence. Some 42 per cent of the stutterers examined by

Ingebregtsen (1936) had stutterers in their immediate families. Meyer (1945) found ten times more stuttering ancestors in the families of stutterers. Freund (1952) reported that 88 immediate relatives of 121 stutterers also stuttered and that other neurotic signs were found among them. Otsuki (1958) claimed that 42 per cent of his stuttering subjects showed familial incidence. Streifler and Gumpertz (1955) discovered stuttering in the immediate relatives of 56 per cent of their stutterers. In France, De Ajuriaguerra, Diakine, Gobineau, Narlian, and Stambak (1958) found that 31 of their 92 stutterers had family histories of stuttering. Luchsinger (1959) found a family history of stuttering in 33 per cent of his 272 Swiss stutterers. Hirschberg (1965) found 51 per cent of 151 Hungarian stutterers to have family histories of stuttering. Mussafia (1964) found 39 per cent of 241 Belgian stutterers to have stuttering in their immediate families. Daskalov (1962) gives a figure of 32 per cent for the familial history of stuttering in 850 Russian stutterers.

One of the first hereditary studies using control groups of normal speakers was performed by Wepman (1939). He found that 71 per cent of 127 stutterers reported stuttering in the immediate family as compared to only 13 per cent of the controls. Bryngelson and Rutherford (1937) reported that 46 per cent of 74 stutterers had stuttering relatives as compared with only 18 per cent of the 74 controls. In a further compilation of data Bryngelson (1935) compared 152 stutterers with their controls and found that stuttering occurred in 51 per cent of the stutterer's families but in only 13 per cent of the normal speakers. Pierce and Lipcon (1959), in a careful study, compared the family histories of 36 Naval stuttering recruits with 36 matched normal speakers and found that 20 of the stutterers had family members who stuttered but none of the normal speakers had family members who stuttered. Johnson, (1959) in his onset of stuttering study found that over five times as many parents of stutterers reported stuttering in their immediate families as compared with that reported by parents of the normal speaking children, the difference being significant beyond the one percent level of confidence. Stutterers had five times as many stuttering fathers, for example, as did their normal speaking controls.

Probably the most carefully done research was that performed by Andrews and Harris (1964). They reported that the risk of stuttering was 5.8 per cent for mothers, 19.1 per cent for fathers; 8.4 per cent for sisters; and 20 per cent for brothers. When their stutterers were compared with the controls, 38 per cent of the stutterers had family histories of stuttering as compared with only 1.4 per cent for the controls. We have been able to find only a single study in all the literature which reports no greater incidence of stuttering in the families of stutterers than in the families of normal speakers. It is a questionnaire study of college students by Sheehan and Martyn (1966). They found no statistically significant differences in reported instances of familial stuttering between recovered stutterers and those who had not recovered. Though no data whatsoever are given, the authors also state that there were no differences in familial history of stuttering between either group of stutterers and their normal speaking controls.

The role of imitation or morbid family attitudes has often been used to explain the tendency for stuttering to run in families. This does not seem to be supported by most of the researches. Nelson (1939) investigated the familial tendency (siblings, parents, grandparents) to stutter in two groups of 204 each, one composed of stutterers and the other of normal speakers. No significant difference in incidence was found between the percentages of those from either group who had had close association with other stutterers. There were 58 stutterers who had stutterers in their immediate families but who had never had personal contact with them. In another study, by Andrews and Harris (1964), 13 of 80 stutterers as compared with only one of 80 controls had a positive family history of stuttering. In addition, 17 of 80 other stutterers had a positive family history with prolonged contact with another stuttering member of the family, but there were no normal speakers in this category. In a much quoted investigation, Gray (1940) compiled the family trees of two branches of a stuttering family for five generations. The Iowa branch had eight stutterers, three former stutterers, and 16 nonstutterers; the Kansas branch had only one stutterer and 16 nonstutterers. The differences in frequency of stuttering (although even the Kansas branch with its one stutterer represents an incidence of 4 per cent which is greater than in the general population) was attributed to semantogenesis—as a family curse.

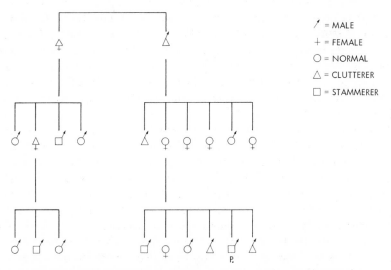

Figure 14. Mixed heredity of cluttering and stuttering. *(From D. A. Weiss: Cluttering, p. 52.)*

Two other family tree studies are available. The first is by Gedda, Branconi, and Bruno (1960). Two male twins who stuttered had a paternal uncle, a maternal grandfather and a great uncle who stuttered. Another such study is given by Weiss (1964) which is illustrated in Figure 14. Weissova and Handzel (1962) report a fascinating study of a family characterized by parathyroid gland insufficiency and stuttering. The father and all three sons had the same parathyroid gland deficiency and also stuttered.

One of the ways to overcome the objection that a family tradition of stuttering or social imitation may explain the familial trends of stuttering is to study the incidence of the disorder in twins. Stuttering has often been cited as occurring frequently in twinning families. In one of the first twin studies, Seemann (1937) found that of 14 monozygotic (identical) twins, nine of them were stutterers, whereas of five dizygotic (fraternal) twins only one child stuttered. Luchsinger (1944) found that if stuttering occurs in monozygotics it occurs in both, whereas in dizygotics it occurs in only one. Nelson, Hunter, and Walter (1945) found that of 200 twin pairs, 20 per cent stuttered, a much higher incidence than in the normal population. They also found that of the identical twins, 14 per cent stuttered as compared with 22 per cent of the fraternal twins. However, Graf (1955), in a study conducted in Iowa found only 21 of 1104 twins who stuttered, an incidence of 1.9 per cent, only about twice as high as in the normal population.

It has been suggested repeatedly by various authors that the family strain of stuttering is strongly associated with cluttering. Freund (1952) studied the families of 95 stutterers and the families of 26 "stutterer-clutterers." In the first group he found 36 stammerers (over a third) and 12 tachylalics (individuals with very hasty speech). Of the stutterer-clutterers, there were 12 stutterers (almost one half) and ten others who had tachylalia. Berry (1937) found that there was a tendency for stuttering to occur more in families containing twins and also that in families containing both twins and siblings, it occurred more frequently among the twins. Luchsinger and Arnold (1965) gave family trees showing the high prevalence of both stuttering and cluttering in these families. Pfändler (1952) summarizes the genetic studies on stuttering and cluttering and concludes, as we do, that it is very difficult to disregard this evidence of some constitutional factor.

In addition to these researches we can add an unpublished study of our own. Over the course of years, we have been collecting data on the children of the stutterers with whom we have worked. In the course of their therapy, some of them met and later married other stutterers receiving treatment. We can report that in all but one of 14 married pairs of stutterers (in which both mates stuttered) at least one child stuttered. Of the total number of their children (29), 20 of them went through a period of stuttering sufficiently severe to have their parents bring them to us for examination and recommendations. This is a tremendously high incidence.

We also recently went through our case files selecting at random 30 former cases (all males) who married normal speaking women and for whom we were able to find information concerning the children. Of their 54 children, 19 stuttered, although only 2 persisted. The only similar report in the literature is that provided by Andrews and Harris (1964), who found six families with two stutterers among the antecedents and collaterals (grandparents and uncles or aunts) and five families in which a parent and grandparent stuttered. We need careful and extensive research extending over three generations before we can be sure of the mode of transmission, if genetic influences are in fact present. At present we cannot say with certainty whether the tendency to stutter is carried by a dominant or recessive gene or whether polygenesis is involved. It does seem probable that certain strains of stuttering are determined in part by inheritance.

BRAIN DAMAGE

There are many studies on brain damage as a factor in the etiology of stuttering. Much of it, however, consists of individual case studies, reports, or uncontrolled investigations. Moreover, just what sort of effect the brain damage has on the sequencing of speech is rarely if ever made clear. Nevertheless, the persistence of the idea that some organic or neurological substrate, possibly a result of brain damage, underlies at least some stuttering, requires that we examine this material.

In his survey of the early literature before 1900, Maas (1946) mentions case studies by Kussmaul, Cornil, Dejerine, and Pick in which stuttering began in adulthood as the result of injuries to the skull and brain. Froeschels (1919) described the case of a young soldier with aphasia and clonic-tonic stuttering brought on by an injury to the temporal lobe. Szondi (1932) used various neurological tests (and measurements of skull size!) and found that 20 per cent of his stutterers showed "signs" of organic damage. Peacher and Harris (1946) mention cases of stuttering in soldiers brought on by combat injuries to the head. Göllnitz (1955) found evidence of cerebral lesions in many young stutterers. Böhme (1968) found that the incidence of stammering in 802 children and adults with cerebral lesions was 19.3 per cent.

There are many accounts of stuttering onset occurring after head injuries in adults. Froeschels (1931) describes a man who began to stutter at the age of 68 after a stroke. He also reported two other aphasic cases in which the aphasia was followed by stuttering. Warren and Akert (1964) report the occurrence of stuttering following frontal lobe lobotomy or lobectomy. Abbott, Due, and Nosik (1943) give accounts of stuttering resulting from blast injuries. Some of these effects may possibly be similar to those produced by Brickner (1940) and Penfield and Rasmussen (1949) who stimulated the cortex electrically in conscious patients and were able to produce repetitions of sounds and syllables or arrest of phonation in epileptics.

STUTTERING IN APHASIA

The appearance of stuttering, or something closely resembling it, following a cerebral trauma that resulted in aphasia has been repeatedly observed. Some examples are those of Head (1926), Nielson (1942), Eisenson (1947), Granich (1947), and Wepman (1947). More recently Arend, Handzel, and Weiss (1962) describe very carefully the changes in speech in two cases of aphasia; they note that stuttering increased and decreased along with the other aphasic symptoms. One of the most interesting case reports is that by McKnight (1936) in which the author, herself an aphasic, describes in detail the development of her stuttering difficulties. An impressive review of all the literature on aphasia and stuttering by Shtremel (1963) makes it very clear that stuttering may be one of the sequellae of aphasia. Shtremel also presents careful studies of three cases. Two of these developed speech dysparaxias and subsequently stuttering following head contusions. In the third case, the pathology was due to a cerebral tumor which, when removed, eliminated the stuttering. All of the lesions in these cases were in the left parietal lobe.

STUTTERING IN EPILEPSY

A greater incidence of stuttering among epileptics has also been reported but the evidence is not impressive. Harrison (1947) reported a large number of stutterers in an epileptic colony. In similar settings, however, Barbara (1946) found an incidence of 2.4 per cent and Wise, quoted in Freund (1955), found only 1.6 per cent. Streifler and Gumpertz (1955) report a stuttering incidence of one per cent among the epileptics seen in their neurological clinic. A particularly fascinating study is that by Guillame, Mazars, and Mazars (1957) in which three stuttering cases are described as having epileptic or convulsive symptoms. Surgery for the first case excised the focal cortical areas responsible for the epileptic discharges and the stuttering stopped. Anticonvulsant medication reduced the stuttering almost completely in the other two cases. In four stutterers, Jones (1966) found that a similar remission of stuttering occurred following brain surgery to remove brain tumors or other brain pathologies. West's (1958) speculations concerning pyknolepsy as the core of much stuttering have been challenged recently by Hamre and Wingate (1967), who show clearly the basic differences between stuttering behaviors and those of the petit mal type sometimes called pyknolepsy.

OTHER BRAIN DAMAGE

Stuttering has also been attributed to injuries or abnormalities in the functioning of *noncortical areas* of the brain. A much higher incidence of stuttering is reported by Palmer and Osborn (1938), and Rutherford (1946) for the cerebral palsied (in which extrapyramidal pathology is involved). Gerstmann and Schilder (1921) described the onset of stuttering after encephalitis. Goda (1961) gives a case study of a child whose stuttering appeared subsequent to spinal meningitis. Anton Schilling (1956) describes a case in which Rh damage to the brainstem resulted in chorea with severe stuttering appearing later. We could report several others from our own files. However, it was Seeman (1934) who first constructed a theory of the nature and cause of stuttering based on the malfunctioning of the subcortical areas of the brain—specifically that which serve the autonomic nervous system. His neurological theory of stuttering, one which is remarkably sophisticated, and, if its assumptions are correct, does explain the core behavior of stuttering and the way in which it is affected by emotion. In this early article he summarizes the research of others and presents evidence in 85 per cent of 260 stutterers that the respiratory and phonatory and other functions of the striopalladum were disturbed.

Generally speaking, Seeman believes that the sympathetic part of the autonomic nervous system becomes hyperactive, in part because of emotional stress or because of lack of inhibition from the cortex, and that this produces disturbances in all of the fundamental processes on which speech is based, i.e., respiration, phonation, and sequencing. Sovak (1935) gave stutterers adrenalin which increases sympathetic arousal and found that his stutterers got worse, while pilocarpin, which activates the parasympathetic system, caused a reduction in stuttering. Seeman (1941) found that 235 stutterers had shorter phonation times and related this to heightened activity of the sympathetic nervous system. Sovak (1935) presented a series of cases of stutterers who seemed to show increased sympathetic irritability.

Sedlacek (1947–48) studied the solar and oculocardiac reflexes of 229 stutterers. These reflexes (which are set off by sudden pressure on the carotid sinus or solar plexus) cause differential changes in pulse rate according to the presumed irritability of the sympathetic or parasympathetic nervous system. Although Sedlacek found that some of the stutterers (13 per cent) showed normal responses, more of them (34 per cent) showed hyperactive sympathetic systems, and the remainder showed either vagotonic or ambivalent responses. The act of stuttering produced almost the same effect on the pulse as the punch to the solar plexus in 98 per cent of the cases. Other evidence, providing some possible though indirect support for Seeman's theories, is found in the pupillometric studies by Gardner (1937). Gardner photographed the pupils of normal speakers and stutterers during silence and speaking and found that the normal speakers either maintained the usual size of the pupils or constricted them, while 100 per cent of the stutterers showed dilation of the pupils while in the act of stuttering. Dilation or increase in size of pupils, however, usually occurs during emotion or sympathetic stimulation and cannot be viewed only in organic terms.

Luchsinger (1943) repeated Gardner's experiment but also studied the pupillary responses in silence and silent calculation as well as in speech. The normal speakers showed no differences in pupillary diameters, but 14 out of 15 stutterers showed pupillary contraction rather than dilation both in silent calculation and in speaking, thus indicating that something other than an anxiety neurosis must be present. In later studies, Luchsinger (1954; 1959) showed that when dilation did occur, it occurred just prior to stuttering and probably reflected specific word fears. Jost and Sontag's (1944) research with children (along with the genetic research in creating strains of anxious and nonanxious rats) shows that certain strains of stutterers may be more prone to autonomic reactivity than most normal speakers or than other strains of stutterers. We certainly find it difficult to accept, on the basis of the presently available research, the view that most stuttering is caused by lesions in the striopallidum or in its malfunctioning. Nevertheless, there may be future pay dirt in these hills.

DISEASE SEQUELLAE

Berry (1938) surveyed the medical histories of 430 stutterers and 462 controls and found that the stutterers had significantly more diseases of the respiratory system and more convulsive disorders than the controls. Kanner (1942) reports stuttering as part of the sequellae of encephalitis and that in juvenile paresis "There was a seemingly 'logoclonic' repetition of the same word or word fragment." Schilling's (1956) case, cited above in which stuttering developed out of chorea and a lesion in the striatum should be recalled here too. Boland (1951) found more instrument births among 209 stutterers than occur in the general population. Opposed to these earlier studies are the more careful and later ones of Johnson (1959) and Andrews and Harris (1964), who found no differences either in birth injuries or diseases.

ELECTROENCEPHALOGRAPHIC
ABNORMALITIES

A fairly substantial amount of research has dealt with the examination of electroencephalographic (EEG) records of stutterers. As is now well known, the brain as a whole produces rhythmical electrical discharges, beginning in the occipital areas of the cortex and sweeping forward into the frontal areas. At rest, an alpha rhythm of about eight to ten waves per second occurs, and these are large in amplitude. When the brain is stimulated, smaller and faster and more irregular waves occur. These can be picked up and recorded with amplification from electrodes placed on or in the scalp. EEG abnormalities are frequently shown in epilepsy, or other disorders due to brain damage or malfunctioning, in the form of brief bursts of electrical potential (spikes), slow wave patterns, focal areas of abnormality, bilateral phase differences, and various forms of dysrhythmias.

Reports of abnormal EEGs must be considered with caution since about ten to 15 per cent of presumably normal individuals show them, especially when triggered by overbreathing (hyperventilation) or by intermittent flashes of light (photic stimulation). Unfortunately, the techniques used in recording and in evaluating abnormality have varied from investigator to investigator. Some researchers used hyperventilation or photic stimulation; others did not. Some investigators recorded from one cortical hemisphere; others from both. Some used monopolar electrodes; others used bipolar ones. Although more EEG abnormalities seem to be found among the younger than the older subjects, the age of the stutterers was frequently disregarded. Far too often no control groups were used.

It should also be mentioned that the absence of EEG abnormality (when scalp electrodes are used) may not indicate the true state of affairs since Kiloh and Osselton (1961) report that intense epileptic discharges may be missed by surface or scalp electrodes but may be picked up by electrodes inserted only one millimeter below the cortical surface. In many of the studies, it is difficult to determine just what the criteria of abnormality are. Moreover visual inspection of EEG records may fail to reveal true differences which appear when autocorrelation or crosscorrelation techniques are applied. Finally, the authors' interpretations of their data often leave the seeker of the truth completely baffled. With these considerations in mind we now report the experiments roughly in the order in which they were published.

Travis and Knott (1936) found no major differences in EEGs between their 17 stutterers and 19 controls in silence or speech. Two of their cases, however, showed spikes which occurred after the moments of stuttering. Travis and Malamud (1937) compared EEGs of normal speakers, stutterers, and schizophrenics and found no major differences. Freestone (1942) compared 20 adult stutterers with their controls. The stutterers showed larger waves during stuttering than during fluent speech and more waves in free speech than in silence. The shift from silence to speech in terms of interruption to the alpha waves was more marked in the normals. Freestone attributed these findings to the stutterers' tendency to undergo states of reduced consciousness.

Lindsley (1940) examined the EEGs of 65 normal children and two severe stutterers, recording them from both hemispheres of the cortex. He found that, in the stutterers, periods of asynchronization between the EEGs on the right and left hemisphere in the occipital and parietal areas and unilateral

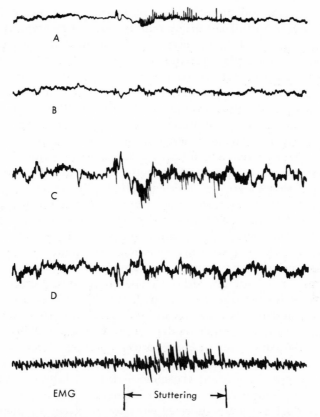

Figure 15. Electroencephalographic recording made during stuttering on the word "problem." A. Left Central; B. Right Central; C. Left Temporal; D. Right Temporal; E. Integrated EMG.

blockings or phase reversals preceded almost every recorded stuttering episode. Rheinberger, Karlin, and Berman (1943) found no differences in EEGs between a very small sample of stutterers and controls. Douglass (1943) compared the EEGs of 20 stutterers and normal speakers and found no differences between stuttering and fluent speech in the stutterers, but he did find some unilateral blocking of the alpha rhythm in silence which did not appear in the normals. His findings were corroborated by Knott and Tjossem (1943) with a similar group of subjects. Scarborough (1943), recording from only the left hemisphere, found no differences between stutterers and normals.

Luchsinger and Landolt (1951), in the first of many European studies, compared the EEGs of stutterers and clutterers and found that almost 90 per cent of the latter group showed abnormalities but that the stutterers generally had normal encephalograms. Dew (1952) recorded the EEGs of stutterers awake and asleep, and reported that stutterers showed fewer alpha waves in sleep. Landolt and Luchsinger (1954) and Luchsinger and Landolt (1951) found that there were many more abnormal EEGs in clutterers than in stutterers and more in stutterer-clutterers (96 per cent) than in "pure" stutterers. In this last group only two of 21 had atypical EEGs. Streifler and Gumpertz (1955), however, could not find any such marked differences between their stutterers and clutterers. In about 35 per cent of both their groups, pathological EEG records were obtained, and the authors reported that of 100 normal speakers, only 15 per cent had similar EEG abnormalities. Murphy (1952) examined the EEGs of 30 male adult stutterers and their controls under conditions of rest, and during frustration and recovery in a listening task, and measured the amount of alpha wave activity from both hemispheres. No differences appeared in silence, both groups showing synchronous alpha waves in both hemispheres. However, the stuttering group showed greater interhemispheric differences in reactivity to frustration, and they were slower to recover normal EEG displays. Bente, Schönhärl, and Krump (1956) report that 59 per cent of their German stutterers showed EEG abnormalities. Busse and Clark (1957) found only three of 27 stuttering children with EEG abnormalities. Knott, Correll, and Shepherd (1959), using photic stimulation, found no EEG differences between stutterers and nonstutterers, although one group of stutterers showed the kind of EEG activity characteristic of high anxiety subjects. Pierce and Lipcon (1959) compared the EEG recordings of 36 stuttering Naval recruits with their controls and found no differences. Graham and Brumlik (1961), using hyperventilation and sleep, reported more EEG abnormality in their stutterers than in their controls and also that the five of their more severe stutterers showed the greatest EEG abnormalities. Schilling (1960) found a correlation of abnormal EEG activity with diaphragmatic tremors and abnormalities during silence in children who stuttered. In another study, Schilling (1962), found that 31 per cent of a large number of stutterers had definitely abnormal electroencephalograms, and 27 per cent borderline abnormalities. Five per cent of them showed spikes although none were manifest epileptics. Moravek and Langova (1962) found more EEG abnormalities in clutterers than in stutterers and more in stutterers than in normal speakers.

Langova and Moravek (1964) found abnormal encephalograms in 16 per cent of stutterers, 39 per cent of stutterer-clutterers, and 50 per cent of "pure" clutterers. Schönhärl and Bente (1960) analyzed 400 EEG records of stutterers. Of these, 54 per cent showed dysrhythmias or spike disturbances. They found that the younger stutterers, aged 5-12, showed more generalized abnormalities. This age difference, indicating that younger stutterers (9-10 years) have more EEG abnormalities than older ones (11-15 years), has also been demonstrated by Fritzell, Petersen, and Sellden (1965) in Sweden. They found too that stutterers as a group have fewer normal electroencephalograms than their controls. Sutu, Mironescu, Cocinschi, Tirziu, and Miscoia (1969) showed that the EEG abnormalities in young stutterers were present before they developed avoidance, struggle, or neurotic behaviors. Hirschberg (1965), in Hungary, found that 60 per cent of 91 stutterers had abnormal EEGs. Negative EEGs were found for only 36 cases. EEGs characteristic of seizures were found in 15 subjects. Cali, Pisani, and Tagliareni (1965) procured EEG records from 58 Italian stutterers ages 3-16. Among them they found only 16 normal tracings. Of the 42 abnormal records, most again were found in the younger age groups. Six of these had focal asymmetries and dysrhythmias of the epileptic type although the children were not epileptic.

In Austria, Schmoigl and Ladisch (1967), excluding all cases in which a cluttering component seemed present, found abnormal EEGs in 70 per cent of 50 stutterers. Six per cent had spikes in their recordings. In this country, Fox (1966) compared 13 adult stutterers with their matched controls during normal speech, simulated stuttering, and silence with eyes opened and when closed. She found no major differences. However, Sayles (1966), in a very careful investigation using hyperventilation, intermittent photic stimulation, and sleep with 23 stutterers and their controls found highly significant differences between the groups in amount of EEG abnormalities. Thirty per cent of his stutterers showed EEG abnormalities as compared with only eight per cent of the normal speakers. Stromsta (1964) compared bilateral EEG recordings of 15 adult stutterers and their controls using both autocorrelation and crosscorrelation. No differences appeared when autocorrelation was employed, but the two groups could be significantly differentiated by crosscorrelation. The normal speakers showed more synchrony in the alpha rhythms in the two sides of the cortex than the stutterers.

It is difficult to summarize these findings. Fourteen of the experiments found EEG abnormalities in stutterers and eight did not, although such a simple count is next to worthless since the studies vary so widely in methodology. Our impression, after critically evaluating and comparing them, is that a rather strong case has been made for the presence of atypical EEGs in a larger number of stutterers than would be expected by chance and that younger stutterers are more likely to show them than older ones. It also seems tenable that their significance for stuttering may lie in their interference with the bilateral gating of the efferent and afferent nervous impulses required for smooth motoric speech. What produces these abnormal EEGs is less clear, but they may imply some sort of neurological damage or malfunctioning.

CEREBRAL DOMINANCE

The theory that a lack of cerebral dominance creates a mistiming of the motor impulses to the bilateral speech muscles and thus produces stuttering was first formulated by Stier (1911) and by Sachs (1924), but it received its early acceptance through the writings of Orton (1927) and Travis (1931). More recently it lost its former popularity largely because of research which cast doubt on the scanty evidence that stutterers showed mixed sidedness or had been shifted in their handedness. We now know that peripheral sidedness or handedness does not always reflect central lateral dominance and now, for the first time, we have new ways of identifying the latter. Accordingly, the cerebral dominance theory of stuttering, so often slaughtered, is again showing signs of new life.

We begin with the study of R. K. Jones (1966) which we mentioned earlier. Jones, a neurosurgeon, was preparing to operate on four patients who had stuttered severely since childhood but who had recently developed brain pathology, and he had decided to use a new technique pioneered by Wada (1949). The technique consisted of injecting sodium amytol directly into first the right and then the left carotid arteries while the patient is conscious and talking. As Wada and Rasmussen (1960) demonstrated, when this drug is introduced into the system in this way, a temporary aphasia results, provided the artery serving the dominant hemisphere of the brain is the one injected. To his surprise, Jones found that all four of these stutterers developed transient aphasia when the drug was injected into *either* the right or left carotid arteries, thus indicating that they had a bilateral cortical control of speech, that there were "speech centers" in both hemispheres. Jones then performed his surgery on the damaged hemisphere and found that complete remission of stuttering took place in all his patients. After recovery, he administered the sodium amytol as before and discovered that now the exstutterers became aphasic only when one artery was injected (the one serving the nonoperated hemisphere). They no longer had cortical representation for speech in both hemispheres but only in one. Jones remarks that "the results on stammering of a one-sided operation for unrelated lesions in these four patients were quite startling and can only be explained by the view that stammering is associated with an interference by one hemisphere with the speech performance of the other." No recurrence of stuttering was noted after periods ranging from 15 months to three years.

Another earlier study by Guillaume, Mazars, and Mazars (1957) had reported a similar complete recovery from stuttering in an epileptic after surgical removal of an epileptogenic focus in the right temporal lobe. They write:

> During this operation, when we were starting the resection of the fusiform gyrus, we were astonished to hear the subject articulate with extraordinary ease and to express his surprise at no longer stuttering. Following this intervention, the patient was entirely cured of his epileptic attacks and his stammer.

Another related case study from Russia is provided by Shtremel (1963) in which a normal speaking adult began to stutter and showed aphasic symptoms at the age of 51. After surgical removal of a tumor ("as large as a Mandarin orange") the stuttering disappeared, although some aphasic difficulties remained.

The fact of cerebral dominance is indisputable. In the majority of people, including some of those who are left-handed, the left cerebral hemisphere appears to be the one dominant in the integration of speaking. Penfield and Rasmussen (1949) and Penfield and Roberts (1959) show that approximately two thirds of left-handed persons have speech localized in the left hemisphere as have right-handed persons. According to Goodglass and Quadfasel (1964) about 60 per cent of left-handed aphasics had their pathology in the left hemisphere rather than in the right.

Benson and Geschwind (1968) review studies which show that there are anatomical asymmetries on the upper surface of the left temporal lobe which might be responsible for left hemispheric dominance, and they even suggest that some lefthandedness might be the result of early lesions in the left hemisphere causing a shift to an unnatural right brain dominance. According to Zangwill (1960) in early childhood, the usual left hemispheric dominance for speech does not seem to be fully developed or stabilized and if cerebral insults occur in one hemisphere, the other may assume the speech function. This has been shown rather clearly by Basser (1962). If the brain damage occurs before the onset of speech, it does not seem to matter whether the injury is in either the left or right hemispheres so far as the later acquisition of speech is concerned. After the onset of speech, however, and especially in adulthood, injuries to the left hemisphere disturb speech greatly. Damage to the right hemisphere does not. Nevertheless, using the Wada techniques, Branch, Milner, and Rasmussen (1964) and others have shown that in certain adult persons, usually the left-handed or ambidextrous, both cerebral hemispheres may contain integrating mechanisms for speech. Hécaen and de Ajuriaguerra (1963) and Zangwill (1960) feel that this hemispheric ambilaterality may be a hereditary trait.

According to modern cerebral dominance theory, stutterers (or a subpopulation thereof) do not have a single hemispheric representation for speech. They have ambilateral dominance like some of the left-handers and ambidextrous persons described by Branch, Milner, and Rasmussen (1964). Without a single dominant center to organize the timing of the bilateral impulses to the peripheral paired speech muscles, the motor sequences tend to be disorganized or interrupted. From this point of view, the cessation of stuttering, once one of the competing hemispheric control centers is damaged by surgery, perhaps becomes understandable. Also, the onset of stuttering, occurring as it does during the years when a single hemispheric center for the control of speech has not yet been developed, or stabilized, also makes some minor sense. If girls mature faster than boys, they might develop a unilateral dominance earlier, and so show less stuttering. Unfortunately, we do not yet have any definitive corroboration of this dual hemispheric control of speech. We have only the hints provided by Jones and the other cases studied. If a large number of stutterers could be given the Wada carotid injection test, the doubt could be resolved, but this may never be done since the technique has a morbidity of about three per cent. Even in his declining years this author would not be willing to play that Russian roulette in the interest of science!

PERIPHERAL SIDEDNESS IN STUTTERERS

It might be appropriate, however, to review the research to determine whether or not stutterers show a greater percentage of left-handedness and ambidexterity than normals, since these seem to accompany known hemispheric ambilaterality more than right-handedness. The whole literature on handedness is full of hazards as well as hints, probably because hand preference can be influenced by many environmental factors. The downfall of the Orton-Travis theory came because it was tested in terms of handedness, a peripheral and motor function, and because some of its advocates blamed stuttering on a forced shift in handedness, a most irrelevant concept since hemispheric dominance does not always reflect itself in peripheral sidedness.

One hates to start digging again in the old boneyard of the laterality research on stuttering.* Let us see what we can unearth. First of all, dominance is peripherally represented not only by hand preference but also by foot, ear, and eye preference, all of which have been included under the term sidedness. (In addition to these motor aspects of cerebral dominance, there is also some evidence of laterality differences in perception.) Hand preference has been the one motor aspect most commonly investigated. Our first question is whether stutterers tend to fall into the categories of left-handed and ambidextrous, since it is in these that central ambilaterality (two-hemispheric control center for speech) has been demonstrated. Unfortunately hand preference is not always easy to determine. As Van Riper (1935) and Subirana (1964) showed, few individuals are completely right-handed or left-handed. Using some overly demanding criteria, the latter author found only eight per cent to be completely right-handed and only one single individual out of the 600 subjects he examined was completely left-handed. Most of the reports indicate an incidence of from eight to 15 per cent of left-handedness in the general population.

Some evidence of a hereditary factor exists in handedness (Bryngelson, 1935) and identical twins usually show opposite hand preference. This has been used to explain the occurrence of left-handed individuals, the right-handed individual being thought to be the surviving member of a pair of embryonic twins. Animals are also predominantly right-handed (Peterson, 1931) but left-handed and ambidextrous rats are to be found. (We had a left-handed rat once that starved to death rather than reach for food readily available to its right paw, and we achieved a strain of completely left-handed mice after seven generations of selective breeding.) Adequate measurement of handedness is difficult. Van Riper (1935) devised an angle

---

* It reminds this author too vividly of his early treatment when he tried to become left-handed, wearing a cast on his right arm for months and doing a daily quota of 50 pages of simultaneous talking and writing with his left hand. Subsequently he returned to his original right-handedness after he lost a fat trout while fly fishing, and he has not used his left hand since. No change in his fluency occurred.

board device which is one of the few tests that permit the quantitative measurement of *how* left-handed or *how* right-handed a person is. Although the distribution of hand preference is highly skewed in favor of the right hand by any of the methods used to determine it, most individuals show mixed laterality rather than complete unilaterality. Footedness and eyedness are even more mixed.

The early studies are difficult to evaluate since the data were obtained by questionnaire. Representative of these is one by Ballard (1912) who stated that four times as many stutterers were found among children whose only right-handed activity was in writing as the result of a questionnaire study of 13,000 school children. Another was performed by Quinan (1921; 1938), who reported three times as many stutterers in predominantly left-handed subjects. Bryngelson (1934), using a 20-item hand preference questionnaire with 700 stutterers classified 61 per cent of them as being ambidextrous. Bryngelson and Rutherford (1937) compared 74 stutterers with 74 normal speaking controls. The percentages of right-handed, left-handed, and ambidextrous normal speakers were 75 per cent, 16 per cent, and eight per cent respectively, and for the stutterers the figures were 61 per cent right-handed, four per cent left-handed, and 34 per cent ambidextrous. Bryngelson reported that a very high incidence of shift of handedness in both of these studies had occurred among those stutterers classed as being predominantly right-handed. Hirschberg (1965) stated that of 151 stutterers he found 66 per cent who were right-handed, five per cent left-handed, and four per cent who were ambidextrous. deAjuriaguerra *et al.* (1958) found only 30 per cent of their stutterers as compared with 68 per cent of their normal speakers to be thoroughly right-handed. Also, 51 per cent of the stutterers (ages 11 to 14 years) showed mixed handedness as compared to 21 per cent of the normal speakers.

In an effort to escape the contamination of possible shifts of handedness which may have occurred early in life, several investigators attempted to find other ways of testing handedness than hand preference for writing, shaving, fork-handling, and the like. Orton and Travis (1929) recorded the precedence of the action currents to both forearms in simultaneous contraction; Travis and Herren (1929) repeated this using adduction and abduction of the two hands; Travis (1928) and Jasper (1932) used mirror tracing; Fagan (1932) and Jasper (1932) used simultaneous writing with both hands on a horizontal surface; and Van Riper (1935) employed simultaneous drawing of figures on a winged apparatus which permitted a quantitative measurement of laterality in terms of the angular displacement of the writing surface from the vertical. All of these studies indicated that the performance of a large number of stutterers resembled that of the left-handed or ambidextrous more than it did that shown by right handers.

There are an impressive number of studies using similar procedures which lend doubt to the figures just mentioned. Daniels (1940) gave handedness and speech tests to 1548 college students. Of the 34 left-handers, one was a stutterer; of the 138 who were ambidextrous, four stuttered. Putting it another way, he reported that stuttering was found in 1.1 per cent of the right-handed students, in 2.9 per cent of the ambidextrous, and in 2.9 per cent of the left-handers. Spadino (1941) matched 70 stuttering school children with 70 controls and applied a battery of tests including handedness, eyedness, and footedness. There were no significant differences on any of the tests. Van Dusen (1939) also gave a battery of tests to stutterers and non-stutterers and found no differences. Johnson and King (1942) replicated Van Riper's angle board study and, using a different method of scoring, found no laterality differences between stutterers and nonstutterers. The nonstutterers were unselected with respect to handedness. Pierce and Lipcon (1959), in a small sample, found no differences in handedness between their stutterers and their controls. Streifler and Gumpertz (1955) and Daskalov (1962) in a large sample of 850 stutterers found that the percentage of left-handedness in stutterers approximated that of the normal population. The same lack of differences in laterality between child stutterers and normal speakers was demonstrated by the research of Johnson (1959) and by Andrews and Harris (1964), who did no testing but only questioned the parents of their subjects. In reviewing all this material with due regard to the limitations of methodology it seems apparent that we cannot conclude that stutterers are generally left-handed or ambidextrous, at least insofar as peripheral sidedness is concerned. The question is still unresolved and will remain so until better measures of laterality preference are resolved. This does not mean that differences in *central* ambilaterality do not exist.

SHIFT OF HANDEDNESS

No one has shown that a shift of peripheral handedness can alter central cerebral dominance, and most of the research indicates that the old belief that such a shift can cause stuttering is far from being corroborated. The evidence supporting this belief comes from research which is fairly old. Haefner (1929) found that 24 per cent of 41 children who had been shifted stuttered. Oates (1929) reports an experiment in which 12 subnormal right-handed children were shifted to the left hand; all of them stuttered after five months of such training, and the stuttering disappeared when the training ceased. Fagan (1932) reported that 27 per cent of his stutterers had had their handedness changed; Bryngelson (1935) and Bryngelson and Rutherford (1937) give shift figures ranging from 60 per cent to 70 per cent; Hirschberg (1965) reported that 25 per cent of his stutterers had been shifted.

Opposed is the research of Ojemann (1931) who shifted 23 pure left-handed children in writing and saw no stuttering appear. Daniels (1940) discovered that only one of 20 stutterers had been shifted. Among African stutterers, Aron (1958) found that only two per cent had been shifted in handedness. Daskalov (1962) mentions that none of 114 left-handed individuals began to stutter after being forced to work with the right hand. It should be a simple matter to dispose of this question by simply getting a large population of individuals who have been shifted at various ages and then determining the incidence of stuttering in this group and comparing it with that of a control group which has not been shifted. However, this research has not to our knowledge been performed and so once again we are left with ambiguity instead of ambilaterality.

A very common assertion in this connection has been that the forced shift of handedness when accomplished unpleasantly creates emotional conflicts and these are what causes the stuttering when it does occur. Although plausible, no one has demonstrated that this is true. We have in our files three case studies of boys who deliberately shifted their own handedness to become like their fathers or to become southpaw (left-handed) baseball pitchers and subsequently developed stuttering which then disappeared when they reluctantly went back to right hand usage. In this connection we give a quotation from Bloodstein (1959) who is certainly no advocate of the cerebral dominance theory:

> It is difficult to read certain case reports of children who began to stutter after a shift of handedness, or to study accounts of certain adults who experienced fluency disturbances after enforced use of the nonpreferred hand without being impressed by the possibility that laterality is a factor in some cases (p. 35).

PERCEPTUAL LATERALITY: VISUAL AND TACTILE

The research on handedness and sidedness which we have just been discussing deals with the peripheral evidence of laterality as expressed in motor behavior. The role of laterality on the input side has only recently received any important investigation. Nevertheless we find a few early attempts. Selzer (1933) found a marked lack of visual fusion in his stutterers. A year earlier, Jasper (1932) had investigated the phi phenomenon (the apparent movement between intermittent visual stimuli) between a fixation light and its double images, using right-handed, left-handed, ambidextrous, and stuttering subjects. Right-handed subjects perceive the phi phenomenon movement going to the right; the left-handed see it moving to the left, and the ambidextrous perceive the movement inconsistently in terms of direction. The stutterers performed more like the ambidextrous. Jasper says,

> These results seem to indicate in general that neural organization is expressed in the field of perception as well as in the field of manual preference. The phi phenomenon test of both peripheral and central dominance clearly

demonstrated the lack of unilaterality on the part of stutterers, and it showed a tendency on the part of stutterers to have more ambilaterality than the ambidextrous normal speakers.*

Perceptual laterality has even been demonstrated for tactual experience —primarily pressure. By using sets of Von Frey hairs, the pressure sensitivity of the right and left thumbs has been investigated by Ghent (1961), Weinstein and Sersen (1961), and Kimura (1963). Although lateral dominance has been demonstrated by such means no one has used this test on stutterers.

AUDITORY LATERALITY

Most investigations of laterality in auditory perception have used dichotic listening techniques to demonstrate that when competing messages are presented simultaneously to the two ears, persons with left hemispheric cerebral dominance will be able to recall and perceive the one presented to the right (preferred) ear better than the message presented to the other ear. For those with right central dominance for speech the reverse is found; they too perceive verbal stimuli better when presented to the contralateral ear, showing left ear dominance. The use of the Wada test has corroborated these findings. Other evidence comes from cerebral lesions.

Although each cochlea is represented bilaterally in the cortex, certain anatomical differences have been demonstrated which may account for this lateral dominance. Rosenzweig (1951) for example, administered clicks to a single ear of a cat and measured the resulting cortical potentials, concluding that "At the level of the auditory cortex . . . the population of cortical units representing the contralateral ear is larger than the population representing the ipsilateral ear."

Boone (1959) found that right hemiplegics, given tasks in which they listened with one ear or the other, made many more errors when listening with the left ear than did left hemiplegics with injuries in the right cortical hemispheres. Kimura (1961a) gave patients with known lesions in the right and left temporal lobes stimulation with two digits presented simultaneously to right and left ears. Those with lesions of the left temporal lobe had much poorer digit spans than those with lesions in the right temporal lobe. Bocca and Calearo (1963) and others have shown that tests of discrimination using distorted or interrupted speech as stimuli showed no binaural differences for normal subjects, but significantly depressed scores were found for patients when stimulated in the ear contralateral to the lesion.

Curry (1967) had 25 left-handed and 25 right-handed subjects perform

---

* We spent a year replicating Jasper's experiment and found the same results he did. We feel a real regret that this intriguing finding has been largely forgotten and disregarded.

three dichotic listening tasks, two verbal and one nonverbal. The mean right ear score was higher than the left ear score on the *verbal* tasks, but the left ear score was higher for the nonverbal task, and this held true for both groups, although the difference approached significance only for the right handers. Since other research has indicated that the central organization of verbalization seems to be located usually in the left hemisphere irrespective of peripheral handedness, this may not be too surprising. What might be more important is a recent study by Curry and Gregory (1967) in which 11 of 20 stutterers had higher left ear scores on a dichotic listening task as compared to only five of the normal speaking controls. Moreover the size of the differences between right and left ear scores were significantly smaller for the stutterers. Nonverbal tasks showed no differences. The authors speculate that this may indicate less clear cut cerebral dominance in the stutterers. Kimura (1961b; 1963; 1967), Bryden (1963), Dirks (1964), and Carr (1969) have all shown that when competitive verbal material is fed simultaneously to the two ears, a right ear preference is shown by most speakers. Kimura feels that the "crossed auditory pathways are stronger than the uncrossed and that the dominant temporal lobe (the left one) is more important than the nondominant in the perception of spoken material (Kimura, 1961b, p. 171)." The importance of this research is that we have in this competitive dichotic listening technique a new method for assessing cerebral dominance which looks very promising. The application of the technique in determining the central laterality or ambilaterality of stutterers has just begun.

THE TOMATIS THEORY

This brings us to the lateral dominance theory of Tomatis who explains stuttering as being due to the same sort of perceptual distortion as that produced by delayed auditory feedback. Briefly, Tomatis (1954; 1963) feels that stutterers monitor their speech with the ear opposite that which should be dominant, and that when this is true, the information (feedback) coming in from their vocal output must be shunted intracerebrally before it can be used. He feels that in stutterers there is a lag in transit time due to the stutterer using the wrong "directing" ear. This lag thus produces the same stuttering disruptions that are the result of delayed auditory feedback.

Tomatis (1954) stated that 90 per cent of his stutterers had a hearing loss in the ear which should have been their preferred or directing ear. He claimed that the dominant ear could be ascertained by masking one and then the other ear as the subject is talking. When the rate of speech slows down, it is the directing (dominant) ear that is being masked. To check this, he suggests delaying the feedback to the directing ear until speech slows down. The delay time then presumably equals the intercerebral transference time. Tomatis also claims that this dominant ear is usually on the same side as the dominant eye. Moreover he says that dominance can also be ascertained by masking each ear in turn and then observing changes in voice quality. Tomatis has also devised an "Electronic Ear" which he uses for the treatment of stuttering. Although he has not reported its construction, this device is evidently some sort of binaural hearing aid in which appropriate counter delays are built in. We have been unable to assess his research since its reporting leaves much to be desired.

Some oblique support for Tomatis' theory of stuttering is found in the research of Curry and Gregory (1967) mentioned earlier. Also, Asp (1965), using 15 adult stutterers and their controls, found that the stutterers had significantly longer interaural localization times. He suggests that this time difference might be related to the same sort of fragmenting of speech produced by the delayed auditory feedback apparatus, and that perhaps Tomatis was correct. On the other hand Aimard, Plantier, and Wittlung (1966) challenged Tomatis' statement that the naturally dominant ear of stutterers was hypacusic. Only one of their 14 stutterers showed such a unilateral loss. Also no lateral differences in central auditory perception on a dichotic phonetic integration test was demonstrated in this study. Stromsta (1966) somewhat supported the Tomatis method of discovering the presumably dominant ear. He too found that stutterers and normal speakers both showed significant differences in reading time when one ear was masked.

COORDINATION OF SPEECH MUSCULATURES

Since the motoric sequencing of words is obviously interrupted in the stutterer, it is quite natural to find advocates of the belief that he has his difficulty because he is poorly coordinated. Stuttering has even been called a coordination neurosis. A number of investigators have therefore studied gross body coordination and the coordination of the speech mechanism in stutterers. Many of these studies investigated diadochokinesis and rhythmokinesis, the abilities to move the paired speech musculatures with speed and precision.

An early study by West and Nusbaum (1929) found 25 stutterers sluggish in jaw and eyebrow movements as compared with normal speakers. An apparent overlap with the normal speakers was attributed to "latent stuttering" [sic!]. Blackburn (1931) observed 13 stutterers who were markedly inferior to their controls in regularity and speed of voluntary movements of the tongue, lips, jaw, and diaphragm, but not in arm and hand movements. No such differences in tongue, jaw, or lip movements were noted by Seth (1934), but he did find stutterers inferior in rhythmic movements of the diaphragm. Cross (1936) found no significant difference between 26 stutterers and their controls in the speed and regularity of jaw, lip, and tongue movements, but the stutterers had inferior diaphragmatic control. Hunsley (1937), in a study conceived and directed by Van Riper, investigated the effects of increasing rate on the rhythmic patterning of jaw, lip, tongue, and breathing movements. She found that her 23 stutterers were inferior to their controls in performing these precise silent movement sequences at all levels of rate, and that they showed clonic and tonic blockings.

There are, however, two negative reports. In studies similar to Hunsley's, but using only 15 stutterers and different scoring procedures, Strother and Kriegman (1943; 1944) found no differences of significance. Chworowsky (1952) used the Sylrater to get the diadochokinetic rates of ten Iowa stutterers and their controls for puh, tuh, kuh, and hand-tapping under normal and frustration conditions, finding no differences.

More recently, Rickenberg (1956), in a careful study, procured diadokinetic rates for nine different cv syllables representing lip, tonguetip, and back-tongue coordinations. His 15 stutterers were significantly inferior to their controls for all the syllables. He concludes: "With respect to the rate at which one impulse can be shifted from one group of muscles to its antagonistic group, stutterers are significantly slower than nonstutterers." Zaleski (1965), in Poland, provides the only careful study using a respectable number of subjects—50 stutterers and their controls. Finger tapping and utterance of "pa," "ta," and "ka" were performed while paced metronomically at differing speeds. On both the finger-tapping and speech movements, stutterers were significantly ($p < .01$) inferior to the normal speakers. We should also report here Travis' original study (1934), in which he showed that discrepancies in the arrival times and patterning of action currents in the peripheral bilateral musculatures of speech occurred during stuttering but not during normal speech in stutterers, nor in the speech of normal speakers. Williams (1955) performed a somewhat similar study with different placement of electrodes and using single words and faked stuttering. When instructed to fake stuttering, the normal speakers showed most of the same abnormalities as did the stutterers. These studies need further replication, but both of them can be said to demonstrate that the fine motor coordinations of speech in either "real" or simulated stuttering show disruptions.

After reviewing all these studies, it is difficult not to conclude that stutterers show coordinative deficiency in the timing of their speech musculatures. While there are three negative findings, both on very limited samples, most of the evidence supports the belief that many stutterers have difficulty in such timing.

GROSS MOTOR COORDINATION

Since speech depends on finely coordinated simultaneous and successive muscular contractions and relaxations, it is important to determine if stutterers, or some types of stutterers, are poorly coordinated. The research is not impressive in quality—small groups of assorted stutterers are matched, if indeed they are matched at all, with motley control groups. For example, Kiehn (1935) found that his stutterers were inferior in a water-carrying test. Kasanin (1931) used a selection of tests from the Oseretsky and Kwinte batteries with 50 assorted stuttering children and reported them to have motor development considerably ahead of their chronological age. Westphal (1933) using some unstandardized motor tests with 26 boys and their controls, found that the stutterers were not as efficient in eye-hand coordinations, strength, or manual manipulation. Bilto (1941) used the standardized Brace Motor Ability Tests, the Nielson-Couzens Jump-and-Reach Test, and a measure of eye-hand coordination, and found that more than two-thirds of the stutterers performed below the mean of the nonstutterers on all three but concluded that no marked retardation in gross motor ability was present.

Kopp (1942–43) applied the Oseretsky and other tests to 450 stutterers and concluded that they showed marked motor disabilities. She gives detailed data on only 28 of these in an English article and the reader finds it impossible to evaluate them. Scrutiny of her French article (1936) shows that a large percentage of the stutterers, varying with the test items used, scored low on the Oseretsky tests. No control group was used. In a later study, Kopp (1946) analyzed the results of Oseretsky tests with 50 stuttering children and found retardation in terms of motor age levels especially in "synkinetic movements, in rhythm and coordination." Despert (1943) also reported motor delay in her stutterers.

In contrast, at Iowa, Finkelstein and Weisberger (1954) however found that a small number (15) of stutterers were, if anything, better coordinated than their controls on a different form of the Oseretsky test. In Germany, Schilling and Krüger (1960) examined 300 children, those with normal speech, a group of stutterers, and a group of children with delayed speech, using the Göllnitz modification of the Oseretsky test. Obvious motor retardation (at least a two year delay) was found in five per cent of the normals, in 18 per cent of the stutterers and in 41 per cent of children with delayed speech. Snyder (1958) gave a battery of test items, most of which came from the Minnesota Mechanical Ability test, using three equal groups of 20 stutterers but with varying degrees of severity and 25 controls, individuals with other types of speech disorders. The stutterers were found to be significantly inferior, and the more severe the stuttering, the more marked the lack of coordination.

In Japan, Shiraiwa and Kawakuba (1958) state that their 70 child stutterers had no deficiency in gross motor coordination but that difficulties in fine coordination were found in 60 per cent of their subjects. De Ajuriaguerra *et al.* (1958) and Launay (1960), in France, applied various psychomotor tests to stutterers and their controls and found no differences. Pierce and Lipcon (1959) found significantly more disparate arm movements while walking in their 36 subjects than in their controls, and, though we are reluctant to mention it, Delacato (1963) claimed that ten of 18 of his stutterers could not cross-pattern in creeping smoothly and accurately.

We can only conclude that no definitive conclusions are possible at this time with regard to gross motor coordinations in stutterers. There are just too many discrepancies in the reported results of these studies to enable anyone to be sure.

OTHER FINE COORDINATIONS
NOT RELATED TO SPEECH

Seth (1934) found no differences in the speed of hand or foot movements in stutterers and normal speakers. In a second study, Seth (1958) compared the tapping rates of 15 right-handed normally speaking children with 15 right-handed stuttering children and found the latter inferior in the use of both hands, but especially when using the preferred hand. Cross (1936) compared 31 right-handed and 11 left-handed normal speakers with 26 stutterers in unimanual bulb-squeezing and bimanual (spool packing) activities. There were no differences in the unimanual activities, but stutterers were inferior in the bimanual ones. Murray (1932) found more incoordinations in eye movements in the silent reading of 18 stutterers than in his controls and so did Moser (1938,) but Hamilton (1940) failed to corroborate this on a larger number (71) of stuttering children. In Italy, Baldan (1965) gave the Kwinte Motor Facial Test to 50 normals, 50 with strabismus, and 50 stutterers. Eighty-five per cent of the normal speakers performed normally for their age, but only 57 per cent of the stutterers and 45 per cent of the strabismus cases did so. Baldan also found a very high stuttering incidence of 17.5 per cent in the strabismic population, almost the same as that discovered 30 years earlier by Fink and Bryngelson (1934), who found that nine of 60 unselected strabismus cases were stutterers, an incidence of over 18 per cent.

Further evidence of incoordination in fine movements comes from investigations of nystagmus. Schilling (1959) discovered that 36 of 75 stutterers showed pathological nystagmograms. This was corroborated in another study by Baldan (1965), who used electronystagmography to investigate the vestibular reflexes of 60 Italian stutterers during silence but with eyes either open or closed. He found marked abnormality in the rhythm of the nystagmoid movements in 80 percent of his subjects. Another nystagmographic study by Bruno, Camarda, and Curi (1965) showed similar abnormalities in form and duration in 58 per cent of their 50 stutterers. These were interpreted to mean that the stutterer's basic timing of motor impulses shows poor integration at a very basic level.

In breathing, Schilling (1960), using radiokymography, also found involuntary pathological movements in the diaphragm resembling those of chorea in 16 of 35 stuttering children while silent and at rest. Their histories and EEGs were said to have indicated early brain damage. Somewhat similar results were described by Shiraiwa and Kawakuba (1967).

Gunderson (1949) recorded the involuntary finger tremors of 75 male stutterers in silence, oral reading, silent reading, and extemporaneous speaking. She found more tremor irregularities in the speaking than in the silent situations, a result also reached by Herren (1931) in his study of voluntary rhythmic hand and foot movements.

"STUTTERING" IN
OTHER COORDINATED ACTIVITIES

Stuttering or stuttering-like behaviors have been noted in other activities requiring precise sequential coordination. Denhardt, as early as 1890, described blocking movements and postures similar to stuttering in handwriting or in playing musical instruments. In a recent study Yastrebova (1962) analyzed the correlation of abnormalities in the written and oral speech of stuttering school children, but it is difficult to assess the author's findings. Van Riper (1952) has reported a case of trumpet stuttering, and Froeschels (1943a) described piano and violin stuttering. Scripture (1909) described penmanship stuttering in some detail. Other cases in which written letters were involuntarily disrupted or pens were described as "stuck to the paper" have been cited by Sikorski (1891), Eisenson (1937), Van Dantzig (1939), Froeschels (1943a), and Cabanas (1951). Careful studies of graphic stuttering by Fagan (1932) and by Roman (1959) give support to the thesis that something more is involved in these cases than merely an expectancy neurosis. Some improper timing of sequential movements seems to be present.

MOTOR PERSEVERATION

Eisenson (1958) has described the tendency toward perseveration as one of the constitutional aspects of stuttering, relating it in part to the well known finding that epileptics and other brain-damaged individuals show greater perseveration, both motorically and perceptually, than normals. We will review only the motoric research, since it is this which bears directly upon coordination. The question is whether stutterers, or definite subpopulations of stutterers, show more perseveration in motor activities than normals. Presumably, the greater the coordinative disability, the more difficult it will be to shift from one task to another.

Unfortunately, most of the tasks used in the research involved no speech sequencing, so that the definitive research still remains to be done. Eisenson (1937) compared 30 stutterers with their controls in their ability to change suddenly to a different task while copying letters and doing simple arithmetic problems. The stutterers perseverated longer than the normals. King (1961) tested the ability to alternate between writing and drawing activities (motor perseveration), and he also tested dispositional rigidity (e.g., changing from capital to lower case letters) in 82 stutterers and their controls. He found the stutterers more perseverative than the nonstutterers on most of the tests. Martin (1962), however, using other but similar copying and writing tests with 52 stutterers and 109 controls, found no differences of significance between them. Kapos and Standlee (1958) tested the ability to shift from one task to another in an electromaze and found no evidence of greater perseveration (behavioral rigidity) in 15 stutterers than in the controls. Wingate (1966), using another test of general behavioral rigidity on 12 stutterers and controls, found no differences. We conclude that the case for greater perseveration in stutterers has not been proven.

BIOCHEMICAL FACTORS

A number of researchers have investigated the biochemistry of stutterers, primarily the composition of the blood, urine, and saliva. The rationale for these studies has usually been that these secretions, which are controlled primarily by the autonomic nervous system, might reveal an organic pathology or malfunctioning of that system which could make the person more prone to stutter. To cite but one example, stuttering is characterized by excessive tension and clonic and tonic behaviors. So also is *tetany*, a calciometabolic imbalance that results in hyperirritability of neuromuscular activity causing clonic and tonic spasms. Tetany may also be latent, appearing only under stress. Kopp (1934), in his biochemical study of blood composition in stutterers, interpreted his data as supporting the concept of stuttering as a form of latent tetany. Shackson (1936) interprets the results of his electromyographic study of muscular contraction in stuttering as also indicating a possible latent tetany. Various European authors such as Fremel, (1913) have also held this view. A recent study by B. Weiss (1967) supports the hypothesis that some stutterers show a latent tetany. Employing electromyographic recordings of muscle excitability with hyperventilation and compression, she found evidence of the same changes usually found in latent tetany in a significant proportion of her 78 stutterers. They had normal serum calcium levels however.

Tetany, latent or otherwise, is caused by a deficiency of calcium in the blood. Such deficiencies have been attributed to heredity, to improper diet, or to a malfunction of the parathyroid glands, which monitor the blood

serum balance between diffusable calcium and the plasma proteins.* Most
of the research, however, does not seem to substantiate the belief of Hogewind (1940) and others that a calcium deficit exists in stutterers. If anything, serum calcium levels are slightly higher in stutterers than in normal
speakers, as Hill (1944a) in his excellent review of biochemical factors in
stuttering has made very clear. Almost all the research he cites indicates
that stutterers show normal or higher calcium levels, and it has long been
known that muscular activity and emotional upheaval can elevate these.
Thus any differences may be the result of the stutterer's fear and struggle.
Oblique support for Hill's position is also found in the study by Chapin
and Kessler (1950), who found that 100 stutterers had fewer dental caries
than the controls. If the stutterer has a blood calcium deficit, their teeth,
according to these authors, should reflect that deficit. Further studies seem
to substantiate this negative conclusion. Brown and Shulman (1940) measured the intermuscular tension of stutterers and normal speakers during
silence and found no differences that might indicate a latent tetany. Johnson, Stearns, and Warweg (1933) found no deficiencies in serum calcium or
blood sugar in their stutterers, but no control group was used. Johnson,
Young, Sahs, and Bedell (1959), using hyperventilation to precipitate signs
of tetany, found no significant difference in the amount of stuttering shown
by the stutterers during hyperventilation tetany, although their controls
showed a slight increase in the number of disfluencies in this condition. In
view of all these investigations, latent tetany must be regarded as an unsatisfactory explanation for stuttering, at least in the large majority of cases.
Karlin, Karlin, and Gurren (1965) offer these other negative comments:

> The biochemical approach to stuttering was suggested by the fact that
> stuttering is characterized by tonic and clonic spasms. It was naturally be-
> lieved that stuttering was therefore associated with latent tetany. Tetany is
> characterized by hyperirritability of the nervous system and is usually caused
> by a deficiency of calcium and Vitamin D. However, calcium and vitamin
> studies on stutterers fail to demonstrate abnormal blood levels. These studies
> seem to rule out tetany as a possible cause of stuttering. Furthermore, tetany

---

* In this connection, several writers, notably Knight Dunlap (1934), have stressed the
importance of a diet rich in meat as part of the treatment of stuttering. In a Czecho-
slovakian journal, Weissova and Handzel (1962) present a detailed description of a
familial, and probably hereditary insufficiency of the parathyroid glands in a father and
three sons, all of whom stuttered and showed the usual signs of tetany. In view of the
sex ratio in the incidence of stuttering it is interesting that in women the parathyroids
are 20 per cent larger than in men. Certain relationships between thyroid and parathyroid glandular activity exist but are not as yet thoroughly understood. There are
several reports of stuttering having been precipitated by thyroid medication and terminated when the medication was discontinued (Gordon, 1928; Cabanas, 1954) and we have
had two cases whose stuttering improved remarkably under parahormone therapy. It
should be noted that more parathyroid hormone is secreted when blood calcium falls
below normal limits.

usually occurs much earlier than stuttering and can develop at two months of age. This tendency for its early occurrence makes tetany a highly unlikely cause of stuttering (pp. 101–2).

Most of the investigations of other biochemical constituents of plasma and whole blood have not yielded any significant differences between stutterers and nonstutterers that could not be explained as the result rather than the cause of stuttering, or as caused by the emotional upheaval that accompanies it. We have reviewed again all of the early research considered by Hill (1944a) and agree with his conclusion that for stuttering, "no findings warrant any assumption of any special metabolic or chemical agents which are casual." In the more than 20 years since his review, there have been only a few investigations of the biochemistry of stuttering. In one, by Girone and Bruno (1957) the glycemic (blood sugar) values in 50 stutterers were analyzed and found to be different from the normal values in about half of the subjects although marked glycemic curve differences were found among the stutterers themselves. No control group was used.

It is quite possible that biochemical differences in stutterers may predispose them to have disrupted speech in ways which do not involve tetany. Excessive thyroid medication can induce tremors and so can an overactive thyroid gland. If stuttering is primarily a coordinative disorder, biochemical factors affecting the autonomic nervous system may facilitate emotional arousal to a degree which interferes with integration of the sequencing of movements. The common therapeutic use of sedatives, tranquilizers, or stimulant drugs such as methylphenidate in the medical treatment of stuttering reflects the recognized importance of biochemical factors in the functioning of the central nervous system with respect to stuttering. Perhaps some day, when we know much more than we do now, we may find the pill to prevent stuttering. May it be pink!

COMMENTARY

During the third and fourth decades of our century, psychological explanations predominated. These are not completely satisfactory to the medical mind, however, because the history of medicine has shown many drastic changes in the interpretation of disease. With the progress of medicine, many "functional" ailments have proved to be caused by organic changes with various anatomic, neurological, or biochemical alterations. (Luchsinger and Arnold, 1965, p. 739)

The evolution of opinion about the cause of stuttering has shown a surprising cycle in the last fifty years. Early authorities thought of stuttering as based upon disfunctions localized in the speech organs themselves—the tongue, lips, jaw, larynx. When upon investigation, the criminal was not discovered in those locales, he was pursued into deeper and deeper recesses of the human organism, and farther and farther back into the ancestry, until now many workers in the field seem to say: "Well, we can't catch him anyway; let's give up and confine our attention to repairing the damage to the special functions that he ravaged." (West, 1943, p. 106)

In summary, there is evidence to suggest that complete hemispheric dominance fails to develop in a small per cent of the population. This category of persons is made up of mostly left-handers and persons having bihemispheric motor and/or sensory preferences. In a small per cent of this group, stammering occurs as a manifestation of speech representation which is bilateral. Though bilateral speech representation occurs in persons who do not stammer, stammerers are unfortunate in having this bilateral representation for speech so evenly balanced that incoordination in the speech effort, in the form of stammering, results. (Jones, 1967, p. 199)

I believe that every child is a potential stutterer, and may stutter if given an environment suitable for stuttering. Most of the time the equation of child versus environment is given in positive terms, i.e., the child does not stutter. However, given certain neurological subsoils, such as evenly balanced brain areas in relation to amplitude and form (alpha waves), stuttering may more easily germinate. That is, the human organism is more likely to become frustrated when it has a relatively weak neurological inheritance, or a neurological inheritance which has become arrested in its normal development. However, if one's environment is frustrating enough, one *may* stutter despite a dominant and healthy neurological background. However, it is no guarantee that one will stutter even if he has an inherently equated cortex, and in general, a poor neural make-up. He may grow up in a compensating environment which avoids undue conflicts and frustrations. If this were so, he would not necessarily stutter. But, *everything else being equal, there will be a tendency for those with weak neurological subsoils to succumb to the average social pressures found in every home.* (Freestone, 1942, p. 467)

For centuries there has been going on a search for some anatomical or inner condition which would set the stutterer apart from the normal speaker. Reactions and behavior of the stutterer have been looked upon as being symptomatic of an inner condition. The condition has been assumed to be expressed through disruptions in speech and other behavior. Workers who demand some special, inner physiological or psychological condition are not all of a past generation; even today the mystics remain in great number. (Hill, 1944b, p. 318)

BIBLIOGRAPHY

Abbot, W. E., O. F. Due, and W. A. Nosik, "Subdural Hematoma and Effusion as a Result of Blast Injuries," *Journal of the American Medical Association,* CXXI (1943), 664–65; 739–41.

Abe, N., ["Statistical Observation of Stutterers at the Time of Their Draft in the Army"], *Naval Surgeon Magazine* (Japan), XXIII (1934), 232–34.

Aimard, P., A. Plantier, and M. Wittlung, "Le Bégaiement: Contribution de l'Audition et de l'Intégration phonétique," *Revue Laryngologie,* LXXXVII (1966), 254–56.

Ajuriaguerra, J. de, "Speech Disorders in Childhood." In C. C. Carterette (ed.), *Brain Function III.* Berkeley: University of California Press, 1966.

Ajuriaguerra, J. de, R. Diatkine, S. de Gobineau, and M. Stambak, "Le Bégaiement," *Presse Medicale,* LXVI (1958), 953–56.

Andrews, G., and M. Harris, *The Syndrome of Stuttering.* London: Heinemann, 1964.

Appelt, A., *The Real Cause of Stammering and Its Permanent Cure.* London: Methuen, 1911.

Arend, R., L. Handzel, and B. Weiss, "Dysphatic Stuttering," *Folia Phoniatrica,* XIV (1962), 55–66.

Aron, M., "An Investigation of the Nature and Incidence of Stuttering Among a Bantu Group of School-Going Children," master's thesis, University of the Witwatersrand, South Africa, 1958.

Asp, C. W., "An Investigation of the Localization of Interaural Stimulation by Clicks and the Reading Times of Stutterers and Nonstutterers Under Monaural Sidetone Conditions," *De Therapia Vocis et Loquellae,* II (1965), 353–55.

Baldan, G., ["Study of the Vestibular Function in a Group of Stutterers: Electronystagmographic Researches"], *De Therapia Vocis et Loquellae,* I (1965), 349–51.

Ballard, P. B., "Sinistrality and Speech," *Journal of Experimental Psychology,* I (1912), 298–310.

Barbara, D. A., "A Psychosomatic Approach to the Problem of Stuttering in Psychotics," *American Journal of Psychiatry,* CIII (1946), 188–95.

Basser, L. S., "Hemiplegia of Early Onset and the Faculty of Speech with Special Reference to the Effects of Hemispherectomy," *Brain,* LXXXV (1962), 427–60.

Bell, C., "Philosophical Transaction," II, *Archives of General Medicine* (2nd series), 1832.

Benson, D. F., and N. Geschwind, "Cerebral Dominance and Its Disturbances," *Pediatric Clinics of North America,* XV (1968), 759–69.

Bente, D., E. Schönhärl, and J. Krump, "Elektroencephalographische Befunde bei Stottereren und ihre Bedeutung für die medikamentöse Therapie," *Archive für Ohrenheilkunde,* CLXIX (1956), 513–19.

Benton, A. L., *Right-Left Discrimination and Finger Localization: Development and Pathology.* New York: Hoeber-Harper, 1959.

Berry, M. F., "A Study of the Medical Histories of Stuttering Children," *Speech Monographs,* V (1938), 97–114.

———. "Twinning in Stuttering Families," *Human Biology,* IX (1937), 329–46.

Bignardi, F., and L. Spettoli, ["Stuttering and Contrasted Left-Handedness: Clinical Study"], *Giornale de Psichiatria e di Neuropatologie,* LXXXIII (1955), 357–61.

Bilto, E. W., "A Comparative Study of Certain Physical Abilities of Children with Speech Defects and Children with Normal Speech," *Journal of Speech Disorders,* VI (1941), 187–203.

Blackburn, W. E., "A Study of Voluntary Movements of the Diaphragm, Tongue, Lips, and Jaw in Stutterers and Normal Speakers," *Psychological Monographs,* XLI (1931), 1–13.

Bloodstein, O., *A Handbook on Stuttering for Professional Workers.* Chicago: National Society for Crippled Children and Adults, 1959.

Bluemel, C. S., *Stammering and Cognate Defects of Speech,* Vol. I. New York: Stechert, 1913.

Bocca, E., and C. Calearo, "Central Hearing Processes." In J. Jerger (ed.), *Modern Developments in Audiology.* New York: Academic Press, 1963.

Bocca, E., C. Calearo, and V. Cassinari, "A New Method for Testing Hearing in Temporal Lobe Tumours: Preliminary Report," *Acta Otolaryngologie,* XLIV (1954), 219–21.

Boland, J. L., "Type of Birth as Related to Stuttering," *Journal of Speech and Hearing Disorders,* XVI (1951), 40–43.

Bolin, B. J., "Left-Handedness and Stuttering as Signs Diagnostic of Epileptics," *Journal of Mental Science,* XCIX (1953), 483–88.

Boome, E. J., and M. A. Richardson, *The Nature and Treatment of Stuttering.* New York: Dutton, 1932.

Boone, D. R., "Communication Skills and Intelligence in Right and Left Hemiplegics," *Journal of Speech and Hearing Disorders,* XXIV (1959), 241–48.

Branch, C., B. Milner, and T. Rasmussen, "Intercarotid Sodium Amytol for the Lateralization of Cerebral Speech Dominance," *Journal of Neurosurgery,* XXI (1964), 399–405.

Brickner, R. M., "A Human Cortical Area Producing Repetitive Phenomena When Stimulated," *Journal of Neurophysiology,* III (1940), 128–30.

Brown, S. R., and E. E. Shulman, "Intramuscular Pressure in Stutterers and Non-stutterers," *Speech Monographs,* VII (1940), 63–74.

Bruno, G., V. Camarda, and L. Curi, ["Contribution to the Study of Organic Causal Factors in the Pathogenesis of Stuttering"], *Bolletino delle Malattie dell'Orecchio, della Gola, del Naso,* LXXXIII (1965), 753–58.

Brunt, M., and C. P. Goetzinger, "A Study of Three Tests of Central Function with Normal Hearing Subjects," *Cortex,* IV (1968), 288–97.

Bryant, F. A., "Influence of Heredity in Stuttering," *Journal of Heredity,* VIII (1917), 46–47.

Bryden, M. P., "Ear Preference in Auditory Perception," *Journal of Experimental Psychology,* LXV (1963), 103–5.

Bryngelson, B., "The Problem of Sidedness and Its Relationship to Stuttering," *Proceedings of the American Society for the Study of Disorders of Speech,* IV (1934), 63–70.

———. "A Study of Laterality of Stutterers and Normal Speakers," *Journal of Social Psychology,* XI (1940), 151–55.

———. "Sidedness as an Etiological Factor in Stuttering," *Journal of Genetic Psychology,* XLVII (1935), 204–17.

Bryngelson, B., and T. B. Clark, "Left-Handedness and Stuttering," *Journal of Heredity,* XXIV (1933), 387–90.

Bryngelson, E., and B. Rutherford, "A Comparative Study of Laterality of Stutterers and Nonstutterers," *Journal of Speech Disorders,* II (1937), 15–16.

Busse, E. W., and R. M. Clark, "The Use of the Encephalogram in Diagnosing Speech Disorders in Children," *Folia Phoniatrica,* IX (1957), 182–87.

Cabanas, R., "Report on a Particular Case of Stuttering," *Folia Phoniatrica,* III (1951), 10–13.

———. "Some Findings in Speech and Voice Therapy Among the Mentally Retarded," *Folia Phoniatrica,* VI (1954), 34–37.

Calearo, C., and A. R. Antonelli, "Cortical Hearing Tests and Cerebral Dominance," *Acta Oto-Laryngologica,* LVI (1963), 17–26.

Cali, G., F. Pisani, and F. Tagliareni, ["Stuttering and Electroencephalographic Curves"], *Clinical ORL,* XVII (1965), 316–28.

Carr, B. M., "Ear Effect Variables and Order of Report in Dichotic Listening," *Cortex,* V (1969), 63–68.

Carterette, E. C. (ed.), *Brain Function,* Vol. III. Berkeley: University of California Press, 1966.

Chapin, A. B., and H. E. Kessler, "Dental Caries in Individuals Who Stutter," *Dental Items of Interest,* LXXII (1950), 162–67.

Chworowsky, C. R., "A Comparative Study of Diadochokinetic Rates of Stutterers and Nonstutterers in Speech Related and Nonspeech Related Movements," *Speech Monographs,* XIX (1952), 192 (abstract).

Claiborne, J. H., "Stuttering Relieved by Reversal of Manual Dexterity," *New York Medical Journal,* CV (1917), 577–81; 619–21.

Clark, M. M., *Left Handedness, Laterality Characteristics, and Their Educational Implications.* London: University of London Press, 1957.

Cross, H. M., "The Motor Capacities of Stutterers," *Archives of Speech,* I (1936), 112–32.

Curry, F. K. W., "A Comparison of Left-Handed and Right-Handed Subjects on Verbal and Nonverbal Dichotic Listening Tasks," *Cortex,* III (1967), 343–51.

———. "A Comparison of the Performances of a Right Hemispherectomized Subject and 25 Normals on Four Dichotic Listening Tasks," *Cortex,* IV (1968), 144–53.

Curry, F. K. W., and H. H. Gregory, "A Comparison of Stutterers and Nonstutterers on Three Dichotic Listening Tasks," convention address, A.S.H.A., 1967.

Daniels, E. M., "An Analysis of the Relation Between Handedness and Stuttering with Special Reference to the Orton-Travis Theory of Cerebral Dominance," *Journal of Speech Disorders,* V (1940), 309–26.

Daskalov, D. D., ["On the Problem of the Basic Principles and Methods of Prevention and Treatment of Stammering"], *Zhurnal Nevropatologii i Psikhiatrii imeni S. S. Korsakova,* LIII (1962), 1047–52.

Delacato, C., *The Diagnosis and Treatment of Speech and Reading Problems.* Springfield, Ill.: Thomas, 1963.

Denhardt, R., *Das Stottern: Eine Psychose.* Leipzig, 1890.

Dew, R., "Electroencephalographic Study of Stutterers During Sleep," *Speech Monographs,* XIX (1952), 192–93.

Dirks, E., "Perception of Dichotic and Monaural Verbal Material and Cerebral Dominance for Speech," *Acta Otolaryngologica,* LVIII (1964), 73–80.

Douglass, L. C., "A Study of Bilaterally Recorded Electroencephalograms of Adult Stutterers," *Journal of Experimental Psychology,* XXXII (1943), 247–65.

Dunlap, K., "Possible Dietary Predisposition to Stammering," *Science N.S.,* LXXX (1934), 206.

Eisenson, J., "A Perseverative Theory of Stuttering." In J. Eisenson (ed.), *Stuttering: A Symposium.* New York: Harper, 1958.

———. "Aphasics: Observations and Tentative Conclusions," *Journal of Speech Disorders,* XII (1947), 290–92.

———. "Some Characteristics of the Written Speech of Stutterers," *Journal of Genetic Psychology,* L (1937), 457–58.

Eisenson, J., and E. Pastel, "A Study of the Perseveratory Tendency in Stutterers," *Quarterly Journal of Speech,* XXII (1936), 626–31.

Eisenson, J., and C. N. Winslow, "The Perseverating Tendency in Stutterers in a Perceptual Function," *Journal of Speech Disorders,* III (1938), 195–98.

Fagan, L. B., "Graphic Stuttering," *Psychology Monographs,* XLIII (1932), 67–71.

———. "The Relation of Dextral Training to the Onset of Stuttering. A Report of Cases," *Quarterly Journal of Speech,* XVII (1931), 73–76.

Fink, W. H., and B. Bryngelson, "The Relation of Strabismus to Right or Left Handedness," *Transactions of the American Academy of Ophthomology and Otolaryngology,* IX (1934), 247–66.

Finkelstein, P., and S. E. Weisberger, "The Motor Proficiency of Stutterers," *Journal of Speech and Hearing Disorders,* XIX (1954), 52–57.

Fox, D. R., "Electroencephalographic Analysis During Stuttering and Nonstuttering," *Journal of Speech and Hearing Research,* IX (1966), 488–97.

Freestone, N. W., "A Brainwave Interpretation of Stuttering," *Quarterly Journal of Speech,* XXVIII (1942), 466–70.

Fremel, F., "Stottern und Fazialsphammen," *Wien Medizinische Wochenschrift,* LXIII (1913), 2207–9.

Freshel, E., quoted in A. Kh. Stremel, ["Stuttering in the Left Parietal Lobe Syndrome,"] *Zhurnal Nevropatologii i Psikhiatrii imeni S. S. Korsakova,* LXIII (1963), 828–32.

Freund, H., *Psychopathology and the Problem of Stuttering.* Springfield, Ill.: Thomas, 1966.

———. "Psychosis and Stuttering," *Journal of Nervous and Mental Diseases,* CXXII (1955), 161–72.

———. "Studies in the Interrelationship Between Stuttering and Cluttering," *Folia Phoniatrica,* IV (1952), 146–68.

Fritzell, B., I. Peterson, and U. Sellden, "An EEG Study of Stuttering and Nonstuttering School Children," *De Therapia Vocis et Loquellae,* I (1965), 343–46.

Froeschels, E., "Pathology and Therapy of Stuttering," *Nervous Child,* II (1943a) 148–61.

———. "Stuttering and Nystagmus," *Monatschrift für Ohrenheilkunde,* XLIX (1915), 161–67.

———. "Survey of the Early Literature on Stuttering, Chiefly European," *Nervous Child,* II (1943b), 86–95.

———. "Die Sprachärztliche Therapie im Kriege III Das Stottern," *Monataschrift für Ohrenheilkunde,* LIII (1919), 161–90.

Gardner, W. H., "The Study of the Pupillary Reflex with Special Reference to Stuttering," *Psychological Monographs,* XLIX (1937), 1–31.

Gedda, L., L. Branconi, and G. Bruno, "Su Alcuni Casi di Balbuzie in Coppie Gemellari Mono-e Dizigotiche," *Acta Geneticae Medicale et Gemellologiae,* IX (1960), 407–26.

Gerstmann, J., and P. Schilder, "Studien über Bewegungstörungen über die typenextrapyramidaler pseudobulbar Paralysie," *Zeitschrift für Neurologie und Psychiatrie,* LXXIX (1921), 350–54.

Ghent, L., "Development Changes in Tactual Thresholds on Dominant and Nondominant Sides," *Journal of Comparative Physiology and Psychology,* LIV (1961), 670–73.

Girone, D., and G. Bruno, "Some Characteristics of the Glycemic Curve in Stutterers," *Folia Phoniatrica,* IX (1957), 87–91.

Goda, S., "Stuttering Manifestations Following Spinal Meningitis," *Journal of Speech and Hearing Disorders,* XXVI (1961), 392–93.

Göllnitz, G., *Die Bedeutung der frühkindlichen Hirnschädigung für die Kinderpsychiatrie.* Leipzig: Thieme, 1954.

————. "Zusammenhänge zwischen Stottern und Frühkindlicher Hirnschädigung," *Medecin Klinik,* L (1955), 685–89.

Goodglass, H., and F. A. Quadfasel, "Language Laterality in Left-Handed Aphasics," *Brain,* LXXVII (1964), 521–48.

Gordon, M. B., "Stammering Produced by Thyroid Medication," *American Journal of Medical Science,* CLXXV (1928), 360–65.

Graf, O. I., "Incidence of Stuttering Among Twins." In W. Johnson and R. Lentenneger (eds.), *Stuttering in Children and Adults.* Minneapolis: University of Minnesota Press, 1955.

Graham, J. K., "A Neurologic and Electroencephalographic Study of Adult Stutterers and Matched Normal Speakers." Doctoral dissertation, Northwestern University, 1958.

Graham, J. K., and J. Brumlik, "Neurologic and Encephalographic Abnormalities in Stuttering and Matched Nonstuttering Adults," *Asha,* III (1961) 342 (abstract).

Granich, L., *Aphasia.* New York: Grune and Stratton, 1947.

Gray, M., "The X Family: A Clinical and Laboratory Study of a 'Stuttering' Family," *Journal of Speech Disorders,* V (1940), 343–48.

Guillaume, J., G. Mazars, and Y. Mazars, "Epileptic Mediation in Certain Types of Stammering," *Revue Neurologique,* XCIX (1957), 59–62.

Gunderson, H., "A Quantitative Analysis of Digital Tremor in Male Stutterers." Doctoral dissertation, Teachers College, Columbia University, 1949.

Guttsmann, H., "Erbbiologische, soziologische und organische Faktoren die sprachstörungen Begungstigen," *Archive für Sprach-Stimmheilkunde,* III (1939), 133–36.

Gutzmann, H., *Das Stottern.* Frankfurt: J. Rosenheim, 1898.

————. "Konstitution und Sprachstörung," *Hippokrates,* (Stuttgart), VIII (1937), 369–71.

Haase, C. A., *Das Stottern: Oder Darstellung und Bleuchtung der Wichtigsten über Wesen, Ursache und Heilung, Desselben, Nebst Abhandlung des Hieronmymus Mercurialis "De Balbutie" für Pädagogen und Medicin.* Berlin: Hirschwald, 1846.

Haefner, R., *The Educational Significance of Left-Handedness.* New York: Teachers College, Columbia University Press, 1929.

Hamilton, P. G., "The Visual Characteristics of Stutterers During Silent Reading." Doctoral dissertation, Teachers College, Columbia University, 1940.

Hamre, C. E., and M. E. Wingate, "Pyknolepsy and Stuttering," *Quarterly Journal of Speech,* LIII (1967), 374–77.

Harrison, H. S., "A Study of the Speech of Sixty Institutionalized Epileptics." Master's thesis, Louisiana State University, 1947.

Head, H., *Aphasia and Kindred Disorders of Speech.* London: Macmillan, 1926.

Hécaen, H., "Clinical Symptomatology in Right and Left Hemisphere Lesions." In V. B. Mountcastle (ed.), *Interhemispheric Relations and Cerebral Dominance.* Baltimore: Johns Hopkins Press, 1962.

Hécaen, H., and J. de Ajuriaguerra, *Les Gauchers, Préférance manuelle et Dominance cérébrale.* Paris: Presses Universitaires de France, 1963.

Herren, R. Y., "The Effect of Stuttering on Voluntary Movement," *Journal of Experimental Psychology,*" XIV (1931), 289–98.

――――. "The Relation of Stuttering and Alcohol to Certain Tremor Rates," *Journal of Experimental Psychology,* XV (1932), 87–96.

Hill, H., "Stuttering: I: A Critical Review and Evaluation of Biochemical Investigations," *Journal of Speech Disorders,* IX (1944a), 245–61.

――――. "Stuttering: II: A Review and Integration of Physiological Data," *Journal of Speech Disorders,* IX (1944b), 289–324.

Hirschberg, J., ["Stuttering"], *Orvosi Hetilap,* CVI (1965), 780–84.

Hogewind, F., "Medical Treatment of Stuttering," *Journal of Speech Disorders,* V (1940), 203–8.

Hunsley, Y. L., "Disintegration in the Speech Musculature of Stutterers During the Production of a Nonvocal Temporal Pattern," *Psychological Monographs,* XLIX (1937), 32–49.

Hunt, J., *Stammering and Stuttering, Their Nature and Treatment,* 7th Ed. London: Longmans, Green, 1870.

Ingebretsen, E., "Some Experimental Contributions to the Psychology and Psychopathology of Stutterers," *American Journal of Orthopsychiatry,* VI (1936), 630–50.

Jasper, H. H., "A Laboratory Study of Diagnostic Indices of Bilateral Neuromuscular Organization in Stutterers and Normal Speakers," *Psychological Monographs,* XLIII (1932), 172–74.

Johnson, W., *The Onset of Stuttering.* Minneapolis: University of Minnesota Press, 1959.

Johnson, W., and A. King, "An Angle Board and Hand Usage Study of Stutterers and Nonstutterers," *Journal of Experimental Psychology,* XXXI (1942), 293–311.

Johnson, W., G. Stearns, and E. Warweg, "Chemical Factors and the Stuttering Spasm," *Quarterly Journal of Speech,* XIX (1933), 409–15.

Johnson, W., M. A. Young, A. L. Sahs, and G. N. Bedell, "Effects of Hyperventilation and Tetany on the Speech Fluency of Stutterers and Nonstutterers," *Journal of Speech and Hearing Research,* II (1959), 203–15.

Jones, R. K., "Dyspraxic Ambiphasia—A Neurophysiologic Theory of Stammering," *Transactions American Neurological Association,* XCII (1967), 197–201.

――――. "Observations on Stammering After Localized Cerebral Injury," *Journal of Neurology and Neurosurgery,* XXIX (1966), 192–95.

Jost, H., and L. W. Sontag, "The Genetic Factor in Autonomic Nervous Function," *Psychosomatic Medicine,* VI (1944), 308–10.

Kamiyama, A., [*Handbook for the Study of Stuttering.*] Tokyo: Kongo-Shupan, 1967.

Kanner, L., *Child Psychiatry.* Springfield, Ill.: Thomas, 1942.

Kapos, E., and L. S. Standlee, "Behavioral Rigidity in Adult Stutterers," *Journal of Speech and Hearing Research,* I (1958), 294–96.

Karlin, I. W., "Psychosomatic Theory of Stuttering," *Journal of Speech Disorders,* XII (1947), 319–22.

Karlin, I. W., D. B. Karlin, and L. Gurren, *Development and Diseases of Speech in Childhood.* Springfield, Ill.: Thomas, 1965.

Karlin, I. W., and A. E. Sobol, "A Comparative Study of the Blood Chemistry of Stutterers and Nonstutterers," *Speech Monographs,* VII (1940), 75–84.

Kasanin, H. R. I., "The Motor Development of Children Suffering from Stammering," *American Journal of Diseases of Children,* XLIV (1931), 1123–25.

Kiehn, E., "Untersuchungen über die Fähigkeiten feinabgemessenen Bewegungen (Feinmotorik) bein Stammelnden, Stotternden und Normalen Volkschüllern," *Vox,* XXI, (1935), 32–35.

Kiloh, L. G., and J. W. Osselton, *Clinical Electroencephalography.* London: Butterworth, 1961.

Kimura, D., "Cerebral Dominance and the Perception of Verbal Stimuli," *Canadian Journal of Psychology,* XV (1961a), 166–71.

———. "Functional Asymmetry of the Brain in Dichotic Listening," *Cortex,* III (1967), 163–78.

———. "Some Effects of Temporal Lobe Damage on Auditory Perception," *Canadian Journal of Psychology,* XV (1961b), 156–65.

———. "Speech Lateralization in Young Children as Determined by an Auditory Test," *Journal of Comparative Physiology and Psychology,* LVI (1963), 899–902.

King, P. T., "Perseveration in Stutterers and Nonstutterers," *Journal of Speech and Hearing Research,* IV (1961), 346–57.

Kistler, K., "Linkshändigkeit und Sprachstörungen," *Schweitz-Medizinische Wochenschrift,* XI (1930), 32–34.

Klingbeil, G. M., "The Historical Background of the Modern Speech Clinic," *Journal of Speech Disorders,* IV (1939), 115–32.

Knott, J. R., E. Correll, and J. N. Shepherd, "Frequency Analysis of Electroencephalograms of Stutterers and Nonstutterers," *Journal of Speech and Hearing Research,* II (1959), 74–80.

Knott, J. R.,and T. D. Tjossem, "Bilateral Encephalograms from Normal Speakers and Stutterers," *Journal of Experimental Psychology,* XXXII (1943), 357–62.

Kopp, G. A., "Metabolic Studies of Stutterers: I. Biochemical Study of Blood Composition," *Speech Monographs,* I (1934), 117–32.

Kopp, H., "Les Troubles de la Parole dans leur Rapport avec les Troubles de la Motrice," *L'Evolution Psychiatrique,* II (1936), 77–112.

———. "Psychosomatic Study of Fifty Stuttering Children. III. Oseretsky Tests," *American Journal of Orthopsychiatry,* XVI (1946), 114–19.

———. "The Relationship of Stuttering to Motor Disturbances," *Nervous Child,* II (1942–43), 107–16.

Kussmaul, A., "Die Störungen der Sprache." In H. V. Ziemssen (ed.), *Cyclopaedia Medica,* 1877.

Landolt, H., and R. Luchsinger, ["Language Disorder, Stuttering, and Chronic Organic Psychosyndrome; Electroencephalographic Results and Studies of Pathology of Speech"], *Deutsche Medizinische Wochenschrift,* LXXIX (1954), 1012–15.

Langova, J., and M. Moravek, ["Experimental Study on Stuttering and Stammering"], *Casopis Lekaru Ceskych,* CI (1962), 297–300.

———. "Some Results of Experimental Examinations Among Stutterers and Clutterers," *Folia Phoniatrica,* XVI (1964), 290–96.

Larson, M., "Representative 19th-Century Stuttering Therapists," master's thesis, University of Denver, 1949.

Launay, C., "Troubles Neurologiques dane le Bégaiement," *Journal Franc. d'Otorhinolaryngologie,* IX (1960), 269–79.

Lenneberg, E. H., "Speech Development: Its Anatomical and Physiological Components." In E. C. Cartarette (ed.), *Brain Function III*. Berkeley: University of California Press, 1966.

Lerbert, G., "La Dominance Latérale," *Année Psychologie,* LXVI (1965), 411–38.

Lindsley, D. B., "Bilateral Differences in Brain Potentials from the Two Cerebral Hemispheres in Relation to Laterality and Stuttering," *Journal of Experimental Psychology,* XXVI (1940), 211–25.

Lovett, D. J. W., and L. I. M. Coleman, "The Psychophysics of Communication. III. Discriminatory Awareness in Stutterers and its Measurement by the Critical Flicker Fusion Threshold," *Archives of Neurology and Psychiatry,* LXXIV (1955), 650–52.

Luchsinger, R., "Die Sprache und Stimme von ein-und zweieiigen Zwillingen in Beziehung zur Motorik und zum Erbcharakter," *Archive Julius-Klaus-Stiftung,* XV (1940), 457–62.

————. "Die Vererbung von Sprach-und Stimmstörungen," *Folia Phoniatrica,* XI (1959), 17–64.

————. ["Biological Studies on Monozygotic and Dizygotic Twins Relative to Size and Form of the Larynx"], *Archive Julius Klaus-Stiftung für Vererbungsforschung,* XIX (1944), 3–4.

————. ["Function of Sympathetic Nervous System as Indicated by Pupillary Reactions in Stutterers"], *Schweizer Medizinische Wochenschrift* (July 10, 1943).

————. "Gibt es organische bedingte Stottererfalle?" *Archive für Ohrenheilkunde,* CLXV (1954), 612–14.

————. "Stottern," *Phonetica,* III (1959), 183–89.

Luchsinger, R., and G. E. Arnold, *Voice-Speech-Language,* Belmont, Cal.: Wadsworth, 1965.

Luchsinger, R., and H. Landholt, "Electroencephalographische Untersuchungen bei Stotteren mit und ohne Polterkomponente," *Folia Phoniatria,* III (1951), 135–51.

Maas, O., "On the Etiology of Stuttering," *Journal of Mental Science,* XCII (1946), 357–63.

MacKay, B. G., "Metamorphosis of a Critical Interval: Age Linked Changes in Delay in Auditory Feedback that Produces Maximal Disruption of Speech." *Journal of the Acoustical Society of America,* XLIII (1968), 810–20.

Makuen, G. H., "A Study of 1000 Cases of Stammering with Special Reference to the Etiology and Treatment of the Affection," *Therapeutic Gazette,* XXXVIII (1914), 385–90.

Martin, R., "Stuttering and Perseveration in Children," *Journal of Speech and Hearing Research,* V (1962), 332–39.

McKnight, R. V., "A Self-Analysis of a Case of Reading, Writing, and Speaking Disability," *Archives of Speech,* I (1936), 18–47.

Meyer, B. C., "Psychosomatic Aspects of Stuttering," *Journal of Nervous and Mental Illness,* CI (1945), 127–57.

Moravek, M., and J. Langova, "Some Electrophysiological Findings Among Stutterers and Clutterers," *Folia Phoniatrica,* XIV (1962), 305–16.

Moser, H. M., "A Qualitative Analysis of Eye-Movements During Stuttering," *Journal of Speech Disorders,* III (1938), 131–39.

Murphy, A. T., Jr., "An Electroencephalographic Study of Frustration in Stutterers." Doctoral dissertation, University of Southern California, 1952.

Murray, E., "Disintegration of Breathing and Eye Movements in Stutterers During Silent Reading and Reasoning," *Journal of Speech Disorders,* XLIII (1932), 218–75.

Mussafia, M., "The Role of Heredity in Language Disorders," *Folia Phoniatrica,* XVI (1964), 228–38.

Mygind, H., "Über die Ursuchen des Stotterns," *Archive für Laryngologie una Rhinologie,* VIII (1898), 294–307.

Nelson, S., "Personal Contact as a Factor in the Transfer of Stuttering," *Human Biology,* XI (1939), 393–401.

Nielsen, J. M., "Epitome of Agnosia, Apraxia, and Aphasia with Proposed Physiologic-Anatomic Nomenclature," *Journal of Speech Disorders,* VII (1942), 105–41.

Oates, D. W. "Left-Handedness in Relation to Speech Defects, Intelligence and Achievement," *Forum of Education,* VII (1929), 91–105.

Ojemann, R. H., "Studies in Handedness; III. Relation of Handedness to Speech," *Journal of Educational Psychology,* XXII (1931), 120–26.

Orton, S. T., "Studies in Stuttering," *Archives of Neurology and Psychiatry,* XVIII (1927), 671–72.

———. *Reading, Writing, and Speech Problems in Childhood.* New York: Norton, 1937.

Orton, S. T., and L. E. Travis, "Studies in Stuttering; IV. Studies of Action Currents in Stutterers," *Archives of Neurology and Psychiatry,* XXI (1929), 61–68.

Otsuki, H., ["Study on Stuttering: Statistical Observations"], *Otorhinolaryngology Clinic,* V (1958), 1150–51.

Palmer, M. F., and C. D. Osborn, "One Thousand Consecutive Cases of Speech Defects," *Transactions of the Kansas Academy of Science,* IV (1938), 116.

Peacher, W. C., and W. E. Harris, "Speech Disorders in World War II: Stuttering," *Journal of Speech Disorders,* XI (1946), 303–8.

Penfield, W., and T. Rasmussen, "Vocalization and Arrest of Speech," *Archives of Neurology and Psychiatry,* LXI (1949), 21–27.

Penfield, W., and L. Roberts, *Speech and Brain Mechanisms.* Princeton: Princeton University Press, 1959.

Peterson, G. M., "A Preliminary Report on Right and Left Handedness in the Rat," *Journal of Comparative Psychology,* XII (1931), 243–50.

Pfändler, U., "Les Vices de la Parole dans l'optique du Géneticien," *Problema Acta Phoniatrie Logopedie,* I (1952), 35–40.

Pierce, C. M., and H. H. Lipcon, "Stuttering: Clinical and Electroencephalographic Findings," *Military Medicine,* XII (1959). 511–19.

Potter, S., *Speech and Its Defects.* Philadelphia: Blakeston, 1882.

Quinan, C., "Sinistrality in Relation to High Blood Pressure and Defects of Speech," *Archives of Internal Medicine,* XXVII (1921), 255–61.

———. "Stammering and Left-Handedness—A Graphic Study," *Journal of Experimental Psychology,* XXII (1938), 90–96.

Rheinberger, M. B., W. I. Karlin, and A. B. Berman, "Electroencephalographic and Laterality Studies of Stuttering and Nonstuttering Children," *Nervous Child,* II (1943), 117–33.

Rickenberg, H. E., "Diadochokinesis in Stutterers and Nonstutterers," *Journal of Medical Society of New Jersey,* LIII (1956), 324–26.

Roman, K. G., "Handwriting and Speech," *Logos,* II (1959), 29–39.

Rosenzweig, M. R., "Representations of the Two Ears at the Auditory Cortex," *American Journal of Physiology,* CLXVII (1951), 147–58.

Rossi, G. F., and G. Rosadini, "Experimental Analysis of Cerebral Dominance in Man." In C. H. Millikan and F. L. Darley (eds.), *Brain Mechanisms Underlying Speech and Language.* New York: Grune and Stratton, 1967.

Rutherford, B., "A Comparative Study of Loudness, Pitch, Rate, Rhythm, and Quality of the Speech of Children Handicapped by Cerebral Palsy," *Journal of Speech Disorders,* IX (1944), 263–71.

Rylander, G., "Personality Analysis Before and After Frontal Lobotomy," *Publications of the Association for Nervous and Mental Diseases,* XXVII (1948), 691–705.

Sachs, M. W., "Zur Aetiologie des Stotterns," *Klinische Wochenschrift,* XXXVII (1924), 113–15.

Sayles, D. G., "Brain Wave Excitability, Perseveration, and Stuttering." Doctoral dissertation, University of Michigan, 1966.

Scarbrough, H. E., "A Quantitative and Qualitative Analysis of the Electroencephalograms of Stutterers and Nonstutterers," *Journal of Experimental Psychology,* XXXII (1943), 156–67.

Schilling, A., ["Electronystamographic Findings as Indication of Central Coordination Defect in Stutterers"], *Archive für Ohren-Nasen- und Kehlkopfheilkunde Vereinigt mit Zeitschrift* CLXXV (1959), 457–61.

———. "Organische Faktoren bei der Entstehung des Stotterns," *HNO,* X (1962), 149–53.

———. ["Radiokymograms of the Diaphragm in Stammerers,"] *Folia Phoniatrica,* XII (1960), 145–53.

———. "Stottern bei Rhesus-bedingter Stammhirnechädigung," *Archive Ohrenheilkunde,* CLXIX (1956), 501.

Schilling, A., and W. Krüger, "Untersuchungen über die Motorik sprachgestörter Kinder nach der motometrischen Skala von Oseretsky-Göllnitz unter Besonderer Berücksichtingung dei Frühkindlichen Hirnschädigung," *HNO,* VIII (1960), 205–9.

Schilling, R., and A. Schilling, ["On the Diagnosis of Early Childhood Brain Injuries in Stutterers"], *Aktuelle Probleme der Phoniatrie und Logopaedie; Supplementa ad Folia Phoniatrica,* I, (1960), 134–40.

Schmoigl, S., and W. Ladisch, "eeg Investigation in Stutterers," *Electroenceph. Clin. Neurophysiol.* XXIII (1967), 184–85.

Schönhärl, E., ["Age-Connected Changes in the Structural Picture of Stuttering"], *HNO,* XII (1964), 152–54.

Schönhärl, E., and D. Bente, "Veränderungen im eeg bei Stottern," *Kongress, Gemeinrhaftstg. allg. Angew. Phonetik.,* Hamburg-Altona, 1960.

Scripture, E. W., "Penmanship Stuttering," *Journal of American Medical Association,* LII (1909), 1480–81.

Scripture, M. K., and O. Glogau, "Speech Conflict as an Etiological Factor in Stuttering," *Journal of Nervous and Mental Disorders,* XLIII (1916), 37–46.

Sedlacek, C., "Reactions of the Autonomic Nervous System in Attacks of Stuttering," *Folia Phoniatrica,* I (1947–1948), 97–103.

Seeman, M., "Speech Pathology in Czechoslovakia." In R. W. Rieber and R. S. Brubaker (eds.), *Speech Pathology.* Philadelphia: Lippincott, 1966.

———. *Sprachstörungen bei Kindern.* Marhold: Halle-Saale, 1959.

————. "Sur la Régulation Neurovegitative de la Durée de la Phonation," *Folia Phoniatrica,* I (1947), 22–37.

————. ["The Significance of Twin Pathology for the Investigation of Speech Disorders"], *Archive gesamte Phonetik,* I, Part II (1937), 88–92.

————. "Über somatische Befunde bei Stottern," *Monatschrift für Orenheilkunde,* LXVIII (1934), 895–912.

————. "Untersuchungen über Phonationsdauer bei Stotterern," *Archive für Sprach- und Stimmphysiologie,* V (1941), 211–13.

Selzer, C. A., "Lateral Dominance and Visual Fusion," *Harvard Monographs in Education,* No. 12 (1933), Cambridge, Mass.: Harvard University Press.

Seth, G., "An Experimental Study of the Control of the Mechanism of Speech and in Particular that of Respiration in the Stutterer," *British Journal of Psychology,* XXIV (1934), 375–88.

————. "Psychomotor Control in Stammering and Normal Subjects: An Experimental Study," *British Journal of Psychology,* XLIX (1958), 139–43.

Shackson, R., "An Action Current Study of Muscle Contraction Latency with Special Reference to Latent Tetany in Stutterers," *Archives of Speech,* I (1936), 87–111.

Sheehan, J., and M. M. Martyn, "Spontaneous Recovery from Stuttering," *Journal of Speech and Hearing Research,* IX (1966), 121–35.

Shiraiwa, T. and J. Kawakuba, ["Study of the Cause of Stuttering"], Abstract No. 185, in G. Kamiyama (ed.), [*A Handbook for the Study of Stuttering.*] Tokyo: Japan, 1967.

Shtremel, A. K., ["Stuttering in Left Parietal Lobe Syndrome"], *Zhurnal Nevropatologii i Psikhiatrii imeni S. S. Korsakova,* LXIII (1963), 828–32.

Ssikorski, J. A., *Über das Stottern.* Berlin: Hirschwald, 1891.

Smith, A., and C. W. Burklund, "Dominant Hemispherectomy: Preliminary Report on Neuropsychological Sequelae," *Science,* CLIII (1966), 1280–82.

Snyder, M. A., "Stuttering and Coordination," *Logos,* I (1958), 36–44.

Sovak, M., "Das vegetative Nervensystem bei Stottern," *Monatschrift für Ohrenheilkunde,* LXIX (1935), 666–80.

Spadino, E. J., *Writing and Laterality Characteristics of Stuttering Children.* New York: Teachers College, Columbia University Press, 1941.

Stier, E., *Untersuchen über Linkshändigkeit und die funktionellen Differenzen der Hirnhälften.* Jena: Fischer, 1911.

Streifler, M., and F. Gumpertz, "Cerebral Potentials in Stuttering and Cluttering," *Confinia Neurologica,* XV (1955), 344–59.

Stromsta, C., "Role of Bone Conducted Sidetone in Stuttering," Terminal Progress Report, Grant NB 03541-02-03, U. S. Public Health Service, 1966.

————. "EEG Power Spectra of Stutterers and Nonstutterers," *Asha,* VI (1964), 418–419 (abstract).

Strother, C. R., and L. S. Kriegman, "Diadochokinesis in Stutterers and Nonstutterers," *Journal of Speech Disorders,* VIII (1943), 325–35.

————. "Rhythmokinesis in Stutterers and Nonstutterers," *Journal of Speech Disorders,* IX (1944), 239–44.

Stutte, H., "Quellenmaterial zur kinderpsychiatrischen Prävention," *Annals Crianca Portuguesa,* XIX (1960), 415–33.

Subirana, A., "The Relationship Between Handedness and Language Function," *International Journal of Neurology,* IV (1964), 215–34.

Subirana, A., J. Corominas, R. Puncernau, L. Oller-Daurella, and J. Monteys, "Nueva Contribucion al Estudio de la Dominancia Cerebral," *Medicamenta,* X (1952), 255–58.

Sutu, A., D. Mironescu, R. Cocinschi, O. Tirziu, and M. Miscoia, "Contributii Clinice si electroencefalografice la Studine Patogenzei Biblielii," *Pediatrica,* VIII (1964), 39–40.

Swift, W. B., "Why Visualization is the Best Method for Stuttering," *Proceedings of the American Speech Correction Association,* II (1932), 89–91.

Szondi, L., "Konstitutionanalyse von 100 Stotterern," *Wien Medizinische Monatschrift,* LXXXII (1932), 922–28.

Tomatis, A., *L'Oreille et le Language.* Paris: Éditions du Seuil, 1963.

———. "Recherches sur la Pathologie du Bégaiement," *Journal Française O R L,* III (1954), 384–90.

Travis, L. E., "A Comparative Study of the Performances of Stutterers and Normal Speakers in Mirror Tracing," *Psychological Monographs,* XXXIX (1928), 45–51.

———. "Brain Potentials and the Temporal Course of Consciousness," *Journal of Experimental Psychology,* XXI (1937), 302–7.

———. "Dissociation of the Homologous Muscle Function in Stuttering," *Archives of Neurology and Psychiatry,* XXXI (1934), 127–33.

———. "Disintegration of Breathing Movements During Stuttering," *Archives of Neurology and Psychiatry,* XVIII (1927), 673–90.

———. *Speech Pathology.* New York: Appleton-Century, 1931.

Travis, L. E., and R. Y. Herren, "Studies in Stuttering: V. A Study of Simultaneous Antitropic Movement of the Hands of Stutterers," *Archives of Neurology and Psychiatry,* XXII (1929), 487–94.

Travis, L. E., and J. R. Knott, "Brain Potentials from Normal Speakers and Stutterers," *Journal of Psychology,* II (1936), 137–50.

Travis, L. E., and D. B. Lindsley, "An Action Current Study of Handedness in Relation to Stuttering," *Journal of Experimental Psychology,* XVI (1933), 359–81.

Travis, L. E., and W. Malamud, "Brain Potentials from Normal Subjects, Stutterers, and Schizophrenic Patients," *American Journal of Psychiatry,* XCIII (1937), 929–36.

Tromner, E., *Das Stottern, die Sprachzwangneurose: II. Versammlung der Deutschen Gesellschaft für Sprach-und Stimmheilkunde.* Leipzig: Kabitzsch, 1929.

Twitmeyer, E. B., "Stammering in Relation to Hemato-Respiratory Factors," *Quarterly Journal of Speech,* XVI (1930), 278–83.

Van Dantzig, B., "Writing, Typing, and Speaking," *Journal of Speech Disorders,* IV (1939), 297–301.

Van Dusen, C. R., "A Laterality Study of Nonstutterers and Stutterers," *Journal of Speech Disorders,* IV (1939), 261–65.

Van Riper, C., "Report of Stuttering on a Musical Instrument," *Journal of Speech and Hearing Disorders,* XVII (1952), 433–34.

———. "The Quantitative Measurement of Laterality," *Journal of Experimental Psychology,* XVII (1935), 327–32.

Wada, J., "A New Method for the Determination of the Side of Cerebral Dominance: A Preliminary Report on the Intracarotid Injection of Sodium Amytol in Man," *Medical Biology,* XIV (1949), 221–22.

Wada, J., and T. Rasmussen, "Intracarotid Injection of Sodium Amytol for the

Lateralization of Cerebral Speech Dominance. Experimental and Clinical Observations," *Journal of Neurosurgery,* XVII (1960), 266–82.

Warren, J. M., and K. Akert (eds.), *The Frontal Granular Cortex and Behavior.* New York: McGraw-Hill, 1964.

Weinstein, E. A., "Affections of Speech with Lesions of the Nondominant Hemisphere." In D. M. Rioch and E. A. Weinstein (eds.) *Disorders of Communication.* Baltimore: Williams and Wilkins, 1964.

Weinstein, S., and E. A. Sersen, "Tactual Sensitivity as a Function of Handedness and Laterality," *Journal of Comparative Physiology and Psychology,* LIV, (1961), 663–67.

Weiss, B., ["Neuromuscular Excitability in Stutterers"], *Folia Phoniatrica,* XIX (1967), 117–24.

Weiss, D. A., *Cluttering.* Englewood Cliffs, N.J.: Prentice-Hall, 1964.

———. "Der Zusammenhang zwischen Poltern und Stottern," *Polia Phoniatrica,* IV (1950), 252–62.

Weissova, B., and L. Handzel, ["Familial Stuttering Caused by Parathyroid Gland Insufficiency"], *Czechoslovakia Otolaryngologie,* XI (1962), 57–61.

Wepman, J. M., "Familial Incidence in Stammering," *Journal of Speech Disorders,* IV (1939), 199–204.

———. "The Organization of Therapy for Aphasia: I. The In-Treatment Center," *Journal of Speech Disorders,* XII (1947), 405–9.

West, R., "An Agnostic's Speculations About Stuttering." In J. Eisenson (ed.), *Stuttering: A Symposium.* New York: Harper, 1958.

———. "The Pathology of Stuttering," *Nervous Child,* II (1943), 96–106.

West, R., and M. Ansberry, *The Rehabilitation of Speech.* New York: Harper, 1968.

West, R., S. Nelson, and M. Berry, "The Heredity of Stuttering," *Quarterly Journal of Speech,* XXV (1939), 23–30.

West, R., and E. Nusbaum, "A Motor Test for Dysphemia," *Quarterly Journal of Speech Education,* XV (1929), 469–79.

Westphal, G., "An Experimental Study of Certain Motor Abilities of Stutterers," *Child Development,* IV (1933), 214–21.

Williams, D. E., "Masseter Muscle Action Current Potentials in Stuttered and Nonstuttered Speech," *Journal of Speech and Hearing Disorders,* XX (1955), 242–61.

Wingate, M. E., "Behavioral Rigidity in Stutterers," *Journal of Speech and Hearing Research,* XIX (1966), 626–30.

Yastrebova, A. V., [*Peculiarities in the Oral and Written Speech of Stuttering Pupils.*] Moscow: Institute of Defectology, 1962.

Zaleski, T., "Rhythmic Skills in Stuttering Children," *De Therapia Vocis et Loquellae,* I (1965), 371–72.

Zangwill, O., "Speech." In J. Field (ed.), *Handbook of Physiology,* Vol. 3. Washington, D. C.: American Physiological Society, 1960.

fourteen

STUTTERING AS THE RESULT
OF DISTURBED FEEDBACK

The various theories of stuttering based on organicity, neurosis, and learning theory have all contributed to our understanding of the disorder. Each of these explanations accounts for part of the disorder's nature, but none, nor all of them combined, seems to be entirely satisfactory. They fail because they do not account adequately for the basic disruption of motor sequences that occur when a word is stuttered. The learning theorists base their explanations of this disruption either on the reinforcement of childhood disfluencies or the breakdown of integrations due to emotion but these are dubious generalities. They do not explain satisfactorily the *form* and intermittency of the core behavior. The organicists (except for Tomatis, 1963) show only that abnormalities in neural or motor functioning exist in some stutterers. And those who see stuttering as a neurosis bypass the core behavior of broken words and do not really make clear why or how they are broken.

FLUENCY DISRUPTION AS
A CYBERNETIC PHENOMENON

Contrasted with these positions is the view that stutterers possess a defective monitoring system for sequential speech. The research is still incomplete but what we have shows that fluency breaks similar to stuttering can be produced in normal speakers by altering the auditory feedback of their speech output. Furthermore, a marked reduction in stuttering can often be achieved by the same process. From these findings, the possible existence of a perceptual disability in stuttering, probably organic in nature, has been inferred.

Unfortunately, our current knowledge of how speech is programmed and controlled is far from satisfactory. The influence of Wiener's (1948) cybernetic theory has led to a number of hypothetical models, such as those by Fairbanks (1954) and Mysak (1966), which describe closed feedback loops as the essential monitoring system for speech. In Fairbanks' well known model we have an effector unit, a sensor unit, a storage unit, a comparator to match input information against the patterns contained in the storage component, and a mixer or controller regulating mechanism which alters the output so as to reduce future error signals. In trying to alter the output, the system may be thrown into oscillation or fixation if too much overload or too much distortion is present in the feedback.

Some controversy exists as to whether or not an on-going motor performance such as speech is monitored continuously or intermittently. The latter seems more tenable although possible neurological mechanisms for continuous monitoring, despite Lashley's (1951) objections, do apparently exist. In any event, motor speech seems to operate like an automatic or semiautomatic servosystem under ordinary conditions. However, since the timing of the simultaneous and successive bilateral musculatures involved in respiration, phonation, and articulation demand an almost incredible precision to produce integrated speech, it is not difficult to understand why distortions or overloads in the feedback signals could cause breakdowns.

Information about the speech output is returned to the central integrating mechanism through six auditory channels, via the right and left feedback routes from (1) airborne side-tone, (2) bone-conducted side-tone, and (3) tissue connected side-tone. Other feedback signals come from the kinesthetic-tactile-proprioceptive sensors on both sides of the body. Stromsta (1962) showed that the auditory feedback signals in these different channels arrive at markedly different times and that the temporal information-processing of speech output by the brain is very complex. Some central mechanisms for integrating all these feedback signals must be present, although their nature is not yet known.

From this cursory sketch, it should be evident that at least there are many possible sources of distortion in the feedback systems used to monitor speech. Asynchrony of feedback signals that arrive in the right and left cortical hemispheres may be involved; differential delays in bone-, tissue and air-conduction of a person's voice might create the distortion in auditory feedback which results in stuttering. These may have an organic basis and yet produce disruption only under stress as reflected in cybernetic noise. Transcerebral transit times, as Tomatis claims, may create a privately owned delayed auditory feedback system within the skull. Auditory feedback may interfere with proprioceptive feedback. All we are saying is that there is ample opportunity built into the system that we use in monitoring our speech for the kinds of signal distortion, interference, or overload which could lead to stuttering. In the succeeding sections of this chapter we will attempt to summarize what little basic information there is about how speech can be disrupted by altering its feedback, and we will try to show how these effects might have some pertinence to stuttering.

DELAYED AUDITORY FEEDBACK (DAF)

Although the phenomenon had long been known, Lee (1951) and Black (1951) were the first to report that when a normal speaker's verbal output was fed back to his ears after a short delay of about one fifth of a second, marked breaks in fluency occurred. Lee called this effect the "artificial stutter." Individuals differ in their vulnerability to this delayed auditory feedback (DAF). Some subjects are relatively unaffected by DAF, while others show marked speech interference. Those who do experience disruption under DAF respond in different ways: sounds and syllables are repeated or prolonged; blocks in phonation are observed; changes in rate, pitch, and vocal intensity occur. Yates (1963b) explains these individual differences in this way:

> . . . whether or not an individual is highly susceptible to DAF . . . depends upon the degree to which he utilizes auditory feedback in monitoring his speech. Individuals who are highly dependent on auditory feedback will be subject to severe breakdown under DAF, while individuals who rely mainly upon bone-conducted or kinesthetic feedback will show less breakdown.

This reasoning has also been accepted by Cohen and Edwards (1965) and other authors.

DAF EFFECTS IN NORMAL SPEAKERS

Although the literature on DAF has become so voluminous as almost to defy review here, some of the major findings for normal speakers under this condition can be summarized. DAF produces repetitions of syllables and prolongations of sounds (Black, 1951; Lee, 1951). Spectrographic analysis of speech under DAF shows a greater prolongation of the vowels (Rawnsley and Harris, 1954) and of glides and continuant sounds (Coblenz and Agnello, 1965). Delayed auditory feedback slows oral reading and speaking rate (Black, 1951; Fairbanks, 1955; Fairbanks and Guttman, 1958).

These authors noted that the substitutions involved in the articulatory errors under DAF were unusual ones and occurred primarily on the stressed syllables. There were many omitted sounds, but the bulk of the errors were repetitive reduplications of sounds and syllables resembling stuttering. According to Beaumont and Foss (1957) there are marked individual differences in the way people react to DAF, and all authors have made similar observations. Some persons show pronounced emotional reactions as measured by the galvanic skin response and other methods, as Haywood (1963) has demonstrated. Others remain relatively unaffected. In some subjects, vocal intensity increases under DAF (Atkinson, 1953; Spilka, 1954). The fundamental pitch of the voice tends to rise (Fairbanks, 1955). These effects may be due to the subjects' attempt to cope with the disruption. Pitch variability decreases and the vibrato becomes uneven (Deutsch and Clarkson, 1959). As a result of these disturbances the intelligibility of speech under delayed feedback becomes somewhat impaired (Atkinson, 1953).

Subjects generally show little adaptation to DAF in repeated readings or at different intervals of delay (Atkinson, 1953; Tiffany and Hanley, 1956). However, when very prolonged exposure to DAF is administered, some temporary adaptation does seem to take place according to Winchester, Gibbons, and Krebs (1959) and Hanley, Tiffany, and Brungard (1958). This decrease in speech disturbance may not be true adaptation however. It may merely mean that the speakers by using certain strategies learn to "beat the machine." They do this by using very slow speaking or sudden shifts of pitch or loudness or sudden speech attempts timed by finger movements or other means. Goldiamond, Atkinson, and Bilger (1962) showed that when subjects were instructed not to listen to the DAF they could read more words per minute than when they were asked to listen to it. In this way attention to proprioceptive feedback probably creates a buffer against the DAF stimuli.

In some few individuals, prolonged exposure to DAF produced residual effects for some hours, but for most subjects, the speech returns to normal fluency as soon as the delay is terminated. Black (1955) found a residual disruption effect lasting about three minutes after the delay was turned off, and Tiffany and Hanley (1956) report that the behavior of those individuals severely affected by delayed feedback seems to persist for a while after the delay is ended. A description of these lingering effects from DAF is illustrated by the following quotation from their article:

> This subject (a normal speaker) had experienced increasing difficulty with the side-tone readings, particularly on one word—pony. Following the delayed side-tone readings, he continued to experience great difficulty with this word even though no side-tone delay was present. He exhibited stuttering-like symptoms as though the experimental readings had produced a kind of specific anxiety for this word. He not only appeared to be more nonfluent than before the side-tone experience but also appeared to show tension and avoidance behavior.

We too have found a few normal adult speakers who showed similar responses, but the effect seems to be more pronounced with certain young children. We have been reluctant to use DAF with children ever since we discovered these long-term effects. Goldfarb and Braunstein (1958), who tested 25 normal speaking children aged 8-10 years under a delayed feedback time of .16 seconds (which would probably not produce maximal disruption), found that there was great speech impairment under the delay. Since children probably have less stable motor configurations for their words than adults, we can understand why DAF might create some havoc. Chase (1958), who found that his subjects could repeat the sound /b/ faster under DAF than when delay was not present, speaks about the facilitating effect of DAF upon syllabic repetitions and gives this personal testimony: "Experimenting with his own vocal responses under delay, the writer has observed that although he does not usually repeat words or speech sounds under delay, once he *voluntarily* repeats various speech elements, it is difficult to stop. Other observers have reported the same experience." This compulsive characteristic of the DAF speech disruptions is commonly experienced by many otherwise normal speakers. Some become quite emotional. A slight relationship between personality characteristics and vulnerability to DAF has been reported by Spilka (1954) and Goldfarb and Braunstein (1958).

Sex differences in the production of artificial stuttering, with the male being more vulnerable than the female to DAF, have been found by Bachrach (1964) and by Mahaffey and Stromsta (1965), but another study by Buxton (1969) found no sex differences. Younger children seem to show more disruptions under DAF than older ones. Although Chase, Sutton, First, and Zubin (1961) reported that younger children showed fewer speech disruptions under DAF than older ones, they used only one delay time. More recent studies by MacKay (1968) and Buxton (1969) both demonstrated that younger children do show more speech difficulty under DAF but that the delay times necessary to produce maximal disruption are much longer. Figure 16 shows MacKay's data. Buxton found that for children aged 4-9 a delay time of .60 second produced the most disruption. For subjects aged 10-26 years, this critical delay was .20 second while for the aged (60-81 years) the delay producing the most disturbance was .40 second.

Individuals differ somewhat in terms of the delay interval required to produce the DAF effect, but the critical delay for most young male adults seems to range from 0.16 to 0.22 second with females showing a longer critical delay time. The best delay time for producing disruption and the intensity of the delayed signal are related, but the most pronounced effects are found when the delayed feedback is at least loud enough to mask the fundamental frequency of the bone-conducted side-tone—50 dB or more above threshold (Butler and Galloway, 1957). Brubaker (1952) also showed that the sound pressure level of the DAF signal must be greater than that of the subject's own speech before disruption occurs. Since, as Butler and Galloway (1957) demonstrated, DAF has more disruptive effects at the higher levels of intensity, most investigators have used sound levels of 80 decibels or more for the delay. Binaural DAF produces more disturbance than monaural. Arens and Popplestone (1959) found that normal speakers with high

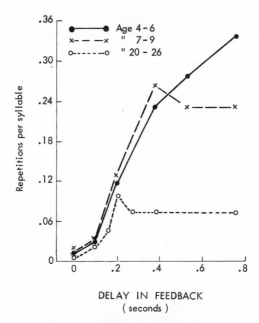

Figure 16. The Frequency of Repetitions (Stutters) Per Syllable as a Function of Feedback Delay for the Three Groups of Subjects of Differing Ages. *(From MacKay, 1968, p. 816, by permission.)*

verbal facility (as measured by Verbal IQ on the Wechsler—a dubious criterion)—were able to resist the DAF better than those with low verbal IQs. Buxton (1969) reported that the faster a speaker's maximum rate of speech, the shorter the delay time that produces the most disruption. Also, rapid speakers in general were less affected by DAF at all delay intervals from .10 to .60 seconds. In this connection, MacKay (1968) also says "The slower the subject's maximum rate, the higher his frequency of stuttering under DAF." By accelerating the feedback electronically so that one's speech is heard even more swiftly than normally, speech rate is improved and so is the fluency according to Peters (1954) and Davidson (1959).

SIMILARITIES OF STUTTERING TO DAF BEHAVIOR

The basic behaviors of stuttering, repetition of syllables and prolongations of sounds, have been found consistently in some normal speakers under delayed auditory feedback. It is also interesting that the spectrograms of repeated syllables of normal speakers under DAF show the same coarticulation defects found in stutterers (Rawnsley and Harris, 1954). If one can assume that the basic disturbance in normal speakers under DAF is temporal disruption in the programming of the motor sequences; i.e., that the time order of events is disturbed, then as Black (1951) and others have suggested, the increase in intensity or pitch or the slowdown in rate may be considered to be secondary reactions to this core experience. Such reactions are commonly found also in young stutterers once they begin to react to their stuttering.

Some authors feel that DAF nonfluencies are not stuttering. Neelley (1961) compared the performances of a group of 23 stutterers with a similar group of normal speakers under a DAF time of 0.14 seconds delay at a level of 75 dB above threshold and again under normal nondelay conditions. He concluded that the DAF speech disruptions of normal speakers as judged by listeners were dissimilar from those of stutterers when stuttering.

The Neelley study has been widely accepted as evidence that DAF speech disruptions are completely different from those shown by stutterers and this is unfortunate. Yates (1963b) has pointed out two extremely important weaknesses in the study "which make Neelley's conclusions quite unacceptable." First of all, Neelley used only one delay time (.14) and one intensity level, and this delay time is not the one that usually produces breakdown of speech in normal adult speakers, but instead it is a delay time that often improves the speech of stutterers. Secondly, Neelley asked his listener judges to distinguish between samples of speech, some from stutterers *speaking under no delay* and some from normal speakers under DAF. His judges of course were able to tell that the samples were different and so Neelley concluded that DAF disruptions bore no resemblance to stuttering ones. Yates' (1963b) remarks in this connection seem quite pertinent:

> But these empirical findings are totally irrelevant to the issue whether speech behaviour under DÁF is determined by the same factors which maintain stammering behaviour. The two groups are in no way meaningfully comparable in these respects. The stammerers in the experiment had presumably spent many years adapting to, and working out ways of dealing with, their perceptual defect (assuming it to exist). The Ss with normal speech were being, on the contrary, subjected to DÁF for the first time. Hence, it is in no way surprising that the speech of Ss subjected to DÁF for the first time is different from that of long-standing stammerers. The problem concerning underlying mechanisms of stammering cannot in fact be resolved by the kind of experiment reported by Neelley. The problem can be solved only by a direct attack on the auditory monitoring skills of stammerers (p. 116).

THE RESPONSES OF
STUTTERERS TO DAF

Recent research has demonstrated that many stutterers respond differently to DAF than normal speakers. Generally their fluency is improved under delay rather than disrupted. This, however, does not seem to be true for all stutterers. The less severe stutterers perform much like normal speakers and have difficulty being fluent. These differences suggest the presence of subpopulations of stutterers or merely the type of monitoring used.

Let us review some of the major findings. Bohr (1963) in South Africa found that stutterers were more fluent under DAF; Zerneri (1966) found two groups among 102 stutterers, one of which (the primarily clonic ones) improved under DAF. Lotzmann (1961), in a German article, found that by varying the delay times until an optimal delay was reached, blockings of all kinds were reduced or completely eliminated. He mentions that the most favorable times for fluency were shorter than those normally used to produce the DAF effect, varying around a delay time of .05 seconds. Lotzmann showed that for 62 stutterers DAF reduced the frequency of stuttering at least by one third, and that a delay of .05 seconds seemed to produce the greatest fluency. Nessel (1958) found that stutterers, unlike normal speakers, were generally unaffected by DAF in oral reading or were able to read faster and with fewer errors. Soderberg (1959) reports that his stutterers, especially the severe ones, showed a significant reduction in the frequency and duration of stuttering under DAF in both oral reading and spontaneous speech. Chase, Sutton, First, and Rubin (1961) also reported a marked improvement under DAF in one third of their stutterers.

Most of the studies reported above used only brief exposures to DAF, but we have a few in which stutterers were given DAF training over longer periods of time. Adamczyck (1959), in Poland, found an improvement in fluency under DAF at 0.25 seconds delay when stutterers were given repeated exposures over a period of three months. Goldiamond (1965) reports that operant conditioning procedures using DAF for several months facilitated fluency. Gross and Nathanson (1966) also used DAF to procure an initial decrease in stuttering and then gradually over a four week period shaped a prescribed slow-blending way of opposing its disruption into normal speech. They reported an increased and sustained improvement in oral reading. Siegenthaler and Brubaker (1957) report that stutterers who learned to monitor their speech through tactile and proprioceptive feedback showed little speech disturbance under DAF and that stutterers in general were less bothered by the delay than were normal speakers.

Two other studies may be of some interest. Stark (1967) used a click activated by lip closure in duplicate series of repeated syllables (mumumumu-muh), then introduced a delay as the subjects were clicking. Both stutterers and nonstutterers experienced equal amounts of disruptions under delay, but the stutterers had greater and more unusual errors. Lip closures lasted longer in the stutterers even when the bone-conducted click was not delayed. The other study, by Cohen and Edwards (1965), had stutterers experience alternations between simultaneous feedback and randomized-interval delayed feedback for 15 sessions of one hour each, three times weekly. No marked reduction in the frequency of stuttering occurred, but the stuttering behaviors changed significantly under this regime. Long, severe blockages disappeared; avoidance and struggle behavior decreased, and most of the stuttering became repetitive and similar to "primary stuttering."

There are, however, some studies which do not show this speech improvement under DAF in stutterers. Ham and Steer (1967), using only ten stutterers and their controls showed no differences in responses under DAF. Logue (1962) and Neelley (1961) also found no significant differences. A critical review of some of these studies by Soderberg (1968) makes clear that some of the discrepancy may be due to the use of noncritical delay times or the small number of subjects. He concludes that, though more carefully designed research is needed, the studies presently available indicate that DAF facilitates fluency in stutterers and that the fluency can be sustained by booster sessions.

In another paper, Soderberg (1969) describes the use of DAF as an aid to help the stutterer learn to stutter with easy repetitions and relaxed prolongations rather than blockages. The recirculation effect described by Chase (1958) may be responsible for this possible therapeutic application. Chase writes:

> It should be noted that facilitation of recirculation for speech units may result in obvious repetitions in speech for some cases, and prolongations of speech in other cases. For example, if facilitation of recirculation functioned at the level of word units, repetitions of words so affected would be noted by the listener. However, if facilitation of recirculation functioned at the level of a unit of speech smaller than a syllable, it might be heard solely as the prolongation of the syllable (p. 589).

Or perhaps even as the prolongation of a sound! It has been our experience that DAF does seem to modify the long hard struggling blocks of the stutterer even when they are not entirely prevented.

DISTORTED SIDETONE

The investigation of stuttering as a perceptual defect has led to an interest in other facets of feedback besides delayed sidetone. One of the most intriguing of these deals with the effects on speech of distorting the person's speech by altering its frequency components or its arrival phases at the two ears. We have already seen that Penfield and Rasmussen (1949) were able to produce arrest of phonation by stimulating certain areas of the cortex while their conscious patients were speaking. Following a lead by Vannier, Saumont, Labarraque, and Husson (1954), Stromsta (1959) showed that it was possible to cause speakers to be unable to continue to phonate—to experience an involuntary stoppage of phonation—while voicing continuous vowels in falsetto. He did this by having his subjects hear themselves through a system which created bilateral distortion of the produced vowel. Extreme pitch variations, lip tremors, and unpleasant changes in voice quality were also observed. In an earlier study, Stromsta (1956) had shown that stutterers as a group seemed to differ from normals in the inter-ear phase relationship of bone-conducted side-tone. This would tend to produce distortion in the feed-back. Since Vannier and his colleagues had produced complete blockage of phonation in normal speakers by altering the phase of the side-tone, Stromsta speculated that the core behavior (in some stutterers at least) might stem from this blockage of phonation. Spectrograms of speech under distorted side-tone not only showed the involuntary blockage of phonatation but also certain formant changes which resembled those found in stuttering. Stromsta suggests that stuttering may be a cybernetic *hunting* type of behavior in which the servo-system seeks, through oscillation and other coping mechanisms, to overcome the effects of the distortion in the stutterer's voice.

ALTERING FEEDBACK
BY MASKING NOISE

It has been known for a long time that a marked reduction in the severity of stuttering follows artificial deafening. Kern (1931) used the beating of loud drums to produce increments in fluency in stutterers. Shane (1955), using a 95 dB masking noise, found that her subjects' stuttering was reduced by 83 per cent under this condition and that eight of her twenty-five stutterers showed no stuttering at all.

Cherry and Sayers (1956) then performed a series of experiments in England showing that pure tones and white noise caused an immediate and in some cases a complete reduction in stuttering. They also demonstrated, by differentially filtering out certain frequency bands, that masking was most effective when the lower range of frequencies (those related to bone conducted sidetone or to the hearing of the fundamental frequency of one's own voice) were masked. May and Hackwood (1968), however, failed to find any differences in stutterer's reading time under high and low masking noise. Cherry and Sayers (1956) also reported a progressive reduction in stuttering as the intensity of the masking noise increased. This was corroborated by Stromsta (1958), who found that the number of stuttering blocks depended on the intensity of the masking sound. Maraist and Hutton (1957) also found that the number of errors (stutterings) decreased as the masking white noise became more intense and that the reading times shortened. Bohr (1963) in South Africa found white noise to reduce the frequency and severity of stuttering. Sutton and Chase (1961) threw some doubt on the belief that masking really altered the basic monitoring of speech by demonstrating that the same reduction in stuttering occurred whether the noise was introduced during speech production or during silent intervals for nine stutterers. Webster and Lubker (1968), however, attributed this discrepancy to the voice-actuated relay system that was used. Baron and Delumeau (1956) in France showed that a total reduction in stuttering occurred when a piece of oil-soaked cotton was placed in one ear, only to reappear in full strength when it was removed, a result which can only be explained in terms of suggestion.

Masking noise has also been used in stuttering therapy. In Russia, Derazne (1966) reported that as early as 1939 he had invented a portable masking device called the "D.C." (Derazne Correctophone) consisting of a low pitched noise generator and earphones. At first this was carried in a knapsack, according to our information, but later miniaturized. Derazne writes:

> In looking over extended results in the treatment of stutterers, we confirmed the fact that it was possible for us to remove stuttering in the majority of our cases. In a small number of cases we noticed recurrences, but this happened as a result of repeated breakdowns of higher nervous function or of a repeated experience of fear, trauma, infectious disease, etc. Those stutterers who had suffered relapses were again treated with the D.C. but for a short period of time (2 or 3 weeks) and consequently resumed normal speech. Our methods did not give positive results in stuttering which was of an organic nature (p. 616).

Parker and Christopherson (1963) designed a portable masker and reported that training in its use produced remarkable improvement in their three stuttering patients. Van Riper (1965) also designed a portable masker and reported a reduction in severity but less of a reduction in frequency in 24 of 25 stutterers when the masker was used intermittently. Difficulties in getting the stutterer to turn on the masker at the appropriate times were demonstrated. Murray (1969), in a careful study, found that masking noise reduced both the frequency and duration of stutterings, but his results showed clearly that continuous masking was more effective than random or intermittent masking when the noise was controlled either by the stutterer or experimenter. An article by Trotter and Lesch (1967) illustrates the effectiveness of the portable masker.

> Some speech pathologists have asked me if I thought the stutter-aid was another distraction device that would eventually become useless. I do not think so. In the two and one half years that I have worn the aid, I estimate that I have turned the aid on between 5000 to 6000 times. My stuttering blocks are shorter or absent as the result (p. 272).

No reported carry-over was experienced. Perkins and Curlee (1969) had three stutterers compare portable masking units which presented either white noise or signal pulses (from 25 to 590 Hz). Both decreased stuttering, but the stutterers did not seem particularly enthusiastic about employing the devices. Little carry-over effect was observed.

Possibly related to the masking effect is the reported low incidence of stuttering among the deaf, a topic we have already discussed in an earlier chapter but some of which we might review briefly here. Backus (1938) found only six totally deaf stutterers in surveying 13,691 children in schools for the deaf. Albright and Malone (1942) in a similar study also failed to discover more than a handful of deaf stutterers in a large population of the hearing handicapped. We ourselves have one authenticated case of an adult male who had stuttered severely from infancy and who immediately stopped stuttering completely after an accident in which he became completely deafened. The cessation of stuttering occurred within three hours of the trauma and shortly after he began to speak.

COMPETING FEEDBACK CHANNELS

That stuttering usually has its onset during the years from 2-4 is not surprising when it is recalled that words are learned motor sequences and that they are first learned and habituated by acoustical matching of the child's output against a model presented by others. When the words are first learned, the auditory channel must be the one through which the essential information flows if the comparison of output with the interiorized model and the consequent reduction of error signals are to be accomplished. However, we need our ears for other important functions—for perceiving our own verbalized thoughts and the thoughts of others. It would be too burdensome if we always had to play our speech by ear—if we were eternally doomed to listen to each sound and syllable of each word to ensure its correctness. In our opinion, the human being, as he always does when overloaded, finds a shorter and easier way. In this case, he turns over the major responsibility for the monitoring of speech to another available information processing system—the kinesthetic-tactual-proprioceptive one—as soon as possible. This change we believe occurs as soon as the auditory system stops giving error signals; as soon as the motor sequences involved in word production seem to be able to be produced correctly without constant auditory scrutiny.

This possible turnover of control to proprioception cannot be viewed as a sudden flip-flop sort of process. The change probably takes place gradually and intermittently at first. For some time there may be some interference between the auditory and proprioceptive signals which could lead to broken words. Or there may be overload. As a child learns to communicate verbally, he must find it difficult to scan his listener visually, to make sure he keeps out phonemic mismatching, to reel off the appropriate motor sequences and to unfold the semantic content he intends. We should not be surprised then to find many children with a history of delayed speech beginning to stutter once they begin to talk—or, for that matter, to find most children being disfluent when they first begin to talk in sentences. Overloaded circuits oscillate and jam. Once the monitoring of the motoric sequencing of words can be turned over to proprioception, much of this overload is reduced. Auditory interference no longer has much impact.

In our opinion it seems tenable that normal speaking adults monitor their speech primarily by somesthesia (touch-kinesthesia-proprioception). We can speak fluently even when we are in the presence of loud masking noise. Adults who suddenly become deaf do not begin to stutter. Indeed, it takes a long time before they begin to show phonemic distortions in their speech and, even after these occur, the speech remains normally fluent. Normal speakers also remain fluent when distortion is introduced into the auditory signals by high pass or low pass filters. What is more illuminating in this regard is that delayed auditory feedback requires great amplification (enough to overcome any self-hearing) before it disrupts our speech. If the motoric sequencing of speech depended primarily upon auditory feedback, we would not expect these results. On the other hand, if the sequencing of speech is monitored primarily by somesthetic feedback, we can readily understand why they occur.

This switching from one sense modality to another in the control of sequential behaviors is not uncommon. We find much the same sort of thing occurring in handwriting where at first visual monitoring is mandatory as the child painstakingly traces his first words. As the motoric patterns become thoroughly learned, kinesthetic and proprioceptive controls take over. We eventually become able to write even in complete darkness though usually vision plays an accessory but subordinate role. Experiments with mirror tracing, where the visual feedback is reversed, show that kinesthesia can serve as a major control.

In speaking, as we have said, we need to use our eyes to scan our listener's reactions and our ears to discover what we are saying and what he may say in return. We do not think of all the words of a sentence first and then speak them later. Our messages unfold and we scan what we are saying in order to know whether or not we have expressed our intent. By turning over the major responsibility for the monitoring of our motor sequences to somasthesia, we doubtless facilitate the auditory scanning of the *meaning* of our messages. In this connection, Broadbent (1958) has offered a theory of perception which has much to offer here as we attempt to explain why some early stuttering tends to occur during the alleged shift from auditory to proprioceptive feedback control of spoken words. Broadbent views the nervous system as acting like a single communication channel of limited capacity. When the input to this channel overloads its capacity, some filtering process occurs so that only selected bits of information having features in common will be allowed to enter the system. If two or more messages with high information value are received through two different internal channels at the same time, the system may jam and the information will not be transmitted into the perceptual system in an orderly way. Although there must be some temporal parallelism in the bits of information being processed through proprioception and audition, it is probably inexact.

Most of the research (Travers, 1964) seems to indicate that when information from more than one sense modality is provided simultaneously in the governing of a given activity, no advantage is gained and inhibitory interference tends to be the more probable result. We do not yet know where this selective filtering mechanism is located, but there are some indications that it resides in the reticular system (Hernandez-Péon, 1959). Moreover it appears that the blocking of one channel is rarely complete and that some information still gets through to the higher cortical centers in attenuated form where again some central inhibitory mechanisms may selectively exclude certain kinds of sensory information (Hernandez-Péon, Scherrer, and Jouvet, 1956).

If it is true, as Webster and Lubker (1968) and others hypothesize, that the disruption in timing which produces stuttering is due to distorted auditory feedback signals, then it would follow that masking should reduce stuttering. The need to disregard DAF signals (to beat the machine) would also stop the stutterer from continually listening to himself and thereby improve his fluency. He would be forced to do what all normal speakers probably do —control his speech primarily by proprioceptive-tactile feedback. By concentrating his attention on the feel of his speech musculatures, the stutterer can create barriers against any auditory interference or distortion which might be present.

From this point of view it is also possible to understand why stutterers seem to be able to speak more fluently while whispering and to be completely fluent when pantomiming speech. In the latter connection we found (in an unpublished study) that stutterers had no stuttering when giving commands by pantomime to skilled lip readers. Also the marked or complete reduction of stuttering produced by using an electrolarynx, a process which requires a high degree of conscious articulation in the pantomiming movements, seems to support this view (Mckenzie, 1955). Several reports are also available which indicate that laryngectomized stutterers who learn esophageal speech (where very careful articulation is mandatory and also probably some disregard of the acoustic features exists) do not show any stuttering when speaking in this way (Oldrey, 1953; Irving and Webb, 1961).*

We were born too soon to understand how the intermorphemic breaks in fluency we call stuttering are really produced, but it seems highly plausible that distortion in the total feedback signal system may be responsible for them. The distortion may reside in the auditory signals alone and be introduced by bilateral phase differences between bone- and air-conducted side-tone, or in the interference produced by auditory and proprioceptive competition, or in overload, or in the central processing of the information. Any of these may disrupt the precise timing of antagonistic or bilateral sets

* There are a few studies that bear obliquely on the relative importance of taction and kinesthesis as compared with audition in the monitoring of speech in the normal speaker. Generally, they show that anesthetizing the articulatory areas produces greater impairment in speech than auditory masking (McCroskey, 1958; Ringel and Steer, 1963). Gross (1964), however, found that such anesthesia had no effect on stutterers.

of muscles and thereby produce stuttering. The basic synergies involved in the coordination of phonation with articulation may be disrupted by bilateral aberrations of the cochleo-recurrential reflex and momentary blockage of utterance many ensue. At the present time we just do not know what happens neurologically when broken words instead of integrated words are produced. Nevertheless, we feel very strongly that this area, which we are just beginning to explore, will teach us much about the essential nature of stuttering.

COMMENTARY

A succession of loops is shown in which speech progresses element by element to make up the phonemes—syllables—words—thoughts which go into a complete sentence. The satisfaction at each stage by a monitoring system is required; otherwise the machine halts, repeats, or reports corrected. Repetition of sentences and words is volitional for emphasis, increased clarity, or correction of gross errors. Repetition of syllables is probably involuntary, or reflex, and it is at this stage that *artificial stutter* is manifested. (Lee, 1951, p. 54)

Observation of clinical patients who are classed as stutterers speaking under delayed feedback indicates that frequently stutterers who have learned to control their speech by nonauditory monitoring methods such as tactile and proprioceptive sensations (i.e., keeping light contacts between the articulators, moving to the next phoneme in a word if speech is blocked, etc.) appear to have little speech disturbance. (Siegenthaler and Brubaker, 1957, pp. 24–31)

. . . the behavior evidenced under a condition of delayed side-tone may be an attempt to return speech to a condition that would produce normal side-tone. This striving toward normality is in line with the observation that people do control the changes, especially the extremes, that occur in their behavior in what might be called a tendency toward behavioral homeostasis. (Atkinson, 1953, p. 386)

The writer has observed that under delay some normal-speaking individuals can be taught to "beat the machine" by concentrating on their oral cavity, particularly their tongue and lip movements, in addition to becoming aware of the proprioceptive feedback resulting from laryngeal functioning. Is this what automatically happens to the stutterer as masking is injected into his ears, or when he whispers? Does he automatically shift to the tactual and proprioceptive aspects of speech monitoring when he cannot monitor his speech auditorally? If stuttering is linked to the way in which the stutterer hears his own vocal utterances, then eliminating or diminishing the use of this monitoring channel may account for his increased fluency. (Gruber, 1965. p. 379)

We noticed that children who tended to repeat words and word groups in their normal speech ceased to do so under conditions of delayed auditory feedback. They slowed down their speech as did the normal children. The delayed feedback evidently shifted the tendency toward repetition to different units. (Chase, 1958, p. 589)

When the side-tone is accelerated through a circuit feeding from a throat microphone and directly to the head-set, the average person speaks much better. The speech is swifter, more precisely articulated and more fluent. (Peters, 1954, p. 488)

One of the most interesting and possibly important findings of the present study was the lack of homogeneity of DAF effect on stutterers. A substantial minority of stutterers responded in respect to additions, substitutions, correct word rate, adaptation, and consistency in a direction opposite to that of the majority. . . . The differences invite further study. (Neelley, 1961, p. 78)

. . . in cases where phantom or whispered speech eventually helps a *system* to *readjust,* it may be due to the complete or incomplete transference of the major speech monitoring function to the tactile or proprioceptive channel and away from the offending auditory circuit. Accordingly, some individuals have been known not to react to auditory delay with stuttering behavior and it has been inferred that these individuals are capable of monitoring with other than the auditory channel.

Further development of the hypotheses will be forthcoming upon more clinical application and research. It should be noted that some of these ideas have been applied to stuttering in one form or another by various clinicians but without adequate explanations of why they were effective. (Mysak, 1960, p. 194)

Elimination of air-conducted sound alone is readily achieved by blocking the ears. The results with this method of interference were neither striking nor consistent. Elimination of both air and bone conducted voice sounds was effected by playing a loud masking tone into both ears of the subject through headphones. The loudness of the tone used approached pain level and complete masking of the subject's awareness of his own speech sound was achieved. The results of this experiment were immediate and consistent. Control of both steady-state speech and of the ability to make immediate starts in speaking was rapidly established. In general, virtually complete elimination of stammering resulted during the experiment. The ability of each subject to make an immediate start in speaking improved to a very considerable extent.

Thus we have found that elimination of air-conducted feedback of the monitored sounds has little effect on the performance of a stammering subject, whereas blocking both air-conduction and bone-conduction pathways of speech feedback results generally in a virtually complete suppression of stammering. Such a method of interference with the appropriate feedback pathways results in virtually complete control of both steady-state and starting-condition utterance of the stammerers we have studied. (Cherry and Sayers, 1956, p. 238)

Of the subjects tested thus far, some develop a quavering slow speech of the type associated with cerebral palsy; others may halt, repeat syllables, raise their voice in pitch or volume, and reveal tension by reddening of the face. . . . Some have challenged the disturbance, but none have as yet defeated it. (Lee, 1951, p. 640)

BIBLIOGRAPHY

Adamczyk, B., ["Use of Instruments for the Production of Artificial Feedback in the Treatment of Stuttering"], *Folia Phoniatrica,* XI (1959), 216–18.

Agnello, J. G., and H. C. Kagan, "Delayed Auditory Feedback and Its Effect on the Manner of Speech Production," Final Report, National Institute of Mental Health, Grant No. 11067–01., 1966.

Albright, M. A., and J. Y. Malone, "The Relationship of Hearing Acuity to Stammering," *Journal of Exceptional Children,* VIII (1942), 186–90.

Arends, C. J., and J. A. Popplestone, "Verbal Facility and Delayed Speech Feedback," *Perceptual and Motor Skills,* IX (1959), 270.

Atkinson, C. J., "Adaptation to Delayed Sidetone," *Journal of Speech and Hearing Disorders,* XVIII (1953), 386–91.

Bachrach, D. L., "Sex Differences in Reactions to Delayed Auditory Feedback," *Perceptual Motor Skills,* XIX (1964), 81–82.

Backus, O., "Incidence of Stuttering Among the Deaf," *Annals of Otology, Rhinology and Laryngology,* XLVII (1938), 632–35.

Baron, F., and G. Delumeau, "An Etiology of Stuttering," *Annals of Otology, Rhinology and Laryngology,* LXXIII (1956), 962–64.

Beaumont, J., and B. Foss, "Individual Differences in Reacting to Delayed Auditory Feedback," *British Journal of Psychology,* XLVIII (1957), 85–89.

Black, J. W., "The Effect of Delayed Sidetone Upon Vocal Rate and Intensity," *Journal of Speech and Hearing Disorders,* XVI (1951), 56–60.

———. "Studies of Delayed Sidetone," *Contributi del Laboratorie di Psicologia,* Nuova Sene, XLIX (1955), Milano: Vita e Pensiero.

Bohr, J. W. F., "The Effects of Electronic and Other External Control Methods on Stuttering: A Review of Some Research Techniques and Suggestions for Further Research," *Journal of South African Logopedic Society,* X (1963), 4–13.

Broadbent, D. E., "Attention and the Perception of Speech," *Scientific American,* CCVI (1962), 143–51.

———. *Perception and Communication.* London: Pergamon Press, 1958.

Brubaker, R., "An Experimental Investigation of Speech Disturbance as a Function of the Intensity of Delayed Auditory Feedback." Doctoral dissertation, University of Illinois, 1952.

Butler, R. A., and F. T. Galloway, "Factoral Analysis of the Delayed Speech Feedback Phenomenon," *Journal of the Acoustical Society of America,* XXIX (1957), 632–35.

Buxton, L. F., "An Investigation of Sex and Age Differences in Speech Behavior

Under Delayed Auditory Feedback." Doctoral dissertation, Ohio State University, 1969.

Chase, R. A., "Comparison of the Effects of Delayed Auditory Feedback on Speech and Key Tapping," *Science,* CXXIX (1959), 903–4.

———. "Effect of Delayed Auditory Feedback on the Repetition of Speech Sounds," *Journal of Speech and Hearing Disorders,* XXIII (1958), 583–90.

Chase, R. A., S. Sutton, D. First, and J. Zubin, "A Developmental Study of Changes in Behavior Under Delayed Auditory Feedback," *Journal of Genetics and Psychology,* XCIX (1961), 101–12.

Cherry, E. C., *On Human Communication.* New York: John Wiley and Sons, 1957.

Cherry, E. C., and B. M. Sayers, "Experiments Upon the Total Inhibition of Stammering by External Control, and Some Clinical Results," *Journal of Psychosomatic Research,* I (1956), 233–46.

Cherry, E. C., B. M. Sayers, and P. Marland, "Some Experiments on the Total Suppression of Stammering; and a Report on Some Clinical Trials," *Bulletin of the British Psychological Society,* XXX (1956), 43–44.

Coblenz, H., and J. G. Agnello, "The Effects of Delayed Auditory Feedback on the Manner of Consonant Production," convention address, A.S.H.A., 1965.

Cohen, J. G., and A. E. Edwards, "The Extraexperimental Effects of Random Sidetones," *Proceedings of the Annual Convention of the American Psychological Association,* I (1965), 211–12.

Davidson, G. O., "Sidetone Delay and Reading Rate, Articulation, and Pitch," *Journal of Speech and Hearing Research,* II (1959), 266–70.

Derazne, J., "Speech Pathology in the U.S.S.R." In R. W. Rieber and R. S. Brubaker (eds.), *Speech Pathology.* Philadelphia: Lippincott, 1966.

Deutch, J., and J. Clarkson, "Musical Feedback," *Scientific American,* CC (1959), 66.

Fairbanks, G., "Systematic Research in Experimental Phonetics–I. A. Theory of the Speech Mechanism as a Servomechanism," *Journal of Speech and Hearing Disorders,* XIX (1954), 133–39.

———. "Selective Vocal Effects of Delayed Auditory Feedback," *Journal of Speech and Hearing Disorders,* XV (1955), 142–53.

Fairbanks, G., and N. Guttman, "Effects of Delayed Auditory Feedback upon Articulation," *Journal of Speech and Hearing Research,* I (1958), 12–22.

Fillenbaum, S., "Delayed Auditory Feedback with Different Delay Times at Each Ear," *Journal of Speech and Hearing Research,* VII (1964), 369–71.

Frankenberger, R., "Disruption of Speech Under Delayed Auditory Feedback: A Function of Syllable Duration and Duration of Delayed Auditory Feedback." Doctoral dissertation, Ohio University, 1968.

Goldfarb, W., and P. Braunstein, "Reactions to Delayed Auditory Feedback in Schizophrenic Children." In P. H. Hock and J. Zubin (eds.), *Psychopathology of Communication.* New York: Grune and Stratton, 1958.

Goldiamond, I., "Stuttering and Fluency as Manipulatable Operant Response Classes. In L. Krasner and L. P. Ullman (eds.), *Research in Behavior Modification.* New York: Holt, 1965.

Goldiamond, I., C. J. Atkinson, and R. C. Bilger, "Stabilization of Behavior and Prolonged Exposure to Delayed Auditory Feedback," *Science,* CXXXVII (1962), 437–38.

Gross, C. M.. "A Study of Certain Effects of Local and Topical Anesthetics on the Speech of Stutterers." Master's thesis, Western Michigan University, 1964.

Gross, M. S., and S. N. Nathanson, "A Study of the Use of a DAF Shaping Procedure for Adult Stutterers," convention address, A.S.H.A., 1966.

Gruber, L., "Sensory Feedback and Stuttering," *Journal of Speech and Hearing Disorders,* XXX (1963), 373–80.

Ham, R., and M. D. Steer, "Certain Effects of Alterations in Auditory Feedback," *Folia Phoniatrica,* XIX (1967), 53–62.

Hanley, C. N., W. R. Tiffany, and J. M. Brungard, "Skin Resistance Changes Accompanying the Sidetone Test for Auditory Malingering," *Journal of Speech and Hearing Research,* I (1958), 286–93.

Harms, M., and J. Malone, "The Relationship of Hearing Acuity to Stammering," *Journal of Speech and Hearing Disorders,* IV (1939), 363–71.

Haywood, H. C., "Differential Effects of Delayed Auditory Feedback on Palmar Sweating, Heart Rate, and Pulse Pressure," *Journal of Speech and Hearing Research,* VI (1963), 181–86.

Hernandez-Péon, R., "Reticular Mechanisms of Sensory Control." In W. A. Rosenblith (ed.), *Sensory Communication.* New York: Wiley, 1961.

Hernandez-Péon, R., H. Scherrer, and M. Jouvet, "Modification of Electric Activity in Cochlear Nucleus During Attention in Unanesthetized Cats," *Science,* CXXIII (1956), 331–32.

Irving, R. W., and M. W. Webb, "Teaching Esophageal Speech to a Pre-Operative Severe Stutterer," *Annals of Otology, Rhinology and Laryngology,* XL (1961), 1069–80.

Karlovich, R. S., and J. T. Graham, "Effects of Pure Tone Synchronous and Delayed Auditory Feedback on Key Tapping Performance to a Programmed Visual Stimulus," *Journal of Speech and Hearing Research,* IX (1966), 596–603.

Kern, A., "Der Einfluss des Hörens auf das Stottern," *Arch. Psychiat.,* 97, (1931), 429–449.

Lashley, K. S., "The Problem of Serial Order in Behavior." In L. A. Jeffress (ed.), *Cerebral Mechanisms in Behavior.* New York: Wiley, 1951.

Lee, B. S., "Artificial Stutter," *Journal of Speech and Hearing Disorders,* XVI (1951), 53–55.

Logue, R., "The Effects of Temporal Alterations in Auditory Feedback upon the Speech Output of Stutterers and Nonstutterers." Master's thesis, Purdue University, 1962.

Lotzmann, G., ["On the Use of Varied Delay Times in Stammerers"], *Folia Phoniatrica,* XIII (1961), 276–310.

MacKay, D. G., "Metamorphosis of a Critical Interval: Age-linked Changes in the Delay in Auditory Feedback that Produces Maximal Disruption of Speech," *Journal of Acoustical Society of America,* XIX (1968), 811–21.

Mahaffey, R. B., and C. Stromsta, "Effects of Peak-Clipped and Center-Clipped Delayed Sidetone," *Asha,* VII (1965), 413–14.

————. "The Effects of Auditory Feedback as a Function of Frequency, Intensity, Time, and Sex," *De Therapia Vocis et Loquellae,* II (1965), 233–35.

Maraist, J. A., and C. Hutton, "Effects of Auditory Masking Upon the Speech of Stutterers," *Journal of Speech and Hearing Disorders,* XXII (1957), 385–89.

Martin, H., "Rehabilitation of the Laryngectomee," *Cancer,* July (1963), 824.

May, A. E., and A. Hackwood, "Some Effects of Masking and Eliminating Low Frequency Feedback on the Speech of Stutterers," *Behaviour Research and Therapy,* VI (1968), 219–24.

McCroskey, R., "The Relative Contribution of Auditory and Tactile Cues in Certain Aspects of Speech," *Southern Speech Journal,* XVI (1958), 86–90.

McKenzie, F. A., "A Stutterer's Experience in Using an Electro-Larynx." In W. Johnson (ed.), *Stuttering in Children and Adults.* Minneapolis: University of Minnesota Press, 1955.

Murray, F. P., "An Investigation of Variably Induced White Noise Upon Moments of Stuttering," *Journal of Communication Disorders,* II (1969), 109–14.

Mysak, E. D., "Servo Theory and Stuttering," *Journal of Speech and Hearing Disorders,* XXV (1960), 188–95.

————. *Speech Pathology and Feedback Theory.* Springfield, Ill.: Thomas, 1966.

Neelley, J. N., "A Study of the Speech Behavior of Stutterers and Nonstutterers Under Normal and Delayed Auditory Feedback," *Journal of Speech and Hearing Disorders, Monograph Supplement,* No. 7 (1961), 63–82.

Nessel, E., "Die Verzögerte Sprachrückkopplung (Lee Effect) bei Stottern," *Folia Phoniatrica,* X (1958), 87–99.

Oldrey, M., in C. Van Riper (ed.), *Speech Therapy: A Book of Readings.* New York: Prentice-Hall, 1953.

Parker, C. S., and F. Christopherson, "Electric Aid in the Treatment of Stammer," *Medical Electronics and Biological Engineering,* I (1963), 121–25.

Penfield, W., and T. Rasmussen, "Vocalization and Arrest of Speech," *Archives of Neurology and Psychiatry,* XLI (1949), 21–27.

Perkins, W. H., and R. F. Curlee, "Clinical Impressions of Portable Masking Unit Effects in Stuttering," *Journal of Speech and Hearing Disorders,* XXXIV (1969), 360–62.

Peters, R. W., "The Effect of Change in Sidetone Delay and Level Upon Rate of Oral Reading of Normal Speakers," *Journal of Speech and Hearing Disorders,* XIX (1954), 483–96.

Rawnsley, A. F., and J. D. Harris, "Comparative Analysis of Normal Speech and Speech with Delayed Sidetone by Means of Sound Spectrograms," Bureau of Medical Research, Project No. NM003–041.56.03, 1954.

Ringel, R. L., and M. D. Steer, "Some Effects of Tactile and Auditory Alterations on Speech Output," *Journal of Speech and Hearing Research,* VI (1963), 369–78.

Shane, M. L. S., "Effect on Stuttering of Alteration in Auditory Feedback." In W. Johnson (ed.), *Stuttering in Children and Adults.* Minneapolis: University of Minnesota Press, 1955.

Siegenthaler, B. M., and R. S. Brubaker, "Suggested Research in Delayed Auditory Feedback," *Pennsylvania Speech Annual,* XIV (1957), 24–31.

Smith, K. U., *Delayed Sensory Feedback and Behavior.* Philadelphia: Sanders, 1962.

Soderberg, G. A., "Delayed Auditory Feedback and the Speech of Stutterers," *Journal of Speech and Hearing Disorders,* XXXIII (1969), 20–29.

————. "Delayed Auditory Feedback and Stuttering," *Journal of Speech and Hearing Disorders,* XXXIII (1968), 260–67.

Spilka, B., "Some Vocal Effects of Different Reading Passages and Time Delays in Speech Feedback," *Journal of Speech and Hearing Disorders,* XIX (1954), 33–47.

Stark, R. E., "Effects of Delayed Auditory Feedback Upon a Speech Related Task in Stutterers," convention address, A.S.H.A., 1967.

Stromsta, C., "The Effects of Altering the Fundamental Frequency of Masking on the Speech Performance of Stutterers," Technical Report, National Institutes of Health, Project B-1331, 1958.

————. "Experimental Blockage of Phonation by Distorted Sidetone," *Journal of Speech and Hearing Research,* II (1959), 286–301.

————. "Averaged Evoked Responses of Stutterers and Nonstutterers as a Function of Interaural Time Relationships," Technical Report. National Institutes of Health, Project NB-03541-03, 1965.

————. "Delays Associated with Certain Sidetone Pathways," *Journal of Acoustical Society of America,* XXXIV (1962), 392–96.

————. "EEG Power Spectra of Stutterers and Nonstutterers," *Asha,* VI, (1964), 418–19.

————. "Interear Phase Disparity of Bone-Conducted Sound Energy in Stutterers and Nonstutterers," Technical Report, National Institutes of Health, Project B-1331-C2, 1961.

————. "A Methodology Related to the Determination of the Phase Angle of Bone Conducted Speech Sound Energy of Stutterers and Nonstutterers," *Dissertation Abstracts,* XVI (1956), 1738–39.

Sutton, S., and R. A. Chase, "White Noise and Stuttering," *Journal of Speech and Hearing Research,* IV (1961), 72.

Tiffany, W. R., and C. Hanley, "Adaptation to Delayed Sidetone," *Journal of Speech and Hearing Disorders,* XXI (1956), 164–72.

Tomatis, A., *L'Oreille et le Langage.* Paris: Éditions du Seuil, 1963.

Travers, R. M. W. (ed.), *Research and Theory Related to Audio-visual Information Transmission.* Bureau of Educational Research, University of Utah, 1964.

Trotter, W. D., and M. M. Lesch, "Personal Experiences with a Stutter-aid," *Journal of Speech and Hearing Disorders,* XXXII (1967), 270–72.

Vannier, J., R. Saumont, L. Labarraque, and R. Husson, "Production Experimentale des Blocages Synaptiques Recurrentials par des Stimulations Auditives Homorythmiques avec Déphasages Réglables," *Revue de Laryngologie,* Supplement I, Bordeau, February, 1954.

Van Riper, C., "Clinical Use of Intermittent Masking Noise in Stuttering Therapy," *Asha,* VI (1965), 381.

Webster, R. L., and R. B. Lubker, "Interrelationships Among Fluency Producing Variables in Stuttered Speech," *Journal of Speech and Hearing Research,* XI (1968), 754–66.

————. "Masking of Auditory Feedback in Stutterers' Speech," *Journal of Speech and Hearing Research,* XI (1968), 219–23.

Wiener, N., *Cybernetics.* New York: Wiley, 1948.

————. *The Human Use of Human Beings.* Boston: Houghton-Mifflin, 1960.

Winchester, R. A., and E. W. Gibbons, "The Effect of Auditory Masking Upon Oral Reading Rate," *Journal of Speech and Hearing Disorders,* XXIII (1958), 250–52.

Winchester, R. A., E. W. Gibbons, and D. F. Krebs, "Adaptation to Sustained Delayed Sidetone," *Journal of Speech and Hearing Disorders,* XXIV (1959), 25–28.

Yates, A. J., "Delayed Auditory Feedback," *Psychological Bulletin,* LX (1963a), 213–32.

————. "Recent Empirical and Theoretical Approaches to the Experimental

Manipulation of Speech in Normal Subjects and in Stammerers," *Behaviour Research and Therapy,* I (1963b), 95–119.

Zerneri, L., ["Attempts to Use Delayed Speech Feedback in Stuttering Therapy"], *Journal Français d' Oto-Rhino-Laryngologie et Chirurgie Maxillo-Faciale,* XV (1966), 415–18.

fifteen

THE NATURE OF STUTTERING:
AN ATTEMPTED SYNTHESIS

Although we know the attempt will not be entirely successful, in this chapter we will try to outline an explanation for the nature of stuttering which will bring together most of the hard information we have about the disorder—and some of the soft. Actually, there is not enough information about the essential nature of stuttering to allow more than a general outline of its patterning. But if we must fail, let us fail forward! Others will mend and build upon the insecure foundations on which this precarious monument to human benightedness is so hesitantly erected.

We should like to suggest that stuttering be considered a disorder of timing. We feel that when a person stutters on a word, there is a temporal disruption of the simultaneous and successive programming of muscular movements required to produce one of the word's integrated sounds, or to emit one of its syllables appropriately or to accomplish the precise linking of sounds and syllables that constitutes its motor pattern. If we ignore for the moment the entire complex overlay of reactions to this experience, we find the essence of the disorder in this fracturing and disruption of the motor sequence of the word. The integrity of a spoken word demands great precision in the timing of its components. When, for any reason, that timing is awry and askew, a temporally distorted word is produced, and when this happens, the speaker has evinced a core stuttering behavior.

There are real advantages to this definition. It escapes much of the foggy confusion in which stuttering has been developed.

In the future, the amount of temporal disruption might be measured objectively; the structures involved in the mistiming might be located; and hopefully, the asynchrony might be traced to its origin.

If stuttering is considered a disorder of timing it is possible to synthesize most of the various points of view concerning the nature of the disorder. Mistiming could be attributed to an organic proclivity, to emotional stress, or to a malfunctioning servo-system. The huge overlay of the variable struggle and avoidance reactions to the experiencing of mistimed words as well as much of the overt and covert phenomenology of the disorder are explained best with the principles of learning and conditioning, for it is probable that stuttering grows and maintains itself largely through differential learning experiences. In short, most of the information we have about stuttering makes sense if its original or core behaviors are temporal disruptions of the motor patterns of words. In the beginning was the word—the broken word!

THE RESEARCH: THE RHYTHM EFFECT

The evidence for this view of stuttering as a disorder of timing is both scanty and oblique, primarily because few researchers have considered it in these terms. Apart from the fact that the temporal sequencing of stuttered words is disordered—a feature so obvious that often it has been overlooked—most of the support for this position comes from the many studies which show that the imposition of a definite rhythm prevents or suppresses stuttering. The history of the treatment of stuttering is replete with accounts of therapists using chanted, rhythmic utterance to facilitate fluency. So far as we can ascertain, it was Thewall, a British physician, in 1764 who first publicly advocated rhythmic speech controls for stutterers although Columbat de L'Isère (1831) is usually credited with the discovery of metronomic speech. It is interesting to read Columbat's rationale for his use of rhythmic speech in the treatment of stuttering:

> It has always been observed that stuttering ceases as though by magic when the afflicted person sings or recites words to musical or poetic rhythms. But no one has tried to explain this phenomenon. . . . Two causes, one the result of the other, may account for the stutterer's fluency in singing. The first is that, since he is able to impose the musical or poetic rhythm upon his speech, the movements of his vocal organs must therefore move with greater accuracy and regularity. The second is that the stutterer by constantly concentrating upon the metrical beat modifies the cerebral excitations so that they proceed more slowly and more orderly. . . . (p. 55)

The first *research* to demonstrate the effect was performed by Johnson and Rosen (1937). They asked 18 stutterers to read in various ways and found that uttering the words in a regular and rhythmic fashion produced by far the fewest stutterings. This was corroborated by Barber (1939) and by Bloodstein (1950). Van Dantzig (1940) showed that when stutterers were asked to time each syllable with a tapping of the finger, they immediately became fluent. In a second study, Barber (1940) used regular visual, auditory, and tactual stimuli to time the speech attempt on consecutively spoken words and found that all of them were equally effective in reducing stuttering. However, she also showed that when the timing stimulus was initiated too fast, more stuttering occurred. Meyer and Mair (1963) demonstrated in two stutterers that when they timed their words with a regularly beating device they became completely fluent but that when the beats were irregular and unpredictable, no reduction in stuttering was obtained. Fransella and Beech (1965) similarly showed that the number of stutterings, produced when speaking in unison with a *rhythmic* metronomic timer, was greatly reduced but that an arhythmic metronome had little effect. Fransella (1967) asked his stutterers to perform the additional task of writing numbers while reading aloud to the rhythmic beat of a metronome and concluded that the rhythmic effect could not be viewed merely as a distraction. In their book, Beech and Fransella (1968) describe another experiment which has significance for our view that stuttering is a disorder of timing. They write:

> Twenty stutterers served as their own controls in the experiment which involved a comparison of the difficulty experienced in reading words which were exposed on a screen for varying lengths of time. For half the words used, the point in time at which they were to be spoken was clearly indicated, while for the other words the utterance was required by unspecified moments during their exposure. The results confirmed the hypothesis, indicating that some means of enabling subjects to determine the moment at which an utterance should occur serves to facilitate fluency.

Finally, Andrews and Harris (1964) report the results of lengthy training in syllable timed speech. Immediate fluency was usually obtained after a few trials, but the permanent carry-over into normal communication was unsatisfactory, probably because normal speaking is not regularly rhythmical. Children responded better than adults. Brandon and Harris (1967) claim that 18 of their 28 stutterers who received intensive training in syllable tapped speech showed a 60 per cent improvement after 18 months. This is hardly spectacular. Wohl (1968) gives a favorable evaluation to the use of an electric metronomic device by stutterers and several such devices have been patented and are presently for sale. In more recent articles in Australian journals, Andrews (1965; 1967) expresses dissatisfaction with syllable timed speech as the sole method of therapy because of the relapse problem. Most stutterers are simply not willing to speak in this unnatural way for any length of time, although a few of them may use a measured form of utterance to tide them over emergencies.

Nevertheless, the rhythm effect has important implications for a theory of stuttering. In our opinion rhythm works because it facilitates the timing of motoric patterns which are prone to asynchrony. The metronomic beat may drive the central mechanism responsible for programming the sound and syllabic coordinations. It may open the reticular or cortical gates with predictable regularity. It has been suggested by Andrews and Harris (1964) that the interval of silence between each timed word or syllable is long enough to overcome any built-in delay which might be operating within the servo-system. It is also possible that each word's motor configuration has a dominant feature about which all the other movements are integrated and that this one serves as a surrogate for the whole sequence. If so, the beat of an accessory timing device coinciding with this feature (whether it be the breath pulse or a jaw movement acting as a prime mover) may thus facilitate the production of a nonfractured word. Most complex motor skills, such as a golf swing, involve such a dominant feature which times the integration of the whole sequence. All these remarks are, of course, the sheerest speculation. We do not know how or why the use of an accessory timing device helps to integrate the motor patterning of a word. We merely know that it does.

THE STUTTERER'S TIMING DEVICES

The stutterer knows this too. Many of his most abnormal behaviors can be regarded as timing devices. He jerks his head or jaw; he protrudes his lips or tongue; he makes a sudden abdominal contraction; he produces a sudden surge of tension in some part of the speech mechanism. Examined closely, they are found to be ballistic movements usually used to time the moment of speech attempt or to effect a release from postponement or fixation. The use of a wide variety of "starters" has long been noted in the phenomenology of stuttering. A case could be made for the position that even the syllabic repetitions so characteristic of stuttering are searching behaviors which seek the precise timing required to utter a unified word.

It is also interesting to consider the common tendency of stutterers to postpone the speech attempt on feared words and to use that pause for tiny covert rehearsals of the motor patterns involved (Van Riper, 1936). Time gaining behaviors are very frequently manifested by stutterers and they are very vulnerable to time pressure. They stutter more frequently when required to speak swiftly (Johnson and Rosen, 1937; Beech and Fransella, 1968). Stutterers often find that if they can postpone long enough on a feared word, it may be spoken fluently. One explanation for this is that the stutterer through covert rehearsal may finally discover the timing he needs, and that when he is deprived of that opportunity for rehearsal, he has little opportunity to search for the timing.

THERAPEUTIC TIMING METHODS

Again, some of the practices used in stuttering therapy may be viewed as efforts to facilitate timing. Froeschels' breath-chewing technique may owe its usefulness to the strong jaw movements with which the sounds and syllables and words are attempted concurrently. Travis and Bryngelson's recommendation of simultaneous talking-and-writing therapy in which the stutterer makes the speech attempt in unison with the dominant stroke of the letter that initiates the written word is another case in point. Also, the use of voluntary stuttering in which the first syllable of the word is deliberately repeated several times before the word is actually attempted seems to be based upon timing and so too does Johnson's "bounce." Many of the breathing and vocalization rituals used in treating stutterers may also be viewed as timing devices for integrating the basic synergies of sound production.

CHORAL OR UNISON SPEECH

When the stutterer speaks in unison with another speaker or group of speakers, he is remarkably fluent. As Johnson and Rosen (1937), and many others have demonstrated, a marked and often total reduction of stuttering occurs under this condition. While various other explanations have been offered—distraction, the masking effect, the reduced propositionality—it is also possible that *in addition* to these factors there is also a timing facilitator involved. As the stutterer utters his words in unison with the other speaker, the latter's utterance may serve as an accessory timing signal. At any rate the effect is dramatic. Many severe stutterers can read in unison with another speaker with almost complete fluency, sometimes even when reading a foreign language they do not understand and even when the other speaker reads very softly. We have repeatedly demonstrated that the model speaker does not even have to say the exact words the stutterer is reading to achieve this fluency. All that is needed is to have the model utter the vowels of the passage or even meaningless sounds in time with the syllables being spoken by the stutterer.*

---

* In this connection, attention should be drawn to the work of Barber (1939) who found that stutterers spoke fluently even when the model speaker read different material. Also, Cherry and Sayers (1956) showed that when reversed speech or gibberish was fed into the ears of the stutterer, he still spoke in unison with it with less stuttering. Wingate (1969) has stated that these findings raise some question about the unison effect as explainable in terms of pace setting. It is possible however that the stutterer may still time his own speech attempts with enough syllabic pulses of this nonidentical speech of the model to facilitate his timing. Also we do not know how much masking effect was present in these experiments. Nevertheless, such findings make us cautious.

SHADOWING

Stutterers can often repeat fluently a word after another speaker has said it. Again there may be many reasons for this, but it is possible that the integrated utterance of the model may provide the timing model the stutterer needs. At any rate, we have a few studies showing that "shadowing," the technique in which the stutterer replicates automatically and immediately what the model speaker is saying, creates a marked or total elimination of stuttering. Colin Cherry in his book on *Human Communication* (1957) describes shadowing as follows:

> A tape recording is made of a reading from a passage of prose and played through headphones to a listener; the listener is instructed to repeat what he hears concurrently, in a subdued or whispered voice. He is then listening and speaking at the same time, but this is found to be an extremely simple task. His spoken repetition tends to be in irregular detached phrases and, with most people and most texts, is given in a singularly emotionless voice as though intoning. It seems as though he is unable to copy the emotional content of the words he hears and, since he is following so close upon the heels of these words, he is unable to see far enough ahead to create his own emotional content. He mouths the words like an automaton and extracts little semantic content, if any. If questioned subsequently, he can say little about the text, especially if it is at all "deep" or difficult. He cannot, for example, act upon a complicated set of instructions if he receives them under such conditions. He is almost in the situation of a parrot which has been taught to speak and can say "Wipe your feet!" or "Go to hell!" without having thoughts of dirty shoes or of damnation (p. 279).

Cherry and Sayers (1956) reported an intensive investigation of the effects of masking noise on stuttering which included a further study of shadowing. They found that when stutterers shadowed the speech of another speaker they had nearly normal fluency. Cherry, Sayers, and Marland (1956) also found an almost total "suppression" of stuttering and suggested that the technique be used more widely in therapy. Walton and Black (1958) applied the method to telephone conversation with some success though this later comment by a subject who participated in the experiment may indicate some of the difficulty in carryover most clinicians have discovered when using shadowing:

> When I came to the hospital I was extremely skeptical of success . . . but on discharge I am quite convinced that I have gotten into a healthier and better method of speech. I am certain that my general level has been maintained at its peak . . . I am still apprehensive about the telephone, but I no longer consider it an unsurmountable difficulty. I am convinced that I can get over it and that my telephone conversation can be brought up to my conversational level.

Kelham and McHale (1966) report striking success using intensive shadowing therapy with 28 stutterers, most of whom were children.

Finally, Sergeant (1961) trained stutterers in "concurrent repetition" of stimulus words. He showed that their fluency and intelligibility improved, but that slower rates of stimulus presentation were needed and also that those stutterers who had a better rhythmic sense profited the most from the shadowing. As in unison speaking, the improvement in fluency brought on by shadowing may be explained in many ways, but the pace-setting characteristic of the procedure should not be ignored.

SINGING

Most stutterers show none of the broken words they usually do when singing, although some of them, including the author, have occasionally experienced some minor difficulty. If is always surprising to the lay listener to discover the stutterer singing perfectly the same words that a moment previously he was unable to utter without great struggle. Nadoleczny (1927) and Witt (1925) showed that less than ten per cent of their cases showed any stuttering while singing. Fletcher (1928), Johnson and Rosen (1937), Bloodstein (1950) and Klemm (1966) also found fluency when the stutterer sang. Wingate (1969) makes a pertinent comment about the phenomenon. He points out that unlike metronomic speech it is not the regularity of the rhythmic beats in singing which accounts for the fluency but some other factor involving time and intonation:

> The influence of singing has been interpreted as a special instance of the effect of rhythm. However, it is questionable whether the effect of singing can be explained adequately in this way. Although a meter of some kind does underlie song, the beat is frequently not clearly evident and the words of the song often do not have a close correspondence to the melody, which expresses the meter. Also, most songs do not have a simple redundant pattern; the tune varies, and many times a syllable may extend beyond one beat of the "time" (meter) or a beat may contain more than one syllable. However—and this is probably of critical significance—syllabic units do correspond to the musical notes. It seems likely that the salutary effect of singing might also be accounted for in terms more fundamental than that it contains a rhythm. Again, we can invoke the interpretation introduced earlier as providing what seems to be a more cogent explanation: in singing, a person intentionally emphasizes vocalization to express a pattern of stresses centering on the syllable nuclei (p. 678).

We agree with Wingate but would emphasize the timing factor inherent in the "pattern of stresses centering on the syllabic nuclei," and the correspondence of the timing of syllables with the musical notes.

PROSODY

In another article Wingate (1966) showed that stuttering adaptation might be explained in part by the practice effect from repeatedly making the same transitional articulatory and phonatory coordinations. This practice effect could be attributed to improvement in timing the motor coordinations involved in the articulatory or the phonatory features of the transitions. Agnello (1966) showed that stutterers had substantial difficulty in producing the complicated transitions required in speaking tongue twisters. Besozzi and Adams (1969) added further support to this position when they found in effect that significantly more adaptation occurred when passages were always read orally than when some of the readings were read silently. Indirect as this evidence is, it points another finger in the direction of stuttering as a disorder characterized by motor mistiming.

SUMMARY

We do not wish to review again all of the studies we summarized in the chapter on organicity which may also be interpreted as supporting this position. However, we might mention the bilateral asynchronization shown in certain EEG studies, especially those by Lindsley (1940) and Stromsta (1964). According to these writers, the bilateral EEGs of nonstutterers seem to be more synchronized than those of stutterers. Moreover, the normal speakers appear to have more or wider excitability gates in their alpha brain waves, which may mean they are more broadly tuned and thus can accept and tolerate more temporal differences in feedback input than can the stutterers. We also find evidence for the timing hypothesis in the modern studies of cerebral dominance (Jones, 1966; Shtremel, 1963), and in those studies indicating that some stutterers show difficulties of motor coordination in the bilateral structures of speech (Hunsley, 1937; Rickenberg, 1956; and Zaleski, 1965). Also, we should not forget the old study by Travis (1934) in which electromyographic recording of action potentials from the masseters showed bilateral discrepancies in arrival times during stuttering which did not appear during normal speech, nor in the speech of the normal speaking controls. Williams' (1955) later research seemed to contradict Travis' results but close inspection of the latter study shows that the replication was far from perfect even with respect to electrode placement.*

---

* In this regard we would like to call attention to the lack of concurrence in arrival times of the "action currents" in Williams' study. He found that only a few words in any of his subjects, stutterers or normal speakers, showed the action currents appearing at about the same time in the paired musculatures. This is most unusual and casts some real doubt upon the methodology and the conclusions.

Finally, we recall the experiment by Stromsta (1956) in which he showed that an intra-ear disparity with respect to bone-conducted side-tone distinguished stutterers from nonstutterers. The latter tended to hear their voices almost simultaneously by bone-conduction at both ears, while the stutterers heard their voices at considerable phase differences at the two ears. We must also remember that the possibility for mistiming of the peripheral muscles may occur in many locations other than the masseters. We hope that definitive research will eventually make the matter clear.

Indeed, we would like to suggest that most of the mistiming may not reside in the simultaneous firing of homologous bilateral muscle groups but rather in the activation of agonist and antagonist sets of musculatures, or in the programming of the synergies of voice, articulation, and respiration. Apart from the many older studies which show breathing abnormalities and the glottographic work of Chevrie-Muller (1963) which demonstrates various asynchronies in vocal fold function in stutterers, we have only the faint glimmerings of the information we need. Using electromyography, we have been investigating the timing of antagonistic muscle groups during stuttering and normal speech but the work is far from publication at this time. We might offer one sample recording showing how, during a long repetitive stuttering moment, one of our stutterers seems to be searching for the timing he finally achieved. The word he was attempting to say was "peep."

Finally, the timing hypothesis is supported by the research that has amply demonstrated that stuttering-like phenomena (in terms of our definition, the disrupted words would constitute stuttering) can be produced

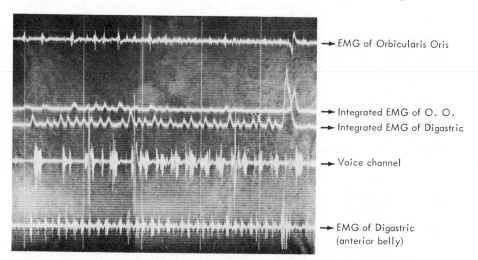

Figure 17. EMG recording showing timing relationships between antagonistic muscle groups during a long repetitive stuttering on the word "peep." Subject displays 7 per second tremor in both lip and digastric. Extreme mandibular jerk preceded final utterance.

in many normal speakers by altering the time relationships of one's self-heard speech. Both the blockage of phonation created by Vannier *et al.* (1954) and by Stromsta (1959) by distorting the side-tone and altering its phase at the two ears, and all the disruptions in speech produced by DAF that we have summarized in the preceding chapter fall into this category of evidence. Fluent speech demands precision in timing.

It is very difficult to evaluate the degree of support all of this scattered and often indirectly focussed research lends to the position that stuttering is a disorder of disrupted timing. It has revealed that the possibility for temporal disruption certainly exists. It has shown that normal speakers' fluency may be disrupted by altering the time relationships of feedback. The imposition of procedures which facilitate the timing of sounds and syllables and words cause the stutterer to become *suddenly* very fluent. Nevertheless we can only conclude that our position is very far from being proven. At the present time it constitutes only a provocative hypothesis, but one which should generate some important research. Although evidence for the hypothesis is far from satisfactory, the same statement could be made about stuttering as a neurosis, as a product of learning, as the effect of organicity, or as the reflection of servo-system instability. Perhaps the major contribution of this view of stuttering is its ability to explain some of the basic phenomena and to synthesize the other concepts of its nature. To this we now address ourselves.

THE POSSIBILITY FOR MISTIMING

The motoric configuration which produces a given word is so complex as to defy detailed description. Over 70 muscles may be involved and each of these must get its appropriate nervous impulses at the required moment in the sequence if the word is to be spoken without disruption. Respiration, phonation, and articulation must be coordinated with amazing precision and each of these component systems requires the reciprocal contraction-relaxation of antagonistic muscle groups. Bilateral synchronization is also necessary since the musculatures involved are located on both the right and left sides of the body. Moreover, in order to achieve successful integration and a smooth flow of unfolding speech sounds, the motor correlates of the component phonemes (the propemes or articulemes) must be pre-programmed so as to provide the necessary coarticulation. In the utterance of a word, the phonemes do not resemble beads on a string or even the links of a chain. Each phoneme is modified by its antecedents and by its consequents as spectrographic analysis shows. They must be blended sequentially. Even as the allophone of /s/ in the word *see* differs spectrographically from the allophone of /s/ in the word *sue*, so also do the motoric equivalents (the distinctive articulatory gestures or allopropes) of these two sounds differ from each other. The postures of the tongue and lips are altered to permit more effective transitions. All of these activities occur in time, the temporal constraints being in milliseconds. If this description of the motoric configurations involved in the production of a word seems unduly elaborate, it is not so at all, but instead it is woefully sketchy. Our purpose has been merely to demonstrate that the possibility for fracturing exists, to show that the mistiming of these simultaneous and successive motor activities could produce a broken word, i.e., cause it to be spoken stutteringly.

THE SYNERGIES OF UTTERANCE

If it seems incredible, in view of this complexity of coordination, that any of us could ever speak a word fluently, we should remember that some of the necessary coordinations are inborn and that we have been spending most of our waking hours perfecting the others. We do not need to be taught how to inhale or to exhale or to produce voice any more than a dog has to learn how to bark, although we may need to discover how to modify these functions to provide the repertoire of sounds we need for effective communication. Long before the child has uttered his first word, he has not only mastered the basic synergistic coordination of respiration, voice, and articulation to produce a wide variety of vowel-like sounds, but also in his babbling he has acquired the ability to produce syllables of many kinds and to repeat them. That these building blocks of motor speech are unfolded and evolved rather than learned seems very plausible, for even deaf babies show them.

This is not to say that all the vowels or all the syllables in our repertoire are unlearned and merely the product of maturation. The author first produced the Swedish vowel /o/ at the age of 60 and he had to *learn* how to do so, but the basic coordinations which produced his early vowels before he was a year old served as models which he could modify to make that strange sound. He did not have to learn to coordinate the basic synergies of breathing and phonation; he did have to explore new movements of the tongue and lips.

HOW THE MOTORIC PATTERNS
OF WORDS ARE LEARNED

In much the same fashion, children master the intricate coordinations involved in producing their first words. They begin with the coordinations they already have and modify them until a recognizable word is emitted. This does not mean that they additively produce a series of phonemic segments like cockleshells all in a row. Instead the child tries the word as a whole, seeking from the first a unified motor sequence, and modifying each successive approximation until the entire acoustic product becomes communicatively acceptable. In so doing, he uses motor patterns he has used before. As the reduplicative nature of the baby's first words (Mama, bye-bye, Daddy), and as a motoric analysis of any of his first approximations will demonstrate, the learning of a new word is a shaping process. At first, there may be only vocalization with appropriate intonation or syllabification. For the new word "Santa Claus" the child may only be able to coordinate a sequence of vowels (æ : a) but the æ is usually nasalized and accented. Then the following series of progressive approximations may occur, but not without temporary regressions:

$$\tilde{æ}{:}a \rightarrow æn\vartheta {:}a \rightarrow \tilde{æ}nt\vartheta \; ta \rightarrow ænt\vartheta \; ka \rightarrow tæn\vartheta \; t \rightarrow sæn\vartheta \; ka \rightarrow sænt\vartheta \; ka z \rightarrow sænt\vartheta \; kl^{\circ}z$$

THE ROLE OF FEEDBACK
IN ACQUIRING NEW WORDS

This shaping process requires feedback. Auditory feedback is particularly important in the learning of a new word, since the child must vary his motor patterns until their product matches the model presented to his ears by his parents. There are many difficulties to be overcome in this shaping, matching process. The auditory model must be discriminated in terms of its distinctive features and held in memory storage so that comparison can take place. The child must be able to discriminate the acoustic variations in his own speech output, and to recognize whether they are coming closer to the model or moving away from it. This is complicated by the fact that he hears himself not only by air borne side-tone but also by bone and tissue transmission of sound all mixed together in a most complicated pattern. Thus, even when his word sounds like the model to others, the child himself hears it somewhat differently. Nevertheless, when the parents indicate that he has produced the word acceptably, this distorted auditory configuration comes to serve as the internalized template of the word. As this is being achieved, the child also comes to discriminate the major features of contact, posture, and movement which characterize the motor sequences of the model, and in this manner the correlated kinesthetic-tactile-proprio-ceptive feedback also becomes patterned. When it does, the child can be said to have learned how to say the word. He now can whisper it or even mouth it in pantomime. The motoric patterning of the word has become stabilized enough to enable him to use it at will.

STABILITY OF THE MOTOR
SEQUENCES OF WORDS

If stuttering consists essentially of broken motor sequences involved in the production of a word, as we have maintained, then some discussion of the stability of these particular motor patterns should be useful. We are not surprised to find the onset of stuttering occurring very early in life in most of our cases. The motor plans for the coordinations required to produce are complex, and there are thousands of words the child must learn. We recognize his early fumbling, stumbling efforts to integrate his speech as natural consequences of the learning process. Parents rarely become concerned when they hear broken words at this time. Stuttering is seldom diagnosed as a disorder when the child is still in the one-word sentence stage of development, even when gaps, repetitions, and prolongations are present. At this time we expect his motor sequences to show some instability. In addition, the amount of interference to communication probably is less apparent when a child has difficulty in emitting a single word than if that word were embedded in a sentence.

STABILITY AS A FUNCTION OF PRACTICE

The stability of a motor sequence, as the research on motor skills demonstrates, depends mainly on three factors: its history of usage (the practice effect), its complexity, and the effectiveness of the feedback systems used to monitor it. Children always show more broken words than adults, but even adults will falter frequently when saying unfamiliar or foreign words that they have not said before. Children who are delayed in speech acquisition often go through a period of stuttering before they achieve the fluent use of language. We might state as another general principle that, at least in children, the more often a word has been correctly spoken in the past the more stable it will be and the less it will tend to be stuttered. Conversely, for all stutterers of any age the more often a word has been spoken stutteringly in the past, the more likely it is to be spoken brokenly in the future. In the latter instance, conditioned disruption may also play a part. In any event, even in children who show no awareness of their stuttering, the general principle holds that the stability of the motor pattern of a word depends in part on practice.

STABILITY AS A FUNCTION OF THE COMPLEXITY OF COORDINATION

Secondly, most of what we know about motor learning suggests that the more complex the word's coordinative pattern, the more difficult it will be to stabilize. The basic research on this is still to be done and it may be difficult to do. We would predict that if positional effects are controlled, i.e., if the first words of sentences are disregarded, more stuttering will occur on polysyllabic words than on monosyllabic ones and on those whose transitional junctures are more complex than on those words in which they are not. About the only evidence we have is that adult stutterers seem to have more hesitation phenomena on longer than on shorter words when the position of the word in the sentence is eliminated as a factor. They have more trouble with tongue twisters. The old example of the word "statistics" as a problem in integration even for normal speakers is also a case in point. To state it generally, *the more complex the motor sequence, the more unstable it tends to be.*

THE ROLE OF FEEDBACK
IN STABILITY

Probably of greater importance is the role of feedback. It is difficult to walk smoothly in the dark. When vision is added to proprioception in the monitoring of this complex motor activity, the coordinations of walking are much better integrated. Yet the blind can learn to walk smoothly, although even then they probably stumble more than those with sight. In speaking, we also have two major feedback systems, the auditory and the proprioceptive,* to help us speak fluently. When either is impaired (e.g., by DAF or by deep anesthesia of the articulatory areas), we speak with more difficulty.

In speaking, we rely to some degree both on auditory and proprioceptive feedback systems. The young child probably needs the auditory feedback to maintain the integrity of his motor patterns of speech more than the adult does. As Mackay (1968) and Buxton (1968) have shown rather clearly, younger children are more affected by DAF than older ones or adults. This is probably to be expected since the child's first words were learned primarily by listening to himself and others, and by matching his output against the acoustic models provided by others. At first the child still needs his ears to assist his mouth if he hopes to speak fluently. But speech can be monitored by proprioception alone once the motor patterns have become stabilized. We can speak fluently even in the presence of loud masking noise, and the person who becomes deaf does not begin to stutter. The fact that we can pantomime a word without vocalization shows also that auditory feedback is not essential to the production of that word once the proprioceptive motor patterns have become well integrated. It seems reasonable therefore to conclude that when a person can reel off the sequential move-

---

* In this discussion we shall frequently use the words proprioceptive and proprioception more loosely and generally than their correct usage would require. We include in these terms not only proprioception but the correlated tactile and kinesthetic features. To have eternally to spell out the whole array whenever we must describe this form of somesthetic feedback seems too awkward.

ments of a word without the aid of self-hearing, the motor pattern of that word has become fairly well stabilized.

A corollary to this might be that the more distortion there is in the auditory feedback the more likely it will be that some stuttering will occur. Unlike adults, whose motor patterns are stabilized enough to let them hear what they are saying rather than how they are saying it, children are doubtless much more vulnerable to auditory feedback distortion. This is probably why children have more broken words. The possibility for such distortion seems almost to have been built into the auditory feedback system. The multiplicity of auditory feedback channels makes disruption likely. Perhaps this is why most of us switch as swiftly as we can to proprioception as the major monitor of speech, and use our self-hearing instead as an accessory control system. As we have made clear in Chapter 14 a strong case can be made that stuttering is the result of auditory interference in the servosystem. Let us tentatively submit therefore another principle: *the more stable the motor sequence of a word, the more feedback distortion it can undergo before it becomes disrupted.* Even under DAF, not all words show breakage or changes in the programming of the sequential movements. This is why no stutterer stutters on every word he utters. The motor patterns of some words are more stable than others.

THE STABILITY HIERARCHY.
LEVELS OF STABILITY

Thus far we have been speaking primarily of broken words, of the disrupted motor sequence patterns at the word level. But there are integrated configurations of sequential movements both within the word and beyond it. Words are made up of syllables and sounds, but our usual utterances are composed of words, phrases, and sentences. Thus there exists at least five levels at which fluency breaks may occur: at the level of the sound, the syllable, the word, the phrase, and the sentence. As motor configurations, however, these levels differ in their vulnerability to disruption and fracturing. To put it another way, they differ in stability, and the hierarchy of stability may be represented from *greatest to least* stability in terms of the following order: sounds, syllables, words, phrases, and sentences.

The stability of the motor integrations at any of these levels probably reflects the past history of usage. Sounds are more stable than syllables, syllables than words, and words than phrases, etc., because they simply have been used more frequently. The total number of phonemic motor patterns are fewer than all the available number of syllables. Thus inevitably they are used more often. Again there are fewer syllables in one's repertoire than there are words, and so the motor patterns of syllables get practiced more often than words do. Also since there are many fewer words than all the different phrases, or sentences which can be assembled, the words must have a longer past history of motor integration (and thus motoric stability) than that for phrases. Phrases have simply occurred less frequently.* The point we are making is that the motor patterns of speech differ in stability and resistance to disruption according to their history of usage and their level of segmental integration.

STABILITY AS RELATED
TO SPEECH DEVELOPMENT.
THE STABILITY OF SOUNDS

Now let us consider this in another way—in terms of the development of speech. The first motor speech patterns to be integrated seem to be the vowel sounds. They appear first as the cries and the cooing comfort sounds of the baby. As any parent knows, they are thoroughly practiced—especially in the dark hours of the night. The basic respiratory, laryngeal, and articulatory coordinations involved in these cries and early sounds are probably patterned in time inherently. Differentiation soon occurs, however, and the baby learns very early to phonate and articulate on exhalation rather than on inhalation and so on. For some time, the primitive sounds of crying and cooing comprise the bulk of the infant's utterance. Sounds are motorically simple compared to cv, vc, or cvc syllables, since little transitional or co-articulation phenomena are required in their production. Decerebrate animals and humans alike are able to produce sounds. The vowel sounds especially seem to be organized around the archetypal breath group. They have strong acoustic power and doubtless activate the first servo-responses of the auditory system. In the life history of the individual, these sounds have the longest usage.

Since vowel sounds are probably the most highly integrated, the most basic of the elementary coordinations involved in speaking, they are the most stable of all the motor patterns used in speech and accordingly they are the most resistant to disruption. It has even been suggested that they are laid down in the cortex or its substructures as reverberatory circuits, deeply engrained in the functioning of the central nervous system. Since the temporal patterns of simultaneous and successive muscular contractions found in vowel utterance seem to be more stable, perhaps this is why less stuttering seems to occur on words beginning with vowels.

---

* Certain phrases such as "bread and butter" or sentences such as "How are you?" have also had similar overlearnings so that they may become as motorically stable as single words. They too can become unitary motor automatisms almost like single words, and their integrations are so stable as even to resist the disruptions of aphasia.

STABILITY OF SYLLABLES

The next most stable motor configuration of speech is that of the syllable, and it characterizes the babbling stage of speech development. That it exists as an integrated and basic motor pattern is demonstrated by the fact all babies babble syllabically. Like the sound, the syllable too can be evoked by electrical stimulation of the cortex. There is some evidence that the syllable, too, may be represented cortically or subcortically by some sort of reverberatory pattern. Penfield and Rasmussen (1949), for example, found that a syllable such as "te" would be repeated and continue involuntarily until the electrical stimulation was turned off. Chase (1958) found that syllable repetition can be facilitated by recycling the delayed feedback at appropriate delays. Syllabic repetition often appears under DAF when words, phrases, and sentences are disrupted. Many of the first words of infants are reiterative, composed of repeated syllables. Also, the diadochokinesis of the same syllable is faster than that of different syllables. Sonograms also show that syllables are unitary configurations, not mere successions of discrete sounds. They are closely conjoined and coarticulated so as to comprise highly integrated patterns. It is also perhaps of some interest here to observe that aphasics who cannot say a polysyllabic word can often tap out the number of syllables which comprise it or produce a jargon word of the same number of syllables.*

HOW SYLLABLES
ARE INTEGRATED

Syllables, as Stetson (1951) and others have shown, occur as entities. They can be distinguished not only through auditory perception but also by examining the variations in air pressure and airflow. They can be distinguished both electromyographically as well as sonographically. Syllables seem to be timed by a sudden breath pulse produced by the contraction of the respiratory muscles. This sudden respiratory contraction may serve as the basic signal in the proprioceptive feedback system controlling the timing of the syllables as a whole. Hardy (1967) simultaneously recorded respiratory muscle action potentials and speech signals and concluded that there was strong evidence of "syllabic pulses by both thoracic and abdominal muscles." Hoshiko (1960) showed electromyographically that the single vowel /a/ or the syllable "pup" both at slow and rapid rates were

---

* We suspect that even among syllables there are differences in the stability of their motor patterns and that the stability hierarchy (from most stability to least) is represented by the following order: v, vc, cv, and cvc. Certainly the relative frequencies of stuttering on these different types of syllables seems to indicate that this is plausible, but again the basic research is still to be done.

initiated by a precisely timed sequence of musculature contractions, always in the following order: internal intercostals, rectus abdominis, and the external intercostals. Again we see how important the time relationships must be in syllable production.

However, it is also possible that a specific lip, jaw, or tongue movement may also function as the surrogate for timing the entire array of simultaneous and successive muscular contractions that comprise the motor pattern of the entire syllable. Lashley (1951) long ago made the observation that there simply was not sufficient transit time to permit the return flow of impulses from the peripheral muscles to serve as feedback signals in the sequencing of the movements needed to speak a word. Lenneberg (1967) makes the same point. However, if one motor gesture may serve as the representative of the whole sequence, we can understand how syllables and words can be monitored by servocontrol.*

The utterance of a syllable demands a series of transitional movements, each one affected by its predecessor and by its successor. They must occur in a precise and definite temporal order. These syllabic sequences are wholes, like the expert fingering of a musical phrase in piano playing. Each movement flows into the next. The expert pianist often uses a head movement, assumes a complex wrist posture or uses some other way of integrating the sequence of his flying fingers. The timing of the successive movements is not done deliberately or individually, but by timing the sequence as a whole. The pianist's nod or gesture or postural change seems to serve as the feedback representative of the entire series of finger movements. It too is a part of the entire motor sequence, but it is the controlling feature. When it is right, the entire sequence flows smoothly. When it is wrong, the sequence is spoiled. We do not know enough about these bits of behavior which serve as the integrating surrogates or prime movers of motor sequences, but we know that they must occur.

Like piano playing, but infinitely more complex, speech too consists of motor sequences. The production of a word or syllable requires motor patterns some of which resemble chords, timed simultaneously; while others follow themselves in time like the notes of a melody. The timing is of the essence, even as it is in piano playing, or swinging a golf club.

The motor integration of a syllable requires coarticulation. Innumerable sonographic studies have demonstrated that separate phonemes are not chained together serially to comprise a syllable, but that a fusion of components occurs instead. The work of Lieberman (1962) and his colleagues of the Haskins group show that the initial consonant of a cv syllable, for example, affects the transition frequencies in the second formant of the succeeding vowel. Moreover, the particular vowel within that syllable also

---

* An alternative explanation views sequential motor patterns as governed by motor commands which are programmed prior to attempt and which obviate the necessity for feedback. See Keele, S. W., "Movement Control in Skilled Motor Performance," *Psychological Bulletin*, 70, (1968) 387-403.

affects the production of the initial consonant. Some preliminary motor "instructions" must therefore have been decided upon before the syllable is uttered. To cite but two of the studies, Daniloff and Moll (1968) demonstrated that coarticulation of lip protrusion may occur and extend over as many as three preceding consonants in a sequence prior to the production of a vowel, as exemplified by such a word as "screw." And MacNeilage and De Clerk (1969), in a more elaborate investigation using cinefluorograms and electromyograms, found that the motor control of a later syllabic component was partially influenced by the characteristics of the preceding one, and that the reverse influence also occurred. The programming of sequential speech must demand an exactitude of timing which seems almost incomprehensible. That the stutterer fails in this timing of coarticulation is evidenced by the studies of Stromsta (1965) and Agnello and Buxton (1966). It is also of interest in this connection that Rawnsley and Harris (1954) found that normal speakers under delayed auditory feedback showed the same lack of normal formant transitions in their repeated syllables. One of the puzzling features about stuttering is its marked reduction during pantomimed speech or whispering. While this could be accounted for on the basis of a simplified synergy (the absence of voice and/or air flow) we may have a clue in the work of Schwartz (1967) who found that the average duration of syllables in whispering was significantly longer than when they were vocalized. Perhaps more time was available to permit synchronization in this case.

We feel that the most important feedback signal in the integration of a word is probably the accented syllable of that word. If that syllable is produced correctly, then the word will be integrated. Stutterers stutter less on unaccented syllables. Why do stutterers repeat the accented syllables over and over again? It is our belief that the syllables that are repeated are not the appropriate ones, not the proper syllables that fit the word wholes. Note how often the repeated syllables end in the schwa or neutral vowel. Stutterers say "Kuh-Kuh-Kuh-Katy." Kuh will never make a Katy. The syllable must be repeated and revised until it carries the transitional components that fit the word pattern. Searchingly the stutterers keep repeating it until by chance, or the decline of anxiety or expectation or for other reasons, they finally produce the *Ka* that belongs to Katy. Note the speed of the syllabic repetition, the instant recoil which often occurs. These stuttering syllabic repetitions are usually not produced at the same tempo as the syllables of the stutterer's nonstuttered speech. They are usually faster, jerkier. Often they are accompanied by other movements that add nothing to the possibility that the word can be spoken as a whole. They become invested *with tension* and this itself must create an abnormal feedback. If words are integrated in their motor sequences by some motoric feature of the dominant syllable, that syllable, that syllabic motor configuration must be normal, not abnormal, if it is to be spoken normally. If it isn't, then the syllable must be said again and again. When this occurs, a reverberatory

oscillation is often created which subsides only when the stutterer feels that the needed timing of coarticulation has been achieved.

The stability of the motor patterns that comprise a syllable are of far reaching importance in stuttering. Their integrity determines whether the person will speak with broken words. Usually they are very well integrated, almost as solidly as the vowel sounds. Yet they too are vulnerable to disruption, especially by auditory interference if the speaker relies too much on self-hearing for the control of speech, and not enough on touch, kinesthesia and proprioception. Syllables can be broken or temporarily distorted. When they are, the person will speak stutteringly.

THE MOTOR INTEGRATION
OF WORDS

As the syllable seems to be on a unitary level of coordinative integration somewhat less stable than that of the sound, so also the word seems to be less stable than the syllable. Let us offer some commentary on the integration of whole words.

Following the babbling stage, the child enters the one-word sentence stage. To recapitulate, he now speaks in motor sequences which require the combination of sounds and syllables into larger units. He remains in this stage for some time before learning to combine these word units into phrases and sentences. During this period, the motor patterns of these single words are practiced repeatedly and are strongly reinforced through communicative facilitation and social rewards. Their sequences of muscular contractions are programmed in time and are monitored both proprioceptively and acoustically by servo processes. That they are units is shown by the pauses and other hesitation phenomena which occur much more often at morphemic boundaries than within the word. In normal speakers there are fewer part-word repetitions or pauses than whole-word repetitions, and more pauses occur before or after the utterance of a word than within its boundaries.

Words become unitary configurations of acoustic and proprioceptive sequences. They are mastered by a series of approximations. The child may omit the final sound at first, or use an incorrect initial sound, but eventually he learns the pattern of movements necessary to produce the unit which his listeners require for communicative interchange. The unitary nature of words is demonstrated by the fact that words can be predicted by the forward guessing devised by Shannon (1951), in which successively presented sounds in the sequence increasingly facilitate the recognition of the target word. Aphasics can often say a single word when they cannot use it in a meaningful phrase or sentence. Meaningful words can be spoken at faster diadochokinetic rates than nonsense words composed of the same sounds and syllables. The specific sequences of motor activities that com-

prise an individual word are practiced so often in the course of a person's life history that they finally become highly automatic and unitary.

THE MOTOR CONFIGURATIONS
OF SUPRAMORPHEMIC SEGMENTS

With few exceptions, the motor patterns for phrases and sentences are not learned as are those for words, nor do they evolve through maturation as the configurations of sounds and syllables do. Although they too form unitary wholes, as shown by the modification of prior words by later ones as well as by the location of pauses and other hesitation phenomena, their bonding is less strong. One almost has to memorize a series of sentences before he can eliminate all the breaks from them. Normal speech is full of fluency breaks of one kind or another. We are not surprised to find that normal speech is full of disfluencies at the morphemic, phrase, or sentence boundaries. These supramorphemic segments demand motor configurations that have rarely been repeated often enough to permit stabilization. They are generated rather than learned. They unfold as a result of constant decision making. This is why society rarely labels fluency breaks at morpheme, phrase, or sentence boundaries as stuttering. We expect some faltering in spontaneous verbal formulation. It seems quite normal to hesitate occasionally in the linking of words to form phrases, or phrases to form sentences, but a different situation exists when breaks occur too often *within* words. We expect the particular motor sequence which creates a word to be integrated, to be rather stable. When we find a speaker with broken words, with too many syllabic repetitions, or one who struggles to utter a sound, we sense abnormality and call it stuttering. It is for this reason that Wendell Johnson's valiant attempt to equate all kinds of disfluencies failed to be convincing even before the research demonstrated that he was wrong.

EFFECTS OF STRESS

We should like to offer the proposition that *the greater the stress, the more likely it is that the sequencing of speech will be disrupted at a more basic level of integration.* Thus, under mild degrees of stress (communicative, emotional, or cybernetic) we will find hesitation phenomena breaking up the smooth flow of the sentence. More stress will disrupt the phrasing: still more the motor patterning of the word; and it usually takes a great deal of stress to break up the integration of the syllable or sound. Although this principle seems to hold generally, it must be modified by consideration of the timing of the stress. If the impact of the stress is vividly sensed within the boundaries of one of these five motor segments, that segment will be the one

disrupted. For example, when a neophyte public speaker becomes overwhelmed by emotion at the moment he begins to speak, he may not even be able to phonate. Or, if he feels the full impact of his emotional storm during the utterance of a phrase, he may not be able to finish his sentence. If a speaker experiences important listener loss and senses it keenly while he is in the middle of uttering a long word, he may repeat preceding words or the syllables of that particular word. Since all the motor patterns of speech are ordered in time, the timing of the stress is bound to play some part in determining which motor patterns will be disrupted. We wish to emphasize however that in the adult normal speaker it takes a lot of stress, and stress that is focused directly at the time the sound, syllable, or word is being produced, before these latter motor units are disrupted.

Under the same amount and impact of stress, children, whose motor patterns are less stable than adults, show more fracturing and disruption at the three more basic levels of integration than adults. As a consequence, they speak stutteringly more often. Moreover, they are probably not only more vulnerable but also more often subjected to communicative stress than adults. They have not yet developed the tolerance for listener interruption or listener loss or other communicative pressures which most of us develop as we grow older. And they probably are interrupted more and disregarded more when they are trying to talk. They are punished too often for what they have to say. Uncertainty whether to speak or to continue speaking abounds. They have not learned to keep their emotions within limits. They are entangled in many conflicts, most of which involve speaking.

Young children are also still in the process of mastering the language—its structure, its rules. They must still cope with perfecting their articulation. Their auditory memory spans are short. Often they forget what they began to say and do not remember what they have already said. Their vocabulary is often inadequate for the coding of the messages they ache to transmit and have understood. Young children have word-finding difficulties. The models of adult speech—so fast, so fluent, so complex—which they try to emulate, are often beyond their formulative capacities or motor abilities. More importantly, this is the period in their lives when children must switch their automatic controls of motor speech from acoustic monitoring to proprioceptive monitoring because they now have to listen to the thoughts they are expressing rather than to the sounds they are uttering.

This account of the stresses to which young children are constantly exposed in trying to integrate their speech is far from comprehensive. Surely there is sufficient stress to account for the prevalence of disfluent speech in childhood and for the onset of stuttering without having to blame it always on a pregenital neurosis or upon anal and oral fixations. Considered simply as a problem in motor learning and coordination, one would expect more disfluency to occur in children. We would expect the more basic integrations involved in sound, syllable, and word production to be disrupted by such stress. Indeed, we would be astonished if stuttering usually

began in adulthood. We are therefore not surprised to find the onset of
the disorder occurring during these early years of overload.

The supramorphemic (phrase and sentence) sequences are probably monitored by *auditory* and *visual* feedback primarily. We listen to what we say
in order to determine whether or not we are saying what we wish to say.
We watch our listener to see if he is comprehending the message we are
sending and to ascertain how he is reacting to it. Our attention is focused
on the coding and decoding of content rather than in scrutinizing our
coordinations. When error signals appear in either the auditory or the
visual feedback circuit, we begin to hunt and search for revisions which
will produce the communication we intended. Most of the hesitation
phenomena which characterize the normal speaker occur as reactions to
failures in message-sending. Many of them are filibuster reactions. They
gain time so that the speaker may revise his output. They are signals to the
listener that he is not to interrupt, that the speaker is still speaking even
if an interruption in communicative flow is apparent. Some of these pauses
are filled; some are unfilled. We halt silently for a moment or, more commonly, we say "ah" or "um" or repeat previous words and phrases until
the revision we need is forthcoming. We hesitate in order to formulate.

To equate these supramorphemic breaks in fluency with the infra-
morphemic ones does not strike us as reasonable. They are of different
kinds, the first being formulative, the other coordinative. They are apparently controlled by different feedbacks. Phrase and sentence integration
requires auditory scanning for appropriate meaningfulness and visual scanning of the listener to see if the decoding process is effective and to ascertain
the listener's reaction to the message. The fluency breaks that occur *within
the boundaries of the word* seem, in contrast, to be failures in motor integration. Primarily, they are responses to the processing of bits of information concerning the tactual, positional, and movement features of the motor
output. They are responses to haptic, kinesthetic, or proprioceptive error
signals.

What are the options open to a speaker when he realizes that the message he is sending is not getting across, or is evoking listener responses that
he does not seek? He may continue his defective verbalizations anyway until
he comes to the end of the sentence and then say more sentences until error
signals no longer return. This is probably what extremely fluent normal
speakers do. But most of us stop, when we get the error signal and use a
filled or unfilled pause to go back to the boundary of an earlier encoding
unit and begin to revise our utterance. We can go ahead, stop, or repeat but
eventually we must alter our output if we want to get our message across.

If we stop, we stop at one of the boundaries of the encoding units. We seldom stop in the middle of a word when we get a bad listener response or realize that we are saying the wrong word. We stop *after* that wrong word and then we say the new word, the different phrase or the changed sentence. In hesitating due to formulative difficulty, if we repeat, we do not repeat sounds or syllables, but the meaningful units of words or phrases. Our search is for meaning.

As we have said, however, there are times when a normal speaker under great stress will break a word. This occurs especially when that stress is pinpointed so that it is felt within the morphemic boundaries as when the speaker is saying a single word or the key word of an unacceptable sentence. For example, we have seen normal speakers start to say a vulgar word, realize suddenly that it is completely unacceptable, and then block. Or they may prolong the first sound as in "S," or repeat the first syllable or part of the syllable ("Shih-shih-"). The stereotype of the suitor begging his beloved to "mm-mare-marry me" is another example. Approach-avoidance conflicts and other kinds of severe emotional stress tend to affect the basic level of integration, the motoric ones, more than they do the upper or formulative ones. Mahl (1957) has shown that filled pauses (*ah's* and repetition of words and phrases) do not occur as often in the stress of psychiatric interviews as they do in ordinary speaking, while the hesitation phenomena he calls *non-ah's*, (the syllabic repetitions and the "stutterings") occur more often under profound emotion. Communicative stress tends to disrupt the upper integrative levels—phrasing and sentencing—while emotional and cybernetic stresses may disrupt the basic motor patterns of the sound, syllable, or word.

EFFECTS OF EMOTIONAL STRESS
ON MOTORIC INTEGRATION
IN THE PRODUCTION
OF SOUND

We do not know the exact mechanism by which emotional stress disrupts motor coordination but that it can do so seems indisputable. When speech becomes hesitant under emotion we suspect that it is in part because the basic synergies involved in the coordination of respiration, phonation, and articulation become disturbed. The precise timing of the simultaneous and successive muscular contractions required for such a basic performance as sound production suffers alteration. That sound will not be forthcoming until the timing is straightened out.

Consider the effect of emotion on just the respiratory component. Emotional states profoundly affect breathing as well as heart beat and other functions. The amplitude of respiration, its rate, and the ratio of inspiration to expiration vary enough under negative emotion to allow these features to be used in polygraphic lie detection. Startle produces the short sudden gasp which can interrupt any other respiratory activity. We automatically hold our breath when danger threatens. The synchronization of abdominal and thoracic musculatures is also affected by emotion. Tremors of the diaphragm (flutter) have often been noted. Respiratory activity becomes dominated by the autonomic nervous system in states of emotional stress, and it is easy to understand why Seeman (1959) could attribute the core behaviors of stuttering to imbalanced functioning of the sympathetic and parasympathetic systems, or why Hill (1945) could view stuttering as basically composed of the physiological startle reaction. This does not, of course, mean that bad breathing habits are the cause of stuttering. We are not so naive as to hold that ancient belief. We are saying merely that emotion can affect breathing so drastically that the basic synergy of respiration, phonation, and articulation may be momentarily disrupted enough to make it hard to utter a sound *at the precise instant* when it should be spoken. Recently, Sears and Davis (1968) have shown very clearly that the variations in respiration required for the changes in phonatory loading which constantly occur during speech are "anticipated by an appropriately phased activation of both intercostal fusimotor and alpha motoneurones." Since the timing of these nervous impulses must be amazingly precise, it is not hard to see that emotional stress could disrupt it.

EFFECT OF STRESS
ON PHONATION

Phonation too may feel the influence of emotion quite apart from its relationship to respiration. In physiologic startle the laryngeal valve is suddenly and tightly closed by the contraction of both the true and often the ventricular vocal folds. Milder emotional states are often reflected in laryngeal tension (globus hystericus). Many of the hyperfunctional voice disorders, such as spastic dysphonia, reflect the common observation that phonation may be impaired by negative emotion. The delicate balancing of antagonistic muscle groups required for phonation can be altered by emotionally induced changes in muscular tension. If it is often difficult to speak under profound emotional stress, the reason may lie in the breakdown of either respiration or phonation or in the disruption of their synchronization.

In this connection, the work of Moravek and Langova (1968) is intriguing. They say:

> We regard the prephonational or initial tonus as the key to the problem of stuttering. By this tonus we mean that phase of speech in which the patient starts to form the voice and where the majority of the phonation muscles are in action, but where the corresponding vocal effect is not achieved. In order to overcome this speech block the stutterer increases his muscular effort but the situation does not improve; in fact it deteriorates.

The importance of this prephonational tonus—which is probably due to inappropriate gamma innervation of the muscle spindles—has also been stressed by Chevrie-Muller (1963) as accounting for some of the aberrant vocal fold activity shown in the glottograms of her stutterers. Long ago, Bryngelson (1932) found similarly minute vocal disturbances just prior to speech attempts which resulted in stuttering.

One possible explanation for these time effects upon phonation is based on the cochleo-recurrential reflex. According to Metz (1946) and Salamon and Starr (1963), the stapedius muscle is activated concurrently with or just prior to onset of speech, perhaps to buffer the auditory system against the overload of one's own voice. These changes in middle ear impedance do not take place once the phonation begins, and thus they cannot be attributed to auditory triggering. Wondering whether there were time differences between middle ear muscle activity in stutterers and nonstutterers, Shearer and Simmons (1965) explored the problem in five stutterers and their controls but found no differences. Only one ear, however, was measured at one time, and perhaps simultaneous determinations of acoustic impedance changes in both ears may yield more significant results.

ARTICULATION: EFFECTS
OF STRESS

Similar disturbances of timing may also be involved in articulation. The Japanese workers Hirose, Kiritani, and Shibata (1968) have shown, for example, that before a vowel sound is phonated, the articulatory muscles responsible for its cavity formation receive their motor impulses about one tenth of a second prior to the onset of phonation. This occurs even while the antecedent sound is being produced and it is independent of rate. While the effects of emotionally produced tension on the timing of articulatory movements have not, to our knowledge, been studied intensively, it seems plausible that such tension could produce some difficulty in utterance. The inability to produce a sound, in some instances, may be the result of the simultaneous contraction of antagonistic muscles, muscles paired functionally in such a way that one set relaxes as its opposing set contracts. Heightened tonus may impede the relaxation of the reciprocal muscle groups. In such a case normal movement may be impossible. Fixations may occur and tremors may appear in the structures being activated so that the fixation is prolonged even further. We find these tremors frequently in our EMG recordings of stuttering moments. Before any muscle contracts, it is placed in readiness by a heightening of tonus. We cock our muscle guns before we pull their triggers, but too much tension may cause the muscles to contract too soon, or too late, or it may cause the antagonists to fail in relaxing enough. Much of the effect of emotional stress on speech

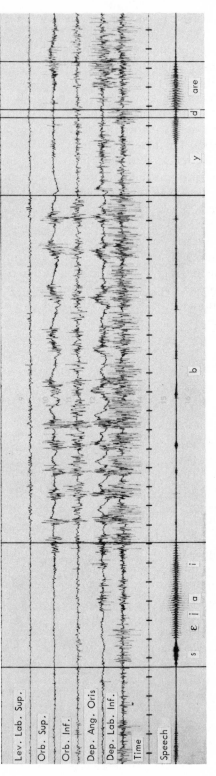

Figure 18. EMG recordings from antagonistic muscle groups during stuttering. (*Courtesy Drs. Rolf Leanderson and A. Persson, Karolinska sjukhiset, Sweden.*)

is probably caused by the mistiming produced by inappropriate changes in muscle tonus of the antagonistic muscle groups.

EFFECTS OF STRESS ON THE INTEGRATION OF SYLLABLES

As we have seen, the motor patterning of the syllable requires not only the synergic coordinations of the vowel sounds which comprise its nucleus, but also a very precise timing of the preparatory articulatory postures needed for coarticulation. Here again emotionally induced changes in tonus could disrupt the reciprocal timing of antagonistic muscles. Moreover, if the motor pattern of the syllable is integrated around or triggered by a breath pulse as Stetson (1951) claimed, the disturbed breathing produced by negative emotion may delay or distort that pulse and so wreck the syllable's timing. And certainly, since the vowel of the syllable depends on phonation, any unnecessary laryngeal closures brought on by emotion could impair syllabic production.

In short, it is not difficult to see that emotional stress might produce alterations in the basic motor patterning of the sound and the syllable and hence to produce the broken words we have called stuttering.

CYBERNETIC STRESS

As we have seen, the motor sequencing of speech is operated and controlled automatically by a most complex servosystem. Like all self-regulating systems whose smooth functioning depends on feedback, trouble can occur in the servosystem governing speech when the system is subjected to overload, or when the signal-to-noise ratio is too low, or for several other reasons. The fact that speech is monitored by scanning information coming in at the same time from several channels (proprioception, auditory, visual) creates a situation which can produce system instability. Time pressure may place exorbitant demands on the system's capacity to process and correct error signals. The possibility of a built in distortion in auditory feedback of stutterers has been stressed by Stromsta (1956) and others. Mysak (1960) writes,

> . . . many stutterers appear to possess over-correcting (underdamped) auditory monitoring systems. Such an oversensitive monitoring channel may feed back tonal flow signals which are so small that they would ordinarily be disregarded. This excessive backflow of inconsequential error-signals over-activates the corrector device and hence speech automaticaticity is disturbed.

Overloaded servosystems tend to go into oscillation or fixation. They may overshoot or undershoot in their attempt to change the output to correct for error. The motoric patterns which serve as the models in the comparator may themselves be indistinct (as in attempting unfamiliar or foreign words, or as experienced by young children still learning the language), and therefore the cybernetic "hunting" may continue even after the motor targets have been hit. Moreover, confirmed stutterers may have competing models against which the feedback is compared: both a stuttering model for the word and the normal speech model. Under fear, only the motor pattern of stuttering may become dominant, and then the regulator will determine that the speech output will conform to its abnormal structure. Multiple feedback loops afford the possibility of instability. Moreover, emotion too can flood the feedback systems with cybernetic noise, with "static," and thereby interfere with the motor integration of speech.

REACTIONS TO DISRUPTIONS
OF MOTOR PATTERNING

It is interesting to observe that most of us react to any break in fluency by trying to reintegrate the sequencing at a lower level. Thus those of us who are highly "sentence-minded" (and stutterers are not, as Beebe [1957] has shown) respond to a formulative disruption by repeating the preceding phrase and only then finishing the sentence. Rarely does such a speaker respond by merely continuing after a formulative gap. He must reintegrate, make the entire communicative sequence a whole again. We find a similar situation when a person momentarily loses the crucial word of a phrase as in "It's a . . . ." "It's a . . . ." "It's a chameleon." He doesn't usually say, "It's a . . . . chameleon" (unless he uses some accessory vocalization as a substitute for the rephrasing). Similarly, if speech is fractured at the word level, most of us respond to the gap by syllabic repetition and we say the word as a whole before we continue. We don't say "Sta . . . stas . . . sta . . ." and then add "tistics." We say the word as a unit before proceeding further. But this characteristic return to more basic levels of integration fails when speech is broken at the level of the syllable. There is no place to go, no lower level, for the characteristic motor features of the phonemes which comprise the syllable overlap each other because of transitional juncturing.

Few normal speakers ever attempt to integrate the syllabic motor sequence by regressing to the sound level. They simply continue to repeat the syllable, varying it slightly, or they pause and make a new attempt on the word as a whole. In the early development of his disorder, the stutterer usually shows this same reaction. He repeats syllables when his words are broken. Only later does he begin to try to break the syllable into its illusory motor components, shattering the unitary sequence in the attempt to put his word together again. And then, of course, he gets into real trouble, trying to integrate breathing, voice, and articulation voluntarily when their complexity of timing demands automaticity. Again, when he finds he cannot integrate the syllable or sound, the stutterer tries to go even further back—to breathe differently; to make a sound, any sound; to move his lips or tongue or jaws voluntarily. The more he fractionates his motor sequences, the farther away he gets from the integrations he needs and the more frustration and panic he experiences. Then struggle and avoidance behaviors arise. It is interesting, in this connection, to find that Stromsta's (1959) normal speakers, when their phonation was suddenly arrested by introducing distortion and interaural phase shifts into their auditory feedback, responded with struggle, heightened tonus, and breathing irregularities very similar to those shown by severe stutterers. All these behaviors seem to be searching behaviors. They were the subjects' attempts (often random) to find the motor patterns needed to produce sound. The stutterer responds in much the same way when his speech is broken at subsyllabic levels.

HOW STUTTERERS CREATE THEIR OWN STRESS AND MOTOR DISRUPTIONS

In our description of its phenomenology we have shown how stuttering, through its generation of fear, shame, and other negative emotional states, tends to produce its own precipitants. When this negative emotion becomes conditioned to verbal or situational cues, the perception of those cues itself creates sufficient stress to disrupt the motor sequencing involved in word production. Here we wish to call attention especially to the way the stutterer's perceptions of approaching difficulty contribute to the fracturing of his words. First of all there is the stutterer's well known tendency to fear certain phonemes. Rarely, if ever, does he fear specific syllables, although the integration of the initial or accented syllable probably presents his major problem.

The result of this perception of "hard" or "Jonah" sounds is that he attempts to utter sounds, not syllables, thereby contributing to the fractionization of the normal motor sequences. Whole words become perceived abnormally, and the initial sound is usually perceived as the dominant feature of its configuration. As models, these abnormal motor sets compete with the normal ones in the feedback monitoring of utterance, and too often they win. Expecting broken words, the stutterer listens for them and of course finds them. Expecting repeated syllables, he uses the schwa vowel in them and so spoils the word. By assuming abnormal trigger postures prior to the speech attempt, he introduces enough interference in the backflow of proprioceptive information to make integration difficult. Anticipating difficulty in phonating, he rehearses the very behaviors which make phonation impossible—the single and multiple closures of the airway. He even tries to speak while holding his breath or gasping. He not only assumes articulatory postures which are abnormal, he often alters the tonus of the antagonistic muscle groups so greatly that tremors are almost bound to be triggered by any attempt to shift from one posture to the next. The stutterer attempts sudden movements rather than smooth ones; he jerks rather than shifts. All of these perceptual and motor responses to the expectancy of stuttering make it more likely that disruption of the motor patterns of words will occur.

INDIVIDUAL DIFFERENCES

Why do some individuals show so many fractured words that they can be said to have the disorder of stuttering? We once hoped that we could identify a single cause of the disruption, but we have unsuccessfully chased that will of the wisp over the hills and far away and in our old age we grow tired. There seem to be just too many different reasons for the breakdown of motoric speech to hope that we will ever find a simple and elegant one-factor explanation for stuttering. Instead we feel that there are multiple factors which probably determine whether or not a person will tend to have too many broken words. Certain of these factors may be absent or insignificant in their impact on a given individual while other factors may be potent enough to wreck his fluency. The timing of the simultaneous and sequential muscular contractions and relaxations which produce an integrated word can be affected by any one or any combination of these influences.

Perhaps some day we will have the technology to measure and compute a composite value which will represent the risk of stuttering. If so, we would probably assign different weights to each of the following factors and doubtless add others to the list: familial incidence; sex; brain damage; abnormal EEGs; bilateral coordination ability; interaural phase differences; intercerebral asynchronies and delays; tremor proneness. If we can dream a little longer we would also measure the individual's proneness toward the various forms of negative emotion, especially anxiety, guilt, and frustration, and his buffering ability to tolerate them. Into the matrix we could also insert measures of facility in free association, verbal intelligence, word-finding ability, and sentence-mindedness. We would include data reflecting the person's vulnerability to a range of delayed auditory feedback times, or some other index of his reliance on proprioceptive versus auditory feedback in the monitoring of his speech. We would need data on both his maximal and habitual syllabic rates and his protensity scores to feed into our evaluative computer. Finally, we would need values for the amount, foci, and kind of communicative stress to which he is subjected daily, the past history of fractured words, the amount of abnormal misperception of word configurations, and perhaps some index of his early speech development.

The point we are making, of course, is that human beings will differ one from the other on this monstrous collage of factors. Each one of them would have his own unique profile and his own composite score. The degree of deviance from the norms for each of these items when summated according to some esoteric formula would indicate the probability of disrupted words in that person's utterance. If we had such composite scores we could probably pick out those persons who were already stuttering and identify those children who would be likely to develop the disorder—without even seeing them or listening to them. Perhaps some day we shall have such a technology, but we shall not wait for that time with bated breath. There is work to be done in the vineyard and we must use the tools of today.

SUMMARY

Let us see how well this view of stuttering fits the known facts about stuttering. First of all, does it have any value in explaining why stuttering is found universally among the human population? All human beings speak, and all speaking requires the production of motoric sequences which must be precisely timed. The normal distribution in motoric facility would produce certain individuals who should have some difficulty in accomplishing that timing. All humans are subject to communicative and emotional stress. Surely there should be some whose motoric configurations in time would show disruption. Why should only about one in one hundred stutter? Perhaps this figure represents the extreme end of the normal distribution in coordinative ability or stress vulnerability. Why does stuttering usually tend to have its onset in early childhood? All motor configurations at this time are less stable. Those involved in word production have had little practice. A shift from auditory to proprioceptive feedback in the monitoring of speech probably occurs at this time. Why should stuttering appear more frequently in certain family strains? Athletic ability seems to show much the same familial pattern. Perhaps the neurological organization for timing bilateral sequential movements may be hereditarily determined in some persons. Why should more males stutter than females? All we can offer here is the research indicating that females seem to require longer delays in auditory feedback before their speech becomes disrupted and they seem to be less vulnerable to delays (or to stress?) than males. Myelinzation of the nerve tracts in the brain seems to occur more swiftly in females. Why do we find the extensive evidence of organicity in stutterers which we reported in Chapter 13? Perhaps because the brain mechanisms for timing sequential movements are indeed faulty in some stutterers.

Why do the behaviors common to all stutterers and those found most frequently in the beginning stutterer consist of syllabic repetitions or prolongations of sounds or silent articulatory postures or phonatory arrest? These are the natural consequences of mistiming. When a motoric sequence is mistimed or interrupted, prolongation or repetition or cessation are about the only responses available. What else?

Why does stuttering show such variability in the adult or confirmed stutterer? The experience of excessively interrupted speech is unpleasant both to the speaker and to the listener. Different stutterers learn to respond in different ways to the experience or fear of broken speech. Those reactions which minimize the social penalties or reduce the frustration will be maintained and automatized. Much of the stutterer's struggle reactions began as searching behaviors seeking the proper timing for reintegration of broken words. They persist because they were followed by utterance. The most powerful reinforcer in the maintenance of stuttering is communicative consummation.

Why do some stutterers become neurotic though most of them do not? Why for that matter do normal speakers? Why do stutterers develop self-concepts in which stuttering plays a major role? Why not?

Why does the stutterer usually show the same loci for stutterings that are found for the disfluencies of normal speakers? The same communicative stresses felt by the latter are also felt by the stutterer; they simply add an extra stress to an already overburdened timing system, but, by so doing, they determine the locus of the stuttering. The major exception—that stutterers have more trouble on the first words of utterances—simply reflects the stutterer's reduced ability to time his synergies or it reflects his fear of displaying his impediment. Why does he stutter more on accented syllables? Because these may be the features which serve as the basic feedback signals for the whole motoric sequence of the word. These above all must be timed appropriately.

Why do different stutterers have different feared words and situations? Because of differential learning experiences. Why do stutterers in general speak better when they are alone? Less communicative stress on the timing mechanism. Why do they stutter more to authority figures? More fear of penalty. Why do they stutter more under time pressure and when required to speak very swiftly? Because they have poor timing mechanisms. Why do they have more trouble when confessing guilt or shame? Emotional stress tends to disrupt all motor sequences. Why can they speak better when speaking in unison or shadowing? Because accessory timing signals are thereby provided. Why do so many of them speak better under masking or DAF? Because most of the mistiming probably has its origin in the processing of auditory feedback from their speech. Both masking and DAF shift the monitoring of motoric sequencing to proprioception.

As we contemplate this cursory summary of our assemblage of the pieces of the puzzle of stuttering, we are miserable. Let us confess it: we have failed. Our attempt to provide an adequate synthesis is far from satisfactory. Yet it is our impression that dimly we see the contours of the pattern of stuttering well enough to know that someone someday shall somehow manage to fit all of its pieces together. Morituri te salutamus! To him our salute! So we end this book with some of the feeling that Moses (also a stutterer) must have experienced when at the end of his days he was taken up on the mountain for a brief glimpse of the promised land, a land he knew he would never enter, but one which the children of his companions assuredly would make their own. Selah!

COMMENTARY

The chief justification for our present theories and methods is that we just don't know any better. . . . To defend an idea in this particular field for more than five years is usually a mark, not of astuteness, but of sheer stagnation. (Johnson, 194, p. 116)

BIBLIOGRAPHY

Agnello, J. G., "Some Acoustic and Pause Characteristics of Nonfluencies in the Speech of Stutterers." Technical Report, National Institute of Mental Health, Grant No. 11067-01, 1966.

Agnello, J. G., and M. A. Buxton, "Effects of Resonance and Time on Stutterers' and Nonstutterers' Speech Under Delayed Auditory Feedback." National Institute of Mental Health, H.E.W. Project No. 11067-01, 1966.

Agnello, J. G., and H. Goehl, "Spectographical Patterns of Disfluencies in the Speech of Stutterers," convention address, A.S.H.A., 1965.

Agnello, J. G., and H. C. Kagan, "Delayed Auditory Feedback and Its Effect on the Manner of Speech Production." Final Report, National Institute of Mental Health, Grant No. 11067-01., 1966.

Andrews, G., "Stuttering: Theoretical and Therapeutic Considerations: II Syllable Timed Speech, Group Psychotherapy, and Recovery from Stuttering," *Australian Psychologist, I* (1967), 64.

———. "The Nature of Stuttering," *Journal Australian College of Speech Therapists,* XV (1965), 6–15.

Andrews, G., and M. Harris, *The Syndrome of Stuttering.* London: Heinemann, 1964.

Barber, V. A., "Studies in the Psychology of Stuttering: XV Chorus Reading as a Distraction in Stuttering," *Journal of Speech Disorders,* IV (1939), 371–83.

———. "Rhythm as a Distraction in Stuttering," *Journal of Speech Disorders,* V (1940), 29–42.

Beebe, H., "Sentence Mindedness," *Folia Phoniatrica,* IX (1957), 44–48.

Beech, H. R., and F. Fransella, *Research and Experiment in Stuttering.* New York: Pergamon, 1968.

Besozzi, T. E., and M. R. Adams, "The Influence of Prosody on Stuttering Adaptation," *Journal of Speech and Hearing Research,* XII (1969), 818–24.

Bloodstein, O., "Hypothetic Conditions Under Which Stuttering is Reduced or Absent," *Journal of Speech and Hearing Disorders,* XV (1950), 142–53.

Brandon, S., and M. Harris, "Stammering—An Experimental Treatment Programme Using Syllable-Timed Speech," *British Journal of Disorders of Communication,* II (1967), 64–68.

Bryngelson, B., "A Phonophotographic Analysis of the Vocal Disturbances in Stuttering," *Psychological Monographs,* XLIII (1932), 1–30.

Buxton, L. F., *An Investigation of Sex and Age Differences in Speech Behaviors Under Delayed Auditory Feedback.* Doctoral dissertation, Ohio State University, 1968.

Chase, R. A., "Effect of Delayed Auditory Feedback on the Repetition of Speech Sounds," *Journal of Speech and Hearing Disorders,* XXIII (1958), 583–90.

Cherry, E. C., *On Human Communication.* New York: Wiley, 1957.

Cherry, E. C., and B. M. Sayers, "Experiments Upon the Total Inhibition of Stammering by External Control, and Some Clinical Results," *Journal of Psychosomatic Research,* I (1956), 233–46.

Cherry, E. C., and P. Marland, "Some Experiments on the Total Suppression of Stammering; and a Report on Some Clinical Trials," *Bulletin of the British Psychological Society,* XXX (1956), 43–44.

Chevrie-Muller, C., ["A Study of Laryngeal Function in Stutterers by the Glotto-Graphic Method"], *Proceedings, VIIᵉ Congrès de la Société Français de Medecine de la Voix et de la Parole,* Paris, 1963.

Colombat de L'Isère, M., Du Bégaiement et de tous les Autres Vices de la Parole Traités par des nouvelles Méthodes. 2ᵉ ed. 1831.

Daniloff, R., and K. Moll, "Coarticulation of Lip Rounding," *Journal of Speech and Hearing Research,* XI (1968), 707–21.

Eisenson, J., and C. Wells, "A Study of the Influence of Communicative Responsibility in a Choral Speech Situation for Stutterers," *Journal of Speech Disorders,* VII (1942), 259–62.

Fletcher, J. M., *The Problem of Stuttering.* New York: Longmans, Green, 1928.

Fransella, F., "Rhythm as a Distractor in the Modification of Stuttering," *Behaviour Research and Therapy,* V (1967), 253–55.

Fransella, F., and H. R. Beech, "An Experimental Analysis of the Effect of Rhythm on the Speech of Stutterers," *Behaviour Research and Therapy,* III (1965), 195–201.

Goldman-Eisler, F., "Sequential Temporal Patterns and Cognitive Processes in Speech," *Language and Speech,* X (1967), 131–40.

Gray, K. C., and D. E. Williams, "Anticipation and Stuttering: A Pupillographic Study," *Journal of Speech and Hearing Research,* XII (1969), 833–39.

Hardy, J. C., "Electromyographic Evidence of 'Syllabic Pulses' in Respiratory Muscles," convention address, A. S.H.A., 1967 (abstract).

Hill, H., "An Interbehavioral Analysis of Several Aspects of Stuttering," *Journal of Speech Disorders,* XXXII (1945), 289–316.

Hirose, H., S. Kiritani, and S. Shibata, "An Electromyographic Study of Articulatory Movements," *Logopedics and Phoniatrics,* Annual Bulletin No. 2, University of Tokyo, 1968.

Holgate, D., and G. Andrews, "The Use of Syllable-Timed Speech and Group Psychotherapy in the Treatment of Adult Stutterers," *Journal of Australian College of Speech Therapists,* XVI (1966), 36–40.

Hoshiko, M. S., "Sequence of Action of Breathing Muscles During Speech." *Journal of Speech and Hearing Research,* III (1960), 291–97.

Hunsley, Y. L., "Dysintegration in the Speech Musculature of Stutterers During the Production of a Nonvocal Temporal Pattern," *Psychological Monographs,* XLIX (1937), 32–49.

Johnson, W., "Some Fundamental Objectives in Special Education," *Journal of Exceptional Children*, X (1944), 115–16.

Johnson, W., and L. Rosen, "Effects of Certain Changes in Speech Patterns upon the Frequency of Stuttering," *Journal of Speech Disorders*, II (1937), 101–4.

Jones, R. K., "Observations on Stammering After Localized Cerebral Injury," *Journal of Neurology and Neurosurgery*, XXIX (1966), 192–95.

Kelham, R., and A. McHale, "The Application of Learning Theory to the Treatment of Stammering," *British Journal of Disorders of Communication*, I (1966), 114–18.

Klemm, M., in H. Freund, *Psychopathology and the Problems of Stuttering*. Springfield, Ill.: C. C. Thomas, 1966, p. 161.

Lashley, K. S., "The Problem of Serial Order in Behavior." In L. L. Jeffress (ed.), *Cerebral Mechanisms in Behavior*. New York: Wiley, 1951.

Lenneberg, E. H., *Biological Foundations of Language*. New York: Wiley, 1967.

Lieberman, P., *Intonation, Perception and Language*. Research Monograph 38, Cambridge: M.I.T. Press, 1967.

Lindsley, D., "Bilateral Differences in Brain Potentials from the Two Hemispheres in Relation to Laterality and Stuttering," *Journal of Experimental Psychology*, XXVI (1940), 211–25.

MacKay, D. G., "Metamorphosis of a Critical Interval: Age Linked Changes in Delay in Auditory Feedback that Produces Maximal Disruption of Speech," *Journal of the Acoustical Society of America*, XLIII (1968), 810–20. ,

MacNeilage, P. F., and J. L. De Clerk, "On the Motor Control of Coarticulation in cvc Monosyllables," *Journal of the Acoustical Society of America*, XLV (1969), 1217–33.

Mahl, G., "Disturbances and Silences in the Patient's Speech in Psychotherapy," *Journal of Abnormal Social Psychology*, XLII (1957), 3–32.

Mahl, G. F., and G. Schultze, "Psychological Research in the Extra Linguistic Area." In T. A. Sebeok (ed.), *Approaches to Semiotics*. The Hague: Mouton, 1964.

Metz, O., "The Acoustic Impedance Measured in Normal and Pathological Ears," *Acta Otolaryngolica*, Supplement 63, 1946.

Meyer, V., and J. M. M. Mair, "A New Technique to Control Stammering: A Preliminary Report," *Behaviour Research and Therapy*, I (1963), 251–54.

Moravek, M., and J. Langova, "Patofyziologie Zachvatu Kojtavsti," *Cas. Lek. Cesk.*, CVII (1968), 536–38.

Mysak, E. D., "Servo Theory and Stuttering," *Journal of Speech and Hearing Disorders*, XXV (1960), 188–95.

Nadoleczny, M., "Stuttering as a Manifestation of a Spastic Coordination Neurosis," *Archive für Psychiatrie*, LXXXII (1927), 235–46.

Pattie, F. A., and B. B. Knight, "Why Does the Speech of Stutterers Improve in Chorus Reading?" *Journal of Abnormal and Social Psychology*, XXXIX (1944), 362–67.

Penfield, W., and T. Rasmussen, "Vocalization and Arrest of Speech," *Archives of Neurology and Psychiatry*, LXI (1949), 21–27.

Rawnsley, A., and J. Harris, "Comparative Analysis of Normal Speech and Speech with Delayed Sidetone by Means of Sound Spectrograms." *United States Navy Medical Research Laboratory Report*, 1954, Project Number NM-003-041.56.03, No. 248.

Rickenberg, H. E., "Diadochokinesis in Stutterers and Nonstutterers," *Journal of Medical Society of New Jersey,* LIII (1956), 324–26.

Salamon, G., and A. Starr, "Electromyography of Middle Ear Muscles in Man During Motor Activities," *Acta Neurologica Scandinavia,* XXXIX (1963), 161–68.

Schwartz, M. F., "Syllable Duration in Oral and Whispered Reading," *Journal of Acoustical Society of America,* XLI (1967), 1367–69.

Sears, T. A., and J. N. Davis, "The Control of Respiratory Muscles During Voluntary Breathing," *Annals of the New York Academy of Sciences,* CLV (1968), 183–90.

Seeman, M., *Sprachstörungen bei Kindern.* Marhold: Halle-Saale, 1959.

Sergeant, R. L., "Concurrent Repetition of a Continuous Flow of Words," *Journal of Speech and Hearing Research,* IV (1961), 373–80.

Shannon, C. E., "Prediction and Entropy of Printed English," *Bell System Technical Journal,* XXX (1951), 50–64.

Shannon, C. E., and W. Weaver, *The Mathematical Theory of Communication.* Urbana, Ill.: University of Illinois Press, 1954.

Shearer, W. M., and F. B. Simmons, "Middle Ear Activity During Speech in Normal Speakers and Stutterers," *Journal of Speech and Hearing Research,* VIII (1965), 203–7.

Shtremel, A. K., ["Stuttering in Left Parietal Lobe Syndrome"], *Zhurnal Nevropatologii i Psikhiatrii imeni S. S. Korsakova,* LXIII (1963), 828–32.

Smith, K. U., M. Mysziewski, M. Mergen, and J. Koehler, "Computer Systems Control of Delayed Auditory Feedback," *Perceptual Motor Skills,* XVII (1963), 343–54.

Stetson, R. H., *Motor Phonetics.* Amsterdam: North Holland, 1951.

Stromsta, C., "A Methodology Related to the Determination of the Phase Angle of Bone-Conducted Speech Sound Energy of Stutterers and Nonstutterers." Doctoral dissertation, Ohio State University, 1956.

———. "Averaged Evoked Responses of Stutterers and Nonstutterers as a Function of Interaural Time Relationships," Technical Report. National Institutes of Health, Project NB-03541-03, 1965.

———. "Delays Associated with Certain Sidetone Pathways," *Journal of Acoustical Society of America,* XXXIV (1962), 392–96.

———. "EEG Power Spectra of Stutterers and Nonstutterers," *Asha,* VI (1964), 418–19.

———. "Experimental Blockage of Phonation by Distorted Sidetone," *Journal of Speech and Hearing Research,* II (1959), 286–301.

Tomatis, A., *L'Oreille et le Langage.* Paris: Éditions du Seuil, 1963.

Travis, L. E., "Dissociation of the Homologous Muscle Function in Stuttering," *Archives of Neurology and Psychiatry,* XXXI (1934), 127–33.

Van Dantzig, M., "Syllable-Tapping: A New Method for the Help of Stammerers," *Journal of Speech Disorders,* V (1940), 127–32.

Vannier, J., R. Saumont, L. Labarroque, and R. Husson, "Production experimentale des Blocages synaptiques récurrentials par des Stimulations auditives homorythmiques avec Déphasages réglables," *Revue de Laryngologie,* Bordeau, 1954.

Van Riper, C., "Study of the Thoracic Breathing of Stutterers During Expectancy and Occurrence of Stuttering Spasms," *Journal of Speech Disorders,* I (1936), 61–72.

Walton, D., and D. A. Black, "The Application of Learning Theory to the Treatment of Stammering," *Journal of Psychosomatic Research,* III (1958), 170–79.

Williams, D. E., "Masseter Muscle Action Current Potentials in Stuttered and Nonstuttered Speech," *Journal of Speech and Hearing Disorders,* XX (1955), 242–61.

Wingate, M. E., "Sound and Pattern in 'Artificial' Fluency," *Journal of Speech and Hearing Research,* XII (1969), 677–86.

————. "Slurvian Skill of Stutterers," *Journal of Speech and Hearing Research,* X (1967), 844–48.

————. "Stuttering Adaptation and Learning, II. Adequacy of Learning Principles in the Interpretation of Stuttering," *Journal of Speech and Hearing Disorders,* XXXI (1966), 211–18.

Witt, M., "Statistische Erhebungen über den Einfluss des Singens und Flüstern auf Stottern," *Vox,* V (1925), 41–43.

Wohl, M. T., "The Electric Metronome—An Evaluative Study," *British Journal of Disorders of Communication,* III (1968), 89–98.

Zaleski, T., "Rhythmic Skills in Stuttering Children," *De Therapia Vocis et Loquellae,* I (1965), 371–72.

subject index

Aborigines, 7
Abulia, 147
Adams personal audit, 273
Adaptation, 240–241, 319
Adults, onset of stuttering, 68–70
Advanced stuttering, 125, 156
Aetius of Amica, 336
Africans, 5
Age of onset, 36, 61–62, 65
Airflow, 23–27
American Indians, 5–8, 41
Anal fixation, 274, 275
Anal interest picture test, 275
Anal trait check list, 275
Anxiety, 174–177, 275
Aphasia, 345
Approach-avoidance conflict, 304–306
Aristotle, 3, 336
Arnott, 336
Asage, 5
Astrie, 337
Attitudes of stutterers, 157, 198
Auditory laterality, 358, 359
Avicenna, 3–4, 337
Avoidance behavior, 141–143

Bacon, Francis, 1, 336
Bannock, 7, 8
Bantu, 6, 46, 47
Battos, Son of Polyonestros, 3
Becquerel, 337
Behavior analysis chart, 214, 232
Bell, Alexander Graham, 286
Bell adjustment inventory, 273

Bernreuter, 273
Bertrand, 336
Bevan, Aneurin, 4
Bibliographies, 11–12, 32–35, 56–61, 91–96, 122–124, 154–156, 190–198, 216–218, 244–248, 262–264, 279–284, 326–334, 368–381, 398–403, 437–441
Biochemical factors, 365–367
Blacky pictures test, 275
Blockages, 133–134
Blood composition, 365
Body image, 201–204
Borneo, 7
Brace motor ability tests, 362
Brain injured, 49–50, 344–347
British Guiana, 7

California test of personality, 273
Cerebral dominance, 338, 351–359
Characteristics of stutterers, 116–117, 125–156, 257–259
Charles I, King of England, 4
Cherokee, 5
Chinese, 5, 205
Chocktaw, 5
Choral speech, 408
Classical conditioning, 298–311
Click sounds, 6
Clonic stuttering, 255–256
Closures, 133, 134
Cluttering, 29, 44, 86, 109, 251, 343, 349
Coarticulation, 23–25, 360–365
Cognitive learning theory, 307–308

Communication conflicts, 86–87
Complemental air, 137–139
Compulsivity, 275
Confirmed stuttering, 125–156
Consistency effect, 312
Convulsions, 79
Coordination difficulties, 360–364, 417
Covert reactions, 157–198
Covert responses, 232–235
Cowichan, 8, 41
Cybernetic theory, 382–396

DAF, 309, 315, 382–403, 417–418
Darwin, Charles, 4, 286
Deafness, 50, 393
Definitions of stuttering, 12–35
Delayed speech development, 108–111
Development of stuttering, 97–124
Developmental stuttering, 39
Diabetics, 50–51
Discomfort relief quotient, 178
Disease and stuttering, 347
Disfluency, 27–29
Disguise reactions, 140
Distinctive features, 20–26
Disturbed feedback, 382–403, 417–418
Domo Mata, 5
Draw-a-person test, 214
Duration of stuttering, 230–232

Early stuttering, 39

443

author index